Essentials in Ophthalmology

Series Editor

Arun D. Singh, Cleveland Clinic Foundation
Cole Eye Institute
Cleveland, OH, USA

Essentials in Ophthalmology aims to promote the rapid and efficient transfer of medical research into clinical practice. It is published in four volumes per year. Covering new developments and innovations in all fields of clinical ophthalmology, it provides the clinician with a review and summary of recent research and its implications for clinical practice. Each volume is focused on a clinically relevant topic and explains how research results impact diagnostics, treatment options and procedures as well as patient management.

The reader-friendly volumes are highly structured with core messages, summaries, tables, diagrams and illustrations and are written by internationally well-known experts in the field. A volume editor supervises the authors in his/her field of expertise in order to ensure that each volume provides cutting-edge information most relevant and useful for clinical ophthalmologists. Contributions to the series are peer reviewed by an editorial board.

More information about this series at https://link.springer.com/bookseries/5332

Mary Qiu
Editor

Neovascular Glaucoma

Current Concepts in Diagnosis and Treatment

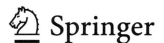 Springer

Editor
Mary Qiu
Ophthalmology and Visual Science
University of Chicago
Chicago, IL, USA

ISSN 1612-3212   ISSN 2196-890X   (electronic)
Essentials in Ophthalmology
ISBN 978-3-031-11722-0   ISBN 978-3-031-11720-6   (eBook)
https://doi.org/10.1007/978-3-031-11720-6

This Springer imprint is published by the registered company Springer Nature Switzerland AG
The registered company address is: Gewerbestrasse 11, 6330 Cham, Switzerland

Contents

Neovascular Glaucoma: An Overview

Pujan Dave and Pradeep Y. Ramulu

Neovascular glaucoma (NVG) is an aggressive secondary glaucoma resulting from iris and anterior chamber angle neovascularization that is most often triggered by underlying retinal ischemia. Because the etiology of angle neovascularization is often the domain of one ophthalmic subspecialty (retina), while the manifestation is the domain of another (glaucoma), the topic is both difficult to treat and to discuss academically. Also, the subject may not have been previously addressed in as much depth as done here based on historical data demonstrating poor visual outcomes in NVG eyes. The current book, which reviews the causes of NVG, while also updating us on latest methods of addressing neovascularization and safely achieving IOP-lowering, is therefore a welcome and much-needed contribution.

The earliest report of what we now understand to be NVG was documented in 1871, which described an eye with elevated intraocular pressure (IOP) in the setting of intraocular hemorrhage [1]. Decades later in 1906, angiogenesis of the iris was histologically described by Coats in a patient with a central retinal vein occlusion (CRVO), and similar abnormal vessel growth was identified on the iris surface of patients with dia-

betes in years to come [2]. A variety of names, including hemorrhagic glaucoma, rubeotic glaucoma, and congestive glaucoma, were used to describe this condition until the introduction of term "neovascular glaucoma" by Weiss in 1963 based on an improved understanding of the pathophysiology of the condition [3, 4].

In contrast to other more common glaucomas (primary open angle, pseudoexfoliation, pigment dispersion, etc.) that have similar approaches to management, NVG requires a unique treatment paradigm involving not only the control of elevated IOP, but also the control of pro-angiogenic conditions that promote neovascularization. The management of NVG has evolved significantly since its early descriptions as we have discovered new approaches to control retinal ischemia and surgically manage elevated intraocular pressure. Though NVG accounts for a minority of all glaucomas, it is aggressive and frequently refractory to medical management, requiring surgical intervention.

An overlooked, but very important, aspect of NVG management is close monitoring for its development in high-risk patients [5]. While we as practitioners are often presented with the challenge of treating eyes where NVG has clearly manifested, we less often ask the question of what we might do better to avoid having patients develop NVG. It is well established that high-risk patients most commonly include those with ischemic CRVO, diabetic retinopathy, and ocular

P. Dave · P. Y. Ramulu (✉)
Wilmer Eye Institute, Johns Hopkins University,
Baltimore, MD, USA
e-mail: pramulu@jhmi.edu

© The Author(s), under exclusive license to Springer Nature Switzerland AG 2022
M. Qiu (ed.), *Neovascular Glaucoma*, Essentials in Ophthalmology,
https://doi.org/10.1007/978-3-031-11720-6_1

ischemic syndrome, but, as discussed later in this textbook, there are many other conditions in which NVG can develop. Early recognition and treatment of underlying etiologies may prevent development of NVG, or arrest and reverse the process at its earliest stages. In the past, panretinal photocoagulation (PRP) was the only option for the prevention and treatment of neovascularization, with variable success depending on the underlying condition and timing of the treatment. The advent of intravitreal antivascular endothelial growth factor (anti-VEGF) treatment, however, has drastically changed our approach and outcomes, and has become the mainstay of treatment alongside PRP for all causes of ocular neovascularization.

Unfortunately, despite these interventions, many patients develop high IOP that necessitates specific IOP lowering treatment. Medical management includes topical IOP lowering agents commonly used for glaucoma management (e.g., carbonic anhydrase inhibitors, alpha-2 agonists, etc.) and oral carbonic anhydrase inhibitors when topical treatment is not sufficient. Topical corticosteroids are used in some patients to control intraocular inflammation. When medical management does not lower the IOP enough to prevent optic nerve damage, which is much more common with NVG than with other forms of glaucoma, surgery becomes necessary to control the IOP. Traditionally, surgical management of NVG includes either implantation of aqueous shunts and diode laser cyclophotocoagulation (CPC). Historically, trabeculectomy has a relatively high failure rate in NVG even with use of antimetabolites and is therefore not routinely performed [6].

Much of our knowledge about the best surgical outcomes for NVG comes from studies that were performed before the routine use of anti-VEGF medications. Moreover, the arrival and popularization of micro-incisional glaucoma surgery (MIGS) have transformed surgical glau-

coma management, and it has not yet been extensively studied whether these novel angle-based surgeries would be effective for NVG. Given the revolutionary effect of combination anti-VEGF and PRP treatment on regression of neovascularization, some patients with NVG may obtain IOP control with MIGS alone as opposed to traditional glaucoma surgery. Certainly, aqueous shunts and diode laser CPC will remain important for particular cases, but angle-based surgeries may modify NVG management in the anti-VEGF era. This book will also review the most recent data regarding the outcomes of procedures that filter aqueous humor to the subconjunctival space (i.e., trabeculectomy)—an important question for areas of the world where the cost of certain surgical implants (i.e., aqueous shunts) may be prohibitive.

Our understanding of NVG and its management have progressed tremendously since its first description in the nineteenth century. The disease remains difficult to treat in spite of these advances and ocular morbidity from NVG remains high. It is vital to rigorously evaluate both novel and conventional treatments to optimize management of this particularly challenging and refractory disease. As vascular disease becomes more prevalent, NVG, too, is likely to become more common given the associations between vascular disease and underlying ocular conditions that predispose to NVG. Retina and glaucoma specialists must work closely together to treat this condition with a combination of PRP, anti-VEGF, medical IOP-lowering therapy, traditional glaucoma surgery, and possibly MIGS, catering to each patient's individual clinical needs as our understanding of NVG becomes increasingly refined. We welcome this comprehensive discussion of a very challenging problem, with the goal that we might change our practice to prevent and/or detect NVG earlier, and to achieve better outcomes when it does present.

References

1. Gilbert W. Beiträge zur Lehre vom Glaukom. Graefes Arch Ophthalmol. 1912;82(3):389–474.
2. Coats G. Further cases of thrombosis of the central vein. London: J. & A. Churchill; 1906.
3. Weiss DI, Shaffer RN, Nehrenberg TR. Neovascular glaucoma complicating carotid-cavernous fistula. Arch Ophthalmol. 1963;69(3):304–7.
4. Smith RJ. Rubeotic glaucoma. Br J Ophthalmol. 1981;65(9):606–9.
5. Hayreh SS. Neovascular glaucoma. Prog Retin Eye Res. 2007;26(5):470–85.
6. Mietz H, Raschka B, Krieglstein GK. Risk factors for failures of trabeculectomies performed without antimetabolites. Br J Ophthalmol. 1999;83(7):814–21.

Epidemiology of Neovascular Glaucoma

Saira Khanna and Dolly S. Chang

1 Introduction

Neovascular glaucoma (NVG) is a form of secondary glaucoma characterized by the proliferation of fibrovascular tissue in the anterior chamber producing neovascularization of the iris (NVI) and/or neovascularization of the iridocorneal angle (NVA), which subsequently causes elevation in intraocular pressure (IOP). Retinal ischemia is the underlying etiology in more than 95% of cases and the most common causes of NVG are proliferative diabetic retinopathy (PDR), retinal vein occlusion (RVO), and ocular ischemic syndrome (OIS). NVG has a high risk of causing severe vision impairment and can result in both unilateral and bilateral blindness [1]. Because NVG occurs as the result of poorly controlled diseases, the epidemiology of NVG is closely linked to the epidemiology and treatment of its underlying diseases.

2 Prevalence

The prevalence of NVG in population-based studies has had variable reports ranging from 0.01 to 0.2% [2–6]. In West Bengal, the prevalence was 0.01% [2], 0.03% in China [6], 0.12% in the Singapore Indian Eye Study [4], and 0.2% in Nigeria [3]. Hospital-based prevalence of NVG in Nigeria was reported to be 0.3% [5]. Additionally, data from the European Union estimated that up to 300,000 people in Europe are affected by NVG, and NVG has been estimated to comprise ~3.9–5.8% of all glaucomas and 15.4% of secondary glaucomas [7, 8]. Based on a longitudinal health insurance database from Taiwan, the prevalence of NVG was shown to have increased substantially from 4.4 per 100,000 individuals in 2000 to 12.4 per 100,000 individuals in 2015 [9]. In the United States, no specific prevalence or number of individuals has been reported to have NVG in population-based studies; however, from the 2016 Intelligent Research in Sight (IRIS®) Registry, the prevalence of NVG in the dataset was 0.23 per 100 patients [10].

From hospital-based data review in Taiwan and Saudi Arabia, the overall incidence of NVG has been reported around 4.3–6.6 per 100,000 person-years [9, 11]. In Saudi Arabia, the incidence of NVG was noted to have increased from 3 per 100,000 person-year in 2002 to 12 per 100,000 person-year in 2008. With the introduc-

S. Khanna
Department of Ophthalmology and Visual Science,
The University of Chicago, Chicago, IL, USA

D. S. Chang (✉)
Genentech Research and Early Clinical Development,
South San Francisco, CA, USA

Byers Eye Institute, Stanford University,
Palo Alto, CA, USA

tion of intravitreal antivascular endothelial growth factor (anti-VEGF) therapies around 2008, the incidence of NVG in Taiwan has decreased to 1.0 per 100,000 person-year in 2012, and there has been a reduction in the number of IOP-lowering surgeries [9].

3 Risk Factors

3.1 Age

NVG can affect any age group, depending on the underlying cause of the neovascularization. The most common age group affected by NVG is 60–80 years of age [12]. Based on the underlying etiology for the neovascularization, different age groups are disproportionately affected. Retinoblastoma and Coats' disease are predominant reasons for neovascularization in the pediatric population whereas diabetes and ischemic vascular diseases predispose patients to neovascularization in older patient populations [13].

3.2 Race

There does not appear to be a racial predilection for race for NVG. Any variations in prevalence or incidence in various racial groups are likely attributed to differences in the underlying etiology for the neovascularization. There is no literature investigating if race is a risk factor specifically for NVG. The underlying cause of neovascularization may differ slightly based on race [13–17]. Future investigation is warranted to determine if there is truly a difference in racial predilection in the development of NVG independent of the underlying condition.

3.3 Gender

There does appear to be an overall male preponderance in both the incidence and prevalence of NVG [8, 9, 11, 18] with the occasional study showing that there is no sex predilection [5]. One study showed that the odds ratio of men having NVG compared to women was 2.2 [11] while others demonstrated a statistically significant difference in the prevalence between men and women (62% men compared to 37% women) [8]. Like age and race, this gender predilection may be attributed to the risk of having underlying diseases that lead to NVG in men rather than sex being an independent risk factor, since men are more likely to develop vascular diseases. It is unclear at this time whether there is a gender predisposition of developing NVG once patients have the underlying disease, however, studies examining predictors of developing NVG in PDR and CRVO, gender was not significant [19, 20].

3.4 Socioeconomic Status

Lower education status has been associated with the development and severity of NVG. In a study of NVG patients conducted in Mexico, it was reported that only 20% of the patients had completed education beyond elementary school [18]. Other studies have demonstrated that there are lower odds of glaucoma (not only NVG) with increasing income level and education [9, 21]. In addition, it has been shown that poorer visual outcomes in glaucoma have been associated with lower socioeconomic status [22].

4 Prevalence Based on Etiology

There are underlying etiologies for the development of NVG, and the three most common etiologies include PDR, RVO, and OIS [12, 23–27]. An extensive list of underlying etiologies that have been associated with NVG is shown in Table 1 [26].

4.1 Diabetes Mellitus

Multiple studies have shown that poorly controlled diabetes mellitus is a leading cause of NVG [8, 28, 29]. The incidence of NVI has been reported to be as high as 65% in patients with PDR in a 1998

Table 1 Diseases which may cause neovascularization glaucoma, adopted from Sivak-Callcott et al. [26]

Retinal ischemic diseases
Diabetes
Central retinal vein occlusion
Ocular ischemic syndrome/carotid occlusive disease
Central retinal artery occlusion
Retinal detachment
Leber's congenital amaurosis
Coats' disease
Eales disease
Sickle cell retinopathy
Retinal hemangioma
Persistent hyperplastic primary vitreous
Norrie's disease
Wyburn Mason
Carotid-cavernous fistula
Dural shunt
Stickler's syndrome
X-linked retinoschisis
Takayasu's aortitis
Juxtafoveal telangiectasis
Surgically induced
Carotid endarterectomy
Cataract extraction
Pars plana vitrectomy/lensectomy
Silicone oil
Scleral buckle
Neodymium: yttrium-aluminum-garnet capsulotomy
Laser coreoplasty
Tumors
Iris: melanoma, hemangioma, metastatic lesion
Ciliary body: ring melanoma
Retina: retinoblastoma, large cell lymphoma
Choroid: melanoma
Conjunctiva: squamous cell carcinoma
Radiation
External beam
Charged particle: proton, helium
Plaques
Photoradiation
Inflammatory diseases
Uveitis: chronic iridocyclitis, Behçet's disease
Vogt-Koyanagi-Harada syndrome
Syphilitic retinitis
Sympathetic ophthalmia
Endophthalmitis
Miscellaneous
Vitreous wick syndrome
Interferon alpha

study [27]. In addition, patients with a higher hemoglobin A1c are more likely to develop NVG

[30]. It has been reported that 5% of blindness in diabetics is caused by NVG [31]. It has also been reported that patients with diabetes with unilateral NVG have a 33% risk of developing NVG in the other eye [32]. In eyes with PDR after vitrectomy, up to 7.1% of males developed NVG within 1 year of vitrectomy; male sex, younger age, higher baseline IOP, and having NVG in the fellow eye were reported to be risk factors [20].

4.2 Retinal Vein Occlusions

Approximately one-third of all cases of NVG can be attributed to retinal vein occlusions [33]. In addition, 20% of patients with ischemic central retinal vein occlusions (CRVO) can develop NVG with an estimated 3800 new cases per year [34]. It has been shown that retinal nonperfusion status and uncontrolled intraocular pressure predispose patients to the development of NVG [35]. In most cases, the development of NVG happens within the first 3 months from onset of disease, but may also occur later especially with the rising use of anti-VEGF injections to treat macular edema in patients with retinal vascular occlusion [36]. Risk factors for the development of NVG in RVOs include presence of RAPD, worse visual acuity on presentation, and systemic hypertension [19].

4.3 Ocular Ischemic Syndrome

NVG has been reported in nearly 50% of eyes with ocular ischemic syndrome [37]. In addition, a delay from onset of symptoms to medical evaluation and severity of carotid artery stenosis has been correlated with the development of NVG [38]. These cases are typically unilateral and should always be on the differential for NVG in the elderly population.

5 Conclusion

NVG is a devastating disease and may become increasingly prevalent as systemic comorbidities associated with its development such as diabetes, hypertension, and metabolic syndrome become more widespread. Prevention and treatment of these underlying systemic conditions as well as the ischemic retinal diseases that directly lead to NVG may help reduce both the incidence and prevalence of NVG and the associated ocular morbidity.

References

1. Rani PK, Sen P, Sahoo NK, Senthil S, Chakurkar R, Anup M, et al. Outcomes of neovascular glaucoma in eyes presenting with moderate to good visual potential. Int Ophthalmol [Internet]. 2021 Mar 21 [cited 2021 May 11]; Available from https://doi.org/10.1007/s10792-021-01789-y
2. Paul C, Sengupta S, Choudhury S, Banerjee S, Sleath B. Prevalence of glaucoma in Eastern India: the Hooghly River Glaucoma Study. Indian J Ophthalmol. 2016;64(8):578.
3. Ashaye A, Ashaolu O, Komolafe O, Ajayi BGK, Olawoye O, Olusanya B, et al. Prevalence and types of glaucoma among an indigenous African population in Southwestern Nigeria. Invest Ophthalmol Vis Sci. 2013;54(12):7410.
4. Narayanaswamy A, Baskaran M, Zheng Y, Lavanya R, Wu R, Wong W-L, et al. The prevalence and types of glaucoma in an urban Indian population: the Singapore Indian Eye Study. Invest Ophthalmol Vis Sci. 2013;54(7):4621.
5. Fiebai B, Onua AA. Prevalence, causes and management of neovascular glaucoma: a 5-year review. Open J Ophthalmol. 2018;09(01):1.
6. Baskaran M, Foo RC, Cheng C-Y, Narayanaswamy AK, Zheng Y-F, Wu R, et al. The prevalence and types of glaucoma in an urban Chinese population: the Singapore Chinese Eye Study. JAMA Ophthalmol. 2015;133(8):874–80.
7. Mocanu C, Barăscu D, Marinescu F, Lăcrăţeanu M, Iliuşi F, Simionescu C. Neovascular glaucoma—retrospective study. Oftalmologia. 2005;49(4):58–65.
8. Liao N, Li C, Jiang H, Fang A, Zhou S, Wang Q. Neovascular glaucoma: a retrospective review from a tertiary center in China. BMC Ophthalmol. 2016;16:14.
9. Lin P-A, Lee C-Y, Huang F-C, Huang J-Y, Hung J-H, Yang S-F. Trend of neovascular glaucoma in Taiwan: a 15-year nationwide population-based cohort study. Ophthalmic Epidemiol. 2020;27(5):390–8.
10. IRIS® Registry|Electronic Health Records and Registries|Information on Data Sources|Vision & Eye Health Surveillance System|Vision Health Initiative (VHI)|CDC [Internet]. 2019 [cited 2021 May 19]. Available from https://www.cdc.gov/visionhealth/vehss/data/ehr-registries/iris.html
11. Al-Bahlal A, Khandekar R, Al Rubaie K, Alzahim T, Edward DP, Kozak I. Changing epidemiology of neovascular glaucoma from 2002 to 2012 at King Khaled Eye Specialist Hospital. Saudi Arabia Indian J Ophthalmol. 2017;65(10):969–73.
12. Rodrigues GB, Abe RY, Zangalli C, Sodre SL, Donini FA, Costa DC, et al. Neovascular glaucoma: a review. Int J Retina Vitreous. 2016;2(1):26.
13. Yu X, Sun X, Guo W. The etiologic considerations of neovascular glaucoma. Chin J Ophthalmol Otorhinolaryngol. 2004;5:291–3.
14. Brown GC, Magargal LE, Schachat A, Shah H. Neovascular glaucoma: etiologic considerations. Ophthalmology. 1984;91(4):315–20.
15. Al-Shamsi HN, Dueker DK, Nowilaty SR, Al-Shahwan SA. Neovascular glaucoma at king khaled eye specialist hospital—etiologic considerations. Middle East Afr J Ophthalmol. 2009;16(1):15–9.
16. Woodcock MGL, Richards JC, Murray ADN. The last 11 years of Molteno implantation at the University of Cape Town. Refining our indications and surgical technique. Eye. 2008;22(1):18–25.
17. Liu L, Xu Y, Huang Z, Wang X. Intravitreal ranibizumab injection combined trabeculectomy versus Ahmed valve surgery in the treatment of neovascular glaucoma: assessment of efficacy and complications. BMC Ophthalmol [Internet]. 2016 May 26 [cited 2021 Apr 25];16. Available from https://www.ncbi.nlm.nih.gov/pmc/articles/PMC4882850/
18. Lazcano-Gomez G, Soohoo JR, Lynch A, Bonell LN, Martinez K, Turati M, et al. Neovascular glaucoma: a retrospective review from a tertiary eye care center in Mexico. J Curr Glaucoma Pract. 2017;11(2):48–51.
19. Rong AJ, Swaminathan SS, Vanner EA, Parrish RK. Predictors of neovascular glaucoma in central retinal vein occlusion. Am J Ophthalmol. 2019;204:62–9.
20. Goto A, Inatani M, Inoue T, Awai-Kasaoka N, Takihara Y, Ito Y, et al. Frequency and risk factors for neovascular glaucoma after vitrectomy in eyes with proliferative diabetic retinopathy. J Glaucoma. 2013;22(7):572–6.
21. Oh SA, Ra H, Jee D. Socioeconomic status and glaucoma: associations in high levels of income and education. Curr Eye Res. 2019;44(4):436–41.
22. Raj S, Savla LP, Thattaruthody F, Seth NG, Kaushik S, Pandav SS. Predictors of visual impairment in primary and secondary glaucoma in a tertiary institute in North India. Eur J Ophthalmol. 2020;30(1):175–80.
23. Hayreh SS. Neovascular glaucoma. Prog Retin Eye Res. 2007;26(5):470–85.
24. Senthil S, Dada T, Das T, Kaushik S, Puthuran GV, Philip R, et al. Neovascular glaucoma—a review. Indian J Ophthalmol. 2021;69(3):525–34.
25. Barac IR, Pop MD, Gheorghe AI, Taban C. Neovascular secondary glaucoma, etiology and pathogenesis. Rom J Ophthalmol. 2015;59(1):24–8.
26. Sivak-Callcott JA, O'Day DM, Gass JDM, Tsai JC. Evidence-based recommendations for the diagnosis and treatment of neovascular glaucoma1 1The

authors do not have any proprietary or financial interest in any products or devices discussed in this study. Ophthalmology. 2001;108(10):1767–76.

27. Lee P, Wang CC, Adamis AP. Ocular neovascularization: an epidemiologic review. Surv Ophthalmol. 1998;43(3):245–69.

28. Preda M, Davidescu L, Damian C, Irimia A, Sollosy M. Neovascular glaucoma—prevention. Oftalmologia. 2006;50(2):108–14.

29. Hamard P, Baudouin C. Consensus on neovascular glaucoma. J Fr Ophtalmol. 2000;23(3):289–94.

30. Lee JH, Kim EY, Kim TK, Shin HY, Kim SY, Lee YC, et al. Prognostic factors of neovascular glaucoma in eyes with treated proliferative diabetic retinopathy. J Korean Ophthalmol Soc. 2017;58(4):415–9.

31. Havens SJ, Gulati V. Neovascular Glaucoma. Dev Ophthalmol. 2016;55:196–204.

32. Ohrt V. The frequency of rubeosis iridis in diabetic patients. Acta Ophthalmol. 1971;49(2):301–7.

33. A randomized clinical trial of early panretinal photocoagulation for ischemic central vein occlusion The Central Vein Occlusion Study Group N Report. Ophthalmology. 1995;102(10):1434–44.

34. Natural history and clinical management of central retinal vein occlusion. The Central Vein Occlusion Study Group. Arch Ophthalmol. 1997;115(4):486–91.

35. Chen H-F, Chen M-C, Lai C-C, Yeung L, Wang N-K, Chen HS-L, et al. Neovascular glaucoma after central retinal vein occlusion in pre-existing glaucoma. BMC Ophthalmol [Internet] 2014 Oct 5 [cited 2021 Apr 25];14. Available from https://www.ncbi.nlm.nih.gov/pmc/articles/PMC4193090/

36. Yang H, Yu X, Sun X. Neovascular glaucoma: handling in the future. Taiwan J Ophthalmol. 2018;8(2):60–6.

37. Terelak-Borys B, Skonieczna K, Grabska-Liberek I. Ocular ischemic syndrome—a systematic review. Med Sci Monit. 2012;18(8):RA138–44.

38. Kim YH, Sung MS, Park SW. Clinical features of ocular ischemic syndrome and risk factors for neovascular glaucoma. Korean J Ophthalmol. 2017;31(4):343–50.

Pathophysiology of Neovascular Glaucoma

Qing Wang and Thomas V. Johnson

Neovascular glaucoma (NVG) is a particularly aggressive form of secondary glaucoma that tends to present acutely when patients develop abrupt elevations of intraocular pressure (IOP). NVG is characterized by neovascularization of the anterior segment, fibrovascular proliferation within an initially open anterior chamber angle, and eventual synechial angle closure. Ocular hypertension leads to retinal ganglion cell injury and death, with the characteristic optic nerve head cupping and progressive visual field defects common to all forms of glaucomatous optic neuropathy. Whereas the term neovascular glaucoma was coined in 1963 by Weiss and colleagues [1], its manifestations and associations with retinal vascular disease have been recognized since the second half of the nineteenth century [2]. Nonetheless, NVG remains a visually devastating entity that is challenging to treat and frequently resistant to medical therapy alone. As such, early recognition and treatment of the ocular pathologies that predispose to NVG are critical for minimizing visual morbidity. A clear understanding of the mechanisms that drive anterior segment neovascularization is essential for effective treatment of the disease and for future development of increasingly effective anti-neovascular therapies. In this chapter, we will describe the natural history of, discuss ocular conditions that predispose to, and review the molecular and cellular mechanisms underlying anterior segment neovascularization.

1 Clinical Aspects of Anterior Segment Neovascularization

The iris, as a uveal tissue, is highly vascularized. Ophthalmologists who perform laser iridotomy learn to recognize (and avoid) physiologic iris vessels, which are typically oriented radially and contained within stromal tissue giving them a gray appearance when not covered by pigmented epithelium (Fig. 1b). Physiologic iris vessels possess endothelial cells bound by tight junctions (zonulae occludentes) without fenestrations, thereby maintaining the blood-aqueous barrier. In contrast, iris neovascularization, or rubeosis, is characterized by the presence of abnormal neovessels, which tend to grow in disorganized, meandering trajectories and are most easily visible at the pupil margin (Fig. 1c–d). They are bright red in appearance, and their endothelial cells contain fenestrations leading to increased permeability, which sometimes manifests as anterior chamber flare on slit-lamp examination. Fluorescein iris angiography demonstrates leakage from neovessels [3]. Neovessels are often

Q. Wang · T. V. Johnson (✉)
Glaucoma Center of Excellence, Wilmer Eye Institute, Johns Hopkins University School of Medicine, Baltimore, MD, USA
e-mail: johnson@jhmi.edu

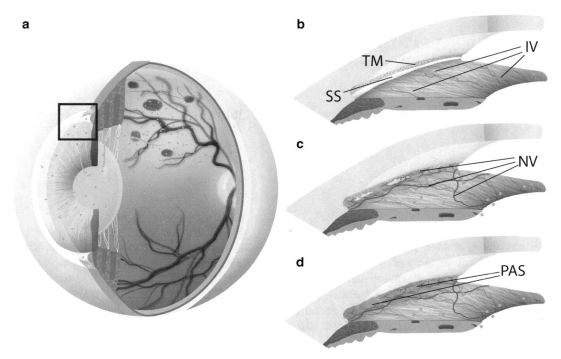

Fig. 1 (**a**) Ischemic retina in the setting of a superior hemiretinal vein occlusion produces vasoproliferative ligands including vascular endothelial growth factor (green dots). These factors diffuse in a gradient toward the anterior segment, enter the aqueous fluid through the posterior chamber, flow through the pupil into anterior chamber, and finally exit the eye through the trabecular meshwork. Inserts (**b–d**) show a magnified view of the iridocorneal angle. (**b**) Normal, physiologic iris vessels (IV) are radially oriented and contained within stromal tissue. The angle is open with a clear distinction between pigmented trabecular meshwork (TM) and scleral spur (SS). (**c**) Iris neovessels (NV) grow in disorganized, meandering trajectories and can be seen at the pupil margin and extending within a fibrovascular membrane into the angle. (**d**) Contraction of the fibrovascular membrane in late neovascularization leads to synechial closure of the angle, as seen by peripheral anterior synechiae (PAS) that sequester the TM. Artwork by Kevin Y Zhang, BS, Wilmer Eye Institute, Johns Hopkins University

accompanied by myofibroblasts, giving rise to a "fibrovascular membrane" that can appear shiny or gray on the iris surface [4]. In some circumstances, fibrovascular membranes can form posterior synechiae to the crystalline lens, or even a posterior chamber intraocular lens, leading to iris bombe. Neovessels are fragile and bleed relatively easily, which can lead to development of hyphema following rapid IOP lowering, as in the context of anterior chamber paracentesis or aqueous shunt implantation.

IOP elevation occurs when neovascularization of the iris begins to extend into the anterior chamber angle. At early stages, the angle remains open and pigmented trabecular meshwork is visible on gonioscopy, though neovessels are visible within the angle (Figs. 1c and 2a, b). Sometimes discrete vessels are difficult to ascertain but the meshwork itself develops a pink or red hue. Eventually fibrovascular proliferation and tissue contraction cause development of adhesions between the iris and the angle tissue, termed peripheral anterior synechiae (PAS). Without intervention to suppress the underlying neovascular drive, PAS lead to widespread synechial angle closure (Figs. 1d and 2a, b). If neovascularization of the angle is recognized prior to extensive synechial closure, prompt treatment is sometimes successful in achieving regression of neovessels and normalization of IOP [5]. Therefore, the importance of gonioscopy in the clinical evaluation of at-risk patients cannot be overemphasized.

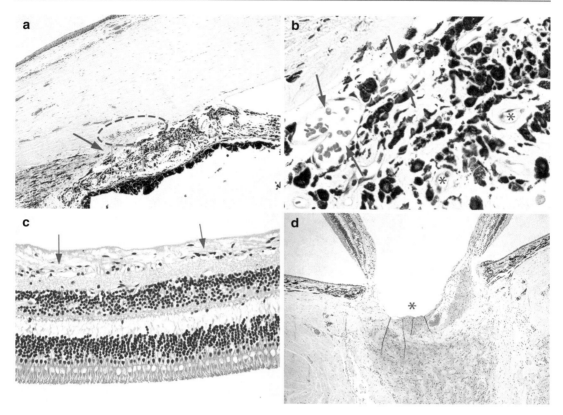

Fig. 2 (**a**) Angle closure due to peripheral anterior synechiae, with red arrow designating the scleral spur and dotted red oval outlining the region of the trabecular meshwork and Schlemm's canal. (**b**) Higher magnification view of the region outlined by the green rectangle in (**a**) shows newly formed thin-walled vessels on the iris surface that are adherent to the sclera (red arrows), and thick-walled vessels in the iris stroma (asterisks). (**c**) Severe retinal ganglion cell loss is present, as well as astrocytic gliosis in the retinal nerve fiber layer (red arrows). (**d**) Severe cupping of the optic nerve head (asterisk), with posterior bowing of the lamina cribrosa. Separation of the peripapillary neural retina from RPE is artifactual. Histology courtesy of Charles G Eberhart, MD, PhD, Director of Neuropathology and Ophthalmic Pathology, Wilmer Eye Institute, Johns Hopkins University

2 Cell Biology of Anterior Segment Neovascularization

Neovessels arise from existing vascular networks through a hierarchical activation of endothelial cells termed sprouting angiogenesis [6, 7], a phenomenon that occurs in both physiologic states, such as development and wound healing, and during pathologic neovascularization including in tumors [8]. In response to vasoproliferative signaling ligands, endothelial *tip cells* extend filopodia away from existing capillary walls [9]. Secondary endothelial *stalk cells* then follow tip cells to generate a vascular lumen thereby producing a vascular sprout [10]. Finally, *phalanx cells* follow stalk cells to line the inner lumen of the new vessel [11]. Pericytes and stromal cells play supportive roles in neovascularization.

Landmark work in cynomolgus monkeys in the late 1980s provided detailed histologic data regarding the cellular events that occur during anterior segment neovascularization [12]. Within 5 days of retinal vein occlusion, tritiated thymidine uptake was significant within vascular endothelial cells, showing increased cellular proliferation. By 4 weeks, thickened vascular membranes formed on the anterior iris surface, with anterior traction at the pupil causing

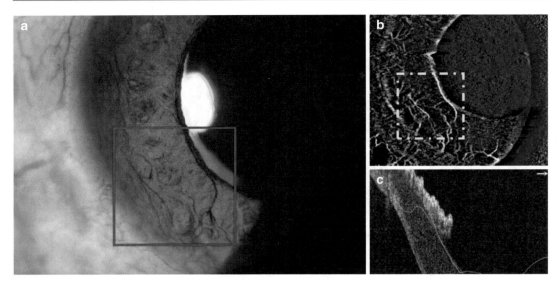

Fig. 3 (**a**) This anterior segment slit-lamp photograph shows prominent iris neovascularization, and fibrovascular traction at the pupil margin has caused ectropion uveae. (**b**) En-face OCT angiography demonstrates flow within these abnormal iris vessels. (**c**) Cross-sectional OCT angiography demonstrates flow (red) through the fibrovascular membrane that is superficial to the iris stroma. The red box in (**a**) corresponds to the yellow box in (**b**). Reprinted from: Lee WD, Devarajan K, Chua J, et al., Optical coherence tomography angiography for the anterior segment. Eye and Vision. 6, 4 (2019). https://doi.org/10.1186/s40662-019-0129-2 under open access CC BY 4.0 License (https://creativecommons.org/licenses/by/4.0/legalcode)

ectropion uveae. At this point, cellular proliferation was primarily seen in iris stromal cells which had discarded their typical intercellular associations with iris melanocytes, adopted a myofibroblast phenotype, and migrated anteriorly to constitute the neovascular membrane. These findings reinforce the idea that NVG is characterized not just by abnormal blood vessels, but rather by a contractile fibrovascular membrane complex (Fig. 3).

3   Posterior Segment Ischemia

Anterior segment neovascularization and fibrovascular proliferation are driven by proangiogenic molecular ligands that diffuse forward from the posterior segment (Fig. 1a). Vascular growth factors are produced by the retina in response to hypoxia, and therefore the ocular conditions that most commonly predispose to NVG are the most frequently occurring retinal vascular diseases: diabetic retinopathy, responsible for approximately one-third NVG cases and

typically, though not exclusively, occurring with the proliferative form of the disease; retinal venous occlusion, responsible for another third of NVG and often manifesting 60–90 days after the onset of venous occlusion; and ocular ischemic syndrome (i.e., carotid artery occlusive disease). The degree of retinal ischemia correlates with the risk for anterior segment neovascularization and NVG, as reflected in the increased risk in ischemic over nonischemic central retinal vein occlusion (CRVO) and in CRVO over hemiretinal vein occlusion [13]. Ocular ischemic syndrome manifests with global limitations of ocular blood flow and therefore anterior segment ischemia also contributes to the development of NVG in this condition. Other rarer conditions also contribute to retinal ischemia and can predispose to NVG including radiation, ocular malignancy, chronic uveitis, retinal vasculitis, and chronic retinal detachment. Because intraocular blood flow is proportional to the difference between mean arterial pressure and IOP, the ocular hypertension resulting from NVG exacerbates retinal ischemia, which in turn, hastens the drive for further anterior segment neovascularization. This positive feedback loop between retinal ischemia and NVG at least partially explains the frequently poor visual outcomes in patients with the disease.

4   Vasoproliferative Factors

The presence of a retina-derived vasoproliferative factor that drives neovascularization in the setting of retinal ischemia was first proposed by Michaelson in 1948 [14]. Candidates vetted in the ensuing hunt for such a growth factor included insulin-like growth factors, fibroblast growth factors, and growth hormone, amongst others. None appeared to serve as a definitive link between retinal ischemic disease and neovascularization until vascular endothelial growth factor (VEGF) emerged [15].

4.1   Vascular Endothelial Growth Factor

First described by Judah Folkman and colleagues in 1970 as a tumor-derived angiogenic factor [16] and purified by Napoleone Ferrara and William Henzel in 1989 [17], VEGF is actually a family of five growth factors composed of VEGFs A-D and placental growth factor. Among the family members, VEGF-A is the most relevant to ischemic ocular disease. VEGF-A is produced in response to hypoxia, under transcriptional regulation of hypoxia-inducible factor (HIF)-1α. Müller glia, retinal pigment epithelial cells, capillary endothelial cell and pericytes, and some retinal neurons all produce VEGF [18, 19]. Whereas VEGF is undetectable in the aqueous humor of normal eyes, its diffusion through the vitreous in pathologic states exposes anterior segment tissues to the growth factor (Fig. 1a). VEGF signal transduction is complex, owing to alternative splicing of transcripts, with $VEGF_{165}$ being the most potent for driving neovascularization. In addition, the dimeric tyrosine kinase VEGF receptors form complexes with numerous other cell surface receptors, thereby altering their sig-

naling function. VEGFR2 is the receptor most relevant for endothelial cell signaling and neovascularization. Within vascular endothelial cells, VEGF simulates proliferation, antiapoptotic signaling, migration, and increased permeability through multiple pathways, including RAS/RAF/ERK/MAPK, PI3K-PBK/AKT, and PLC-γ /Ca^{++}/eNOS [20, 21].

The centrality of VEGF to NVG pathogenesis is supported by especially high growth factor concentrations in the aqueous humor of patients with active iris neovascularization in the setting of diabetic retinopathy, retinal vein occlusion, and retinopathy of prematurity [22]. Indeed, VEGF levels in the aqueous humor of NVG patients are more than 40-fold higher than in patients with primary open angle glaucoma [23]. VEGF is sufficient to cause iris neovascularization, as demonstrated in nonhuman primate models following intravitreal VEGF injection [24]. Prolonged exposure to VEGF over 30 days further induces NVG with IOP elevation and the characteristic anatomical changes described above. The requirement of VEGF in developing NVG was established in primate models with laser-induced retinal venous occlusion, where anti-VEGF antibodies blocked iris neovascularization development [25]. This finding heralded the success of anti-VEGF treatment in treating not only posterior segment disease in retinal ischemic disorders but also early stages of NVG.

The beneficial effects of panretinal photocoagulation (PRP) in reducing iris and angle neovascularization and NVG are well established [26]. In support of VEGF as a mediator of NVG pathogenesis, aqueous VEGF levels are reduced in patients with diabetic retinopathy following PRP treatment in a dose-dependent manner [27].

The therapeutic targeting of VEGF has revolutionized ophthalmology by providing new avenues for treating ocular disease, and NVG is no exception. The first FDA-approved pharmacologic VEGF inhibitor pegaptanib (Macugen®) was a pegylated aptamer (an oligonucleotide) designed specifically to bind and sequester VEGF-A. Subsequently, a series of monoclonal antibodies and antibody-receptor hybrids that recognize and sequester VEGF-A have been developed for the treatment of diabetic retinopathy and age-related macular degeneration, though they are frequently used for other ischemic retinal conditions as well. This has provided data in human patients that corroborate the central role of VEGF in driving NVG pathogenesis. Both intracameral and intravitreal injection of bevacizumab lead to rapid reduction in vascular leakage and regression of iris neovascularization within 48 hours in early disease, and, more importantly, IOP reduction when the angle remains open [3, 5, 28–32]. This is associated with a direct reduction in aqueous VEGF levels [33]. However, in late-stage disease when the angle has already become partially or fully synechially closed, intravitreal bevacizumab is generally not sufficient in achieving adequate IOP control [5]. This observation underscores the critical importance of early diagnosis of NVG. Since intravitreal antibody has a half-life on the order of days, anti-VEGF therapy induces temporary regression of neovascularization and repeated treatment is needed to prevent recurrence of neovascularization. Interestingly, anterior segment angiography shows that while bevacizumab reduces the intense vascular leakage seen with iris and iridocorneal angle neovessels, it does not change the overall vascular structure of the anterior segment, suggesting that these vessels may not fully regress [3, 28].

Ultimately, PRP leads to structural reduction of neovessels in the anterior segment [34] and a more permanent reduction of VEGF signaling by suppressing growth factor production. Moreover, other proangiogenic factors play a role in retinal neovascularization that are not targeted by VEGF-binding antibodies (see below). While evidence for these other factors playing a direct role in anterior segment neovascularization is less readily available, they may explain observations of persistent anterior and/or posterior segment fibrovascular activity in the face of ongoing anti-VEGF treatment. Therefore, while anti-VEGF therapy is useful to induce

short-term anterior segment regression of neovascularization, many clinicians recommend that PRP be a component of the treatment repertoire for NVG [35].

4.2   Platelet-Derived Growth Factor (PDGF)

The platelet-derived growth factors are another family of signaling ligands that regulate cell proliferation and growth, particularly in vasculature and other mesenchymal-derived tissues [36]. PDGF exists as a homo- or heterodimer of four subunits, PDGFs-A-D, acting through two monomeric tyrosine kinase receptors, PDGFR-α and -β. In ocular tissue, PDGF proteins are closely associated with pericytes and the maintenance of the retinal microvasculature. While PDGF expression is increased in retinal hypoxia, their effects are thought to be distinct from and complimentary to VEGF signaling in endothelial cells. PDGF-BB, for example, protects retinal microvasculature from damage caused by metabolic inhibitors [37]. However, in mouse studies, upregulation of retinal PDGF-BB also leads to neovascular proliferation in the posterior segment [38], whereas blockage of PDGF-BB signaling reduces the development of choroidal neovascularization at breaks in Bruch's membrane [39]. Other PDGF family members, particularly PDGF-C and -D have been shown to play a role in ischemia-induced retinopathy [36]. Whereas PDGF has been implicated strongly in AMD, its role in the pathophysiology of NVG is less clear. Expression of PDGF-C is upregulated in aqueous humor of patients with NVG [40]. Moreover, PDGF levels are high in patients with NVG even after treatment with bevacizumab, suggesting that PDGF regulation may be VEGF-independent [41]. Whereas combination therapies targeting VEGF and PDGF are of clinical interest and could potentially be useful in NVG, PDGF inhibitors are not approved for the treatment of ocular disease. Significant interest in

PDGF and other vasoactive targets exist for the treatment of AMD and diabetic retinopathy [42, 43]; however, the failures in 2016 of two phase-3 randomized clinical trials for the anti-PDGF therapy, pegpleranib (Fovista), have unfortunately stalled further development in this arena for the time being [44, 45].

4.3   Other Angiogenic Factors

Angiopoietin-like 4 (ANGPTL4) has emerged as another hypoxia-induced vasoproliferative factor. The aqueous fluid of patients with proliferative diabetic retinopathy recently treated with anti-VEGF is capable of experimentally inducing endothelial tubule formation in vitro, suggesting that there are other factors that contribute to neovascularization. In an expression screen of retinal Müller cells subjected to hypoxia, ANGPTL4 was identified as being upregulated at levels similar to VEGF [46]. Moreover, ANGPTL4 was also upregulated in the vitreous and aqueous fluid of patients with PDR. Neutralizing antibodies against ANGPTL4 inhibited the in vitro angiogenic potential of aqueous fluid from these patients and was additive with the effects of anti-VEGF. Interestingly, aqueous ANGPTL4 is elevated in BRVO patients with macular edema and correlates with retinal nonperfusion area [47].

Like VEGF, *interleukin (IL)-6* (IL-6) is induced by hypoxia. Elevated levels of IL-6 are found in the aqueous humor of patients with CRVO only when anterior segment neovascularization is evident [48]. *Erythropoietin* is a HIF-1α-regulated glycoprotein that is elevated in the vitreous of patients with PDR. In murine models, blockage of erythropoietin has been shown to decrease retinal neovascularization in vivo and inhibit endothelial cell proliferation in in vitro assays [49]. Other pro-angiogenic or profibrotic factors that may play a role in anterior segment neovascularization include: *transforming growth factor (TGF)-β* [50], *fibroblast growth factor (FGF)* [51], *and tumor necrosis factor (TNF)-α* [52].

These proangiogenic factors act in balance with antiangiogenic signaling molecules, chief among them being *pigment epithelium-derived factor (PEDF)* [53, 54]. Indeed, not only are proangiogenic factors produced in retinal ischemic disease, but also PEDF levels decline [55–58], due to hypoxia-induced matrix metalloprotease degradation, further tipping the molecular signaling balance toward neovascularization [59, 60]. PEDF functions by regulating cell cycle progression and apoptosis through Fas, p38 MAPK, and p53 signaling [61–63].

5   From Retina to Aqueous

As vasoproliferative growth factors are primarily produced by tissues of the posterior segment, it follows that diffusion from the vitreous cavity exposes anterior segment tissues to VEGF and other vasogenic growth factors. Indeed, a common route of molecular clearance from the vitreous is through anterior diffusion into the aqueous of the posterior then anterior chamber and subsequent clearance through the trabecular meshwork (Fig. 1a) [64]. A concentration gradient of VEGF has been shown in eyes with diabetic macular edema with highest levels within the posterior premacular vitreous and lowest levels within the anterior peripheral vitreous [65]. In support of that mechanism, neovascularization is first visible at the pupil margin where the highest flux of aqueous humor occurs. One might speculate that diffusion rates of vasoproliferative factors to the front of the eye, and hence the incidence of NVG, would therefore be altered by vitrectomy. VEGF clearance from the vitreous cavity indeed increases after vitrectomy in rabbit eyes [66]. In reality, confounding factors such as severity of retinal disease leading to complications that necessitate vitrectomy (vitreous hemorrhage or traction retinal detachment) hamper the ability to test this hypothesis clinically. However, it has been noted in multiple studies that the likelihood of developing NVG after vitrectomy is greater in aphakic or pseudophakic eyes, than in phakic eyes [67–70], suggesting that the crystalline lens may serve as a barrier to diffusion of vasoproliferative ligands to the front of the eye.

6 Beyond Retinal Ischemia

Despite the focus on the retina as the source of proangiogenic signals, recent investigations have turned toward the anterior segment as a potential secondary source of VEGF. Anterior segment ischemia, induced by cauterization of the long posterior ciliary arteries, induces VEGF production by the ciliary body and anterior segment neovascularization in rabbits [71]. Indeed, immunocytochemistry and in situ hybridization studies have confirmed the nonpigmented ciliary epithelium as a site of VEGF synthesis in NVG [72]. This observation is interesting in the context of patients whose NVG is refractory to PRP and may be particularly relevant in conditions where anterior segment ischemia is a prominent feature, such as OIS. A better understanding of the effects of neovascularization on the ciliary body may also help shed light on why rates of hypotony following cyclophotocoagulation are higher in patients with NVG than with other forms of glaucoma [73].

7 Conclusions

NVG results from posterior segment vasoproliferative signals in the setting of retinal ischemia, leading to anterior segment neovascularization. A mechanistic understanding of proangiogenic growth factor signaling has brought us into the anti-VEGF era of ophthalmology. Other potential treatments are on the horizon that will target anterior segment vasoproliferation in early disease and potentially circumvent NVG development. There is, however, still a role for more traditional treatments, such as PRP, for more sustained control of vasoproliferative signals, and for surgical treatments in the setting of secondary synechial angle closure in chronic NVG.

References

1. Weiss DI, Shaffer RN, Nehrenberg TR. Neovascular glaucoma complicating carotid-cavernous fistula. Arch Ophthalmol. 1963;69:304–7.
2. Barac IR, Pop MD, Gheorghe AI, Taban C. Neovascular secondary glaucoma, etiology and pathogenesis. Rom J Ophthalmol. 2015;59:24–8.
3. Ishibashi S, Tawara A, Sohma R, Kubota T, Toh N. Angiographic Changes in Iris and Iridocorneal Angle Neovascularization After Intravitreal Bevacizumab Injection. Arch Ophthalmol. 2010;128:1539–45.
4. John T, Sassani JW, Eagle RC. The myofibroblastic component of rubeosis iridis. Ophthalmology. 1983;90:721–8.
5. Wakabayashi T, Oshima Y, Sakaguchi H, Ikuno Y, Miki A, Gomi F, Otori Y, Kamei M, Kusaka S, Tano Y. Intravitreal bevacizumab to treat iris neovascularization and neovascular glaucoma secondary to ischemic retinal diseases in 41 consecutive cases. Ophthalmology. 2008;115:1571–1580.e3.
6. Eilken HM, Adams RH. Dynamics of endothelial cell behavior in sprouting angiogenesis. Curr Opin Cell Biol. 2010;22:617–25.
7. Stahl A, Connor KM, Sapieha P, et al. The mouse retina as an angiogenesis model. Invest Ophthalmol Vis Sci. 2010;51:2813–26.
8. Hillen F, Griffioen AW. Tumour vascularization: sprouting angiogenesis and beyond. Cancer Metastasis Rev. 2007;26:489–502.
9. Siemerink MJ, Klaassen I, Noorden CJFV, Schlingemann RO. Endothelial tip cells in ocular angiogenesis potential target for anti-angiogenesis therapy. J Histochem Cytochem. 2013;61:101–15.
10. Iruela-Arispe ML, Davis GE. Cellular and molecular mechanisms of vascular lumen formation. Dev Cell. 2009;16:222–31.
11. Bock KD, Smet FD, Oliveira RLD, Anthonis K, Carmeliet P. Endothelial oxygen sensors regulate tumor vessel abnormalization by instructing phalanx endothelial cells. J Mol Med. 2009;87:561–9.
12. Nork TM, Tso MOM, Duvall J, Hayreh SS. Cellular mechanisms of iris neovascularization secondary to retinal vein occlusion. Arch Ophthalmol. 1989;107:581–6.
13. Hayreh SS, Rojas P, Podhajsky P, Montague P, Woolson RF. Ocular neovascularization with retinal vascular occlusion-III incidence of ocular neovascularization with retinal vein occlusion. Ophthalmology. 1983;90:488–506.
14. Michaelson IC. The mode of development of the vascular system of the retina, with some observations on its significance for certain retinal disease. Trans Ophthalmol Soc U K. 1948;68:137–80.
15. Aiello LP. Vascular endothelial growth factor and the eye: past, present, and future. Arch Ophthalmol. 1996;114:1252–4.
16. Folkman J, Merler E, Abernathy C, Williams G. Isolation of a tumor factor responsible for angiogenesis. J Exp Med. 1971;133:275–88.

17. Ferrara N, Henzel WJ. Pituitary follicular cells secrete a novel heparin-binding growth factor specific for vascular endothelial cells. Biochem Biophys Res Commun. 1989;161:851–8.

18. Shima DT, Gougos A, Miller JW, Tolentino M, Robinson G, Adamis AP, D'Amore PA. Cloning and mRNA expression of vascular endothelial growth factor in ischemic retinas of Macaca fascicularis. Invest Ophthalmol Vis Sci. 1996;37:1334–40.

19. Behzadian MA, Wang XL, Al-Shabrawey M, Shabrawey M, Caldwell RB. Effects of hypoxia on glial cell expression of angiogenesis-regulating factors VEGF and TGF-β. Glia. 1998;24:216–25.

20. Koch S, Claesson-Welsh L. Signal transduction by vascular endothelial growth factor receptors. Cold Spring Harb Perspect Med. 2012;2:a006502.

21. Ho QT, Kuo CJ. Vascular endothelial growth factor: biology and therapeutic applications. Int J Biochem Cell Biol. 2007;39:1349–57.

22. Aiello LP, Avery RL, Arrigg PG, et al. Vascular endothelial growth factor in ocular fluid of patients with diabetic retinopathy and other retinal disorders. New Engl J Med. 1994;331:1480–7.

23. Tripathi RC, Lixa J, Tripathi BJ, Chalam KV, Adamis AP. Increased level of vascular endothelial growth factor in aqueous humor of patients with neovascular glaucoma. Ophthalmology. 1998;105:232–7.

24. Tolentino MJ, Miller JW, Gragoudas ES, Chatzistefanou K, Ferrara N, Adamis AP. Vascular endothelial growth factor is sufficient to produce iris neovascularization and neovascular glaucoma in a nonhuman primate. Arch Ophthalmol. 1996;114:964–70.

25. Adamis AP, Shima DT, Tolentino MJ, Gragoudas ES, Ferrara N, Folkman J, D'Amore PA, Miller JW. Inhibition of vascular endothelial growth factor prevents retinal ischemia—associated iris neovascularization in a nonhuman primate. Arch Ophthalmol. 1996;114:66–71.

26. Wand M, Dueker DK, Aiello LM, Grant WM. Effects of panretinal photocoagulation on rubeosis iridis, angle neovascularization, and neovascular glaucoma. Am J Ophthalmol. 1978;86:332–9.

27. Shinoda K, Ishida S, Kawashima S, Wakabayashi T, Uchita M, Matsuzaki T, Takayama M, Shinmura K, Yamada M. Clinical factors related to the aqueous levels of vascular endothelial growth factor and hepatocyte growth factor in proliferative diabetic retinopathy. Curr Eye Res. 2000;21:655–61.

28. Grisanti S, Biester S, Peters S, Tatar O, Ziemssen F, Bartz-Schmidt KU, Group TTBS. Intracameral bevacizumab for iris rubeosis. Am J Ophthalmol. 2006;142:158–60.

29. Iliev ME, Domig D, Wolf-Schnurrbursch U, Wolf S, Sarra G-M. Intravitreal bevacizumab (avastin®) in the treatment of neovascular glaucoma. Am J Ophthalmol. 2006;142:1054–6.

30. Yazdani S, Hendi K, Pakravan M, Mahdavi M, Yaseri M. Intravitreal bevacizumab for neovascular glaucoma. J Glaucoma. 2009;18:632–7.

31. Oshima Y, Sakaguchi H, Gomi F, Tano Y. Regression of iris neovascularization after intravitreal injection of bevacizumab in patients with proliferative diabetic retinopathy. Am J Ophthalmol. 2006;142:155–157.e1.

32. Mason JO, Albert MA, Mays A, Vail R. Regression of neovascular iris vessels by intravitreal injection of bevacizumab. Retina. 2006;26:839–41.

33. Grover S, Gupta S, Sharma R, Brar VS, Chalam KV. Intracameral bevacizumab effectively reduces aqueous vascular endothelial growth factor concentrations in neovascular glaucoma. Br J Ophthalmol. 2009;93:273.

34. Akagi T, Fujimoto M, Ikeda HO. Anterior segment optical coherence tomography angiography of iris neovascularization after intravitreal ranibizumab and panretinal photocoagulation. JAMA Ophthalmol. 2020;138:e190318.

35. Olmos LC, Sayed MS, Moraczewski AL, Gedde SJ, Rosenfeld PJ, Shi W, Feuer WJ, Lee RK. Long-term outcomes of neovascular glaucoma treated with and without intravitreal bevacizumab. Eye. 2016;30:463–72.

36. Kumar A, Li X. PDGF-C and PDGF-D in ocular diseases. Mol Asp Med. 2018;62:33–43.

37. Kodama T, Oku H, Kawamura H, Sakagami K, Puro DG. Platelet-derived growth factor-BB: a survival factor for the retinal microvasculature during periods of metabolic compromise. Curr Eye Res. 2001;23:93–7.

38. Mori K, Gehlbach P, Ando A, Dyer G, Lipinsky E, Chaudhry AG, Hackett SF, Campochiaro PA. Retina-specific expression of PDGF-B versus PDGF-A: vascular versus nonvascular proliferative retinopathy. Invest Ophthalmol Vis Sci. 2002;43:2001–6.

39. Dong A, Seidel C, Snell D, et al. Antagonism of PDGF-BB suppresses subretinal neovascularization and enhances the effects of blocking VEGF-A. Angiogenesis. 2014;17:553–62.

40. Li Y, Hu D, Lv P, Xing M, Song Z, Li C, Wang Y, Hou X. Expression of platelet-derived growth factor-C in aqueous humor of patients with neovascular glaucoma and its correlation with vascular endothelial growth factor. Eur J Ophthalmol. 2019;30:500–5.

41. Ohira S, Inoue T, Shobayashi K, Iwao K, Fukushima M, Tanihara H. Simultaneous increase in multiple proinflammatory cytokines in the aqueous humor in neovascular glaucoma with and without intravitreal bevacizumab injection aqueous humor cytokines in neovascular glaucoma. Invest Ophthalmol Vis Sci. 2015;56:3541–8.

42. Jaffe GJ, Ciulla TA, Ciardella AP, et al. Dual antagonism of PDGF and VEGF in neovascular age-related macular degeneration a phase IIb, multicenter, randomized controlled trial. Ophthalmology. 2017;124:224–34.

43. Jaffe GJ, Eliott D, Wells JA, Prenner JL, Papp A, Patel S. A phase 1 study of intravitreous E10030 in combination with ranibizumab in neovascular age-related macular degeneration. Ophthalmology. 2016;123:78–85.

44. Dunn EN, Hariprasad SM, Sheth VS. An overview of the Fovista and Rinucumab trials and the fate of anti-PDGF medications. Ophthalmic Surg Lasers Imaging Retina. 2017;48:100–4.
45. Hussain RM, Ciulla TA. Emerging vascular endothelial growth factor antagonists to treat neovascular age-related macular degeneration. Expert Opin Emerg Drugs. 2017;22:235–46.
46. Babapoor-Farrokhran S, Jee K, Puchner B, et al. Angiopoietin-like 4 is a potent angiogenic factor and a novel therapeutic target for patients with proliferative diabetic retinopathy. Proc Natl Acad Sci. 2015;112:E3030–9.
47. Kim JH, Shin JP, Kim IT, Park DH. Aqueous angiopoietin-like 4 levels correlate with nonperfusion area and macular edema in branch retinal vein occlusion. Invest Ophthalmol Vis Sci. 2016;57:6–11.
48. Chen KH, Wu CC, Roy S, Lee SM, Liu JH. Increased interleukin-6 in aqueous humor of neovascular glaucoma. Invest Ophthalmol Vis Sci. 1999;40:2627–32.
49. Watanabe D, Suzuma K, Matsui S, et al. Erythropoietin as a retinal angiogenic factor in proliferative diabetic retinopathy. New Engl J Med. 2005;353:782–92.
50. Yu X-B, Sun X-H, Dahan E, Guo W-Y, Qian S-H, Meng F-R, Song Y-L, Simon GJB. Increased levels of transforming growth factor-beta1 and -beta2 in the aqueous humor of patients with neovascular glaucoma. Ophthalmic Surg Lasers Imaging. 2007;38:6–14.
51. Tripathi RC, Borisuth NSC, Tripathi BJ. Detection, quantification, and significance of basic fibroblast growth factor in the aqueous humor of man, cat, dog and pig. Exp Eye Res. 1992;54:447–54.
52. Gardiner TA, Gibson DS, de Gooyer TE, de la Cruz VF, McDonald DM, Stitt AW. Inhibition of tumor necrosis factor-α improves physiological angiogenesis and reduces pathological neovascularization in ischemic retinopathy. Am J Pathol. 2005;166:637–44.
53. Gao G, Li Y, Zhang D, Gee S, Crosson C, Ma J. Unbalanced expression of VEGF and PEDF in ischemia-induced retinal neovascularization. FEBS Lett. 2001;489:270–6.
54. Ogata N, Nishikawa M, Nishimura T, Mitsuma Y, Matsumura M. Unbalanced vitreous levels of pigment epithelium-derived factor and vascular endothelial growth factor in diabetic retinopathy. Am J Ophthalmol. 2002;134:348–53.
55. Ogata N, Nishikawa M, Nishimura T, Mitsuma Y, Matsumura M. Inverse levels of pigment epithelium-derived factor and vascular endothelial growth factor in the vitreous of eyes with rhegmatogenous retinal detachment and proliferative vitreoretinopathy. Am J Ophthalmol. 2002;133:851–2.
56. Spranger J, Osterhoff M, Reimann M, et al. Loss of the antiangiogenic pigment epithelium-derived factor in patients with angiogenic eye disease. Diabetes. 2001;50:2641–5.
57. Ogata N, Tombran-Tink J, Nishikawa M, Nishimura T, Mitsuma Y, Sakamoto T, Matsumura M. Pigment epithelium-derived factor in the vitreous is low in diabetic retinopathy and high in rhegmatogenous retinal detachment. Am J Ophthalmol. 2001;132:378–82.
58. Holekamp NM, Bouck N, Volpert O. Pigment epithelium-derived factor is deficient in the vitreous of patients with choroidal neovascularization due to age-related macular degeneration11InternetAdvance publication at ajo.com. May 7, 2002. Am J Ophthalmol. 2002;134:220–7.
59. Gao G, Li Y, Gee S, Dudley A, Fant J, Crosson C, Ma J. Down-regulation of vascular endothelial growth factor and up-regulation of pigment epithelium-derived factor: a possible mechanism for the anti-angiogenic activity of plasminogen kringle 5*. J Biol Chem. 2002;277:9492–7.
60. Notari L, Miller A, Martínez A, Amaral J, Ju M, Robinson G, Smith LEH, Becerra SP. Pigment epithelium–derived factor is a substrate for matrix metalloproteinase type 2 and type 9: implications for downregulation in hypoxia. Invest Ophthalmol Vis Sci. 2005;46:2736–47.
61. Volpert OV, Zaichuk T, Zhou W, Reiher F, Ferguson TA, Stuart PM, Amin M, Bouck NP. Inducer-stimulated Fas targets activated endothelium for destruction by anti-angiogenic thrombospondin-1 and pigment epithelium–derived factor. Nat Med. 2002;8:349–57.
62. Chen L, Zhang SS-M, Barnstable CJ, Tombran-Tink J. PEDF induces apoptosis in human endothelial cells by activating p38 MAP kinase-dependent cleavage of multiple caspases. Biochem Bioph Res Commun. 2006;348:1288–95.
63. Ho T-C, Chen S-L, Yang Y-C, Liao C-L, Cheng H-C, Tsao Y-P. PEDF induces p53-mediated apoptosis through PPAR gamma signaling in human umbilical vein endothelial cells. Cardiovasc Res. 2007;76:213–23.
64. del Amo EM, Rimpelä A-K, Heikkinen E, et al. Pharmacokinetic aspects of retinal drug delivery. Prog Retin Eye Res. 2017;57:134–85.
65. Shimada H, Akaza E, Yuzawa M, Kawashima M. Concentration gradient of vascular endothelial growth factor in the vitreous of eyes with diabetic macular edema. Invest Ophthalmol Vis Sci. 2009;50:2953–5.
66. Lee SS, Ghosn C, Yu Z, et al. Vitreous VEGF clearance is increased after vitrectomy. Invest Ophthalmol Vis Sci. 2010;51:2135–8.
67. Aaberg TM. Clinical results in vitrectomy for diabetic traction retinal detachment. Am J Ophthalmol. 1979;88:246–53.
68. Summanen P. Neovascular glaucoma following vitrectomy for diabetic eye disease. Acta Ophthalmol. 1988;66:110–6.
69. Blankenship GW. The lens Influence on diabetic vitrectomy results: report of a prospective randomized study. Arch Ophthalmol. 1980;98:2196–8.
70. Rice TA, Michels RG, Rice EF. Vitrectomy for diabetic traction retinal detachment involving the macula. Am J Ophthalmol. 1983;95:22–33.

71. Tawara A, Kubota T, Hata Y, Sakamoto T, Honda M, Yoshikawa H, Inomata H, Ohnishi Y. Neovascularization in the anterior segment of the rabbit eye by experimental anterior ischemia. Graefes Arch Clin Exp Ophthalmol. 2002;240:144–53.

72. Chalam KV, Brar VS, Murthy RK. Human ciliary epithelium as a source of synthesis and secretion of vascular endothelial growth factor in neovascular glaucoma. JAMA Ophthalmol. 2014;132:1350–4.

73. Ramli N, Htoon HM, Ho CL, Aung T, Perera S. Risk factors for hypotony after transscleral diode cyclophotocoagulation. J Glaucoma. 2012;21:169–73.

Clinical Diagnosis of Neovascular Glaucoma in the Ophthalmology Office

Inas F. Aboobakar and Michael M. Lin

1   Introduction

Neovascular glaucoma (NVG) is a particularly aggressive type of secondary glaucoma that develops in the setting of retinal ischemia and subsequent release of angiogenic factors into the aqueous humor [1]. The most common underlying etiologies for NVG are proliferative diabetic retinopathy (PDR), central retinal vein occlusion (CRVO), and ocular ischemic syndrome (OIS). PDR and CRVO each comprise approximately one-third of NVG cases, and OIS is the most common etiology amongst the remaining one-third of cases [2]. Other rarer causes include various ocular tumors (e.g., retinoblastoma, uveal melanomas, ciliary body medulloepithelioma, and vasoproliferative tumors of the retina), central retinal artery occlusion, sickle cell retinopathy, radiation retinopathy, carotid-cavernous fistulas, and ocular inflammatory disease [3–8]. Systemic conditions that have been associated with the development of neovascular glaucoma include juvenile xanthogranuloma, systemic lupus erythematosus, cryoglobulinemia, and neurofibromatosis type I [9–13].

The earliest stage on the NVG spectrum is when an eye is at high risk for developing anterior segment neovascularization, but there is no visible neovascularization of the iris (NVI) or angle (NVA) and the IOP is normal; this has classically been termed the prerubeosis stage. As the disease progresses, there is visible NVI and/or NVA, but the intraocular pressure (IOP) is still normal and the patient is asymptomatic; this has classically been termed the preglaucoma stage. As the NVA progresses, the development of a fibrovascular membrane in the angle obstructs aqueous outflow and the IOP becomes elevated, though there is no synechial angle closure yet; this has classically been termed the open-angle glaucoma stage. As the fibrovascular tissue in the angle contracts to form peripheral anterior synechiae, there is progressive synechial angle closure and profoundly elevated IOP; this has classically been termed the closed-angle glaucoma stage. Of note, the classical terms "open-angle NVG" and "closed-angle NVG" refer to anterior segment neovascularization with elevated IOP with or without true glaucomatous optic neuropathy. However, the historical convention is to refer to these stages as "NVG," so for the purpose of this chapter, this terminology will be used. Future consensus panels are needed to determine whether neovascular "ocular hypertension" may be a more descriptive term in the setting of elevated IOP without true glaucomatous optic neuropathy.

I. F. Aboobakar · M. M. Lin (✉)
Massachusetts Eye and Ear, Harvard Medical School, Boston, MA, USA
e-mail: michael_lin@meei.harvard.edu

© The Author(s), under exclusive license to Springer Nature Switzerland AG 2022
M. Qiu (ed.), *Neovascular Glaucoma*, Essentials in Ophthalmology,
https://doi.org/10.1007/978-3-031-11720-6_4

In this chapter, we discuss the clinical evaluation of patients who are at high risk of developing NVG and the diagnosis of NVG in the outpatient clinic setting, including critical components of the patient history, physical examination, and ancillary testing.

2 Clinical History

A thorough systemic and medical history is critical to identify possible etiologies for the development of NVG. This includes assessing for vascular risk factors (diabetes, hypertension, hyperlipidemia, coronary artery disease, cerebrovascular accident, and carotid occlusive disease), coagulopathies, and vasculitides. The patient's past ocular history may reveal possible conditions that can lead to the development of NVG, including PDR or CRVO. It is important to assess what previous treatments the patient has had for underlying retinal ischemic disorders (e.g., panretinal photocoagulation or anti-VEGF injections) and whether the patient has ever been diagnosed with high IOP or glaucoma in the past.

It is also critical to assess the patient's symptoms as well as their onset and duration. History of sudden onset vision loss a few months prior to presentation may raise CRVO higher on the differential, while episodes of transient vision loss (amaurosis fugax) may suggest ocular ischemic syndrome as an underlying etiology. In the early stages of NVG, patients may be asymptomatic. Conversely, patients who present in the angle-closure stage with acute elevations in IOP typically have associated eye pain, decreased vision, headaches, nausea/vomiting, and halos around lights. Hemodialysis may acutely increase IOP and lead to intermittent pain or blurry vision during dialysis sessions.

3 Examination

The diagnosis of NVG is mainly clinical, and a complete ophthalmologic examination is therefore critical. A special challenge in examination is that while many patients with PDR, CRVO,

and other NVG-predisposing conditions are managed by retina specialists who typically examine eyes after dilation, key parts of the examination such as evaluating for NVI are best performed before dilation. Moreover, retina specialists may not be as likely to perform or be comfortable with gonioscopy as glaucoma specialists. Many patients with early NVG are asymptomatic, and their disease may only be detected if an astute clinician was performing routine screening gonioscopy on high-risk patients. Important components of the examination for eyes at risk of NVG or with NVG are highlighted below.

3.1 Visual Acuity

It is critical to check visual acuity at every clinic visit and to compare to the baseline. Patients with NVG often have poor visual acuity due to corneal edema in the setting of acutely elevated IOP, underlying retinal pathology (e.g., vitreous hemorrhage, macular edema, macular ischemia), or glaucomatous optic neuropathy. However, visual acuity can range widely in all stages of NVG, with some patients with closed-angle NVG maintaining 20/20 central vision after IOP is stabilized and underlying retinal disease is treated.

3.2 Pupil Examination

The pupils should be assessed for a relative afferent pupillary defect (RAPD), as this can be a sign of asymmetric optic nerve damage. In patients with CRVO, studies have demonstrated that patients with an RAPD are at increased risk for developing NVI [14]. However, the presence of an RAPD does not necessarily indicate glaucomatous optic neuropathy, as the underlying retinal disease such as CRVO could cause RAPD even in the absence of NVG.

3.3 Intraocular Pressure (IOP)

In the earliest stages of the disease process, the IOP may still be normal even though there is visible NVA on gonioscopy. As the disease progresses, the IOP rises even though the angle may still appear to be open; these eyes are often responsive to medical IOP-lowering therapy since the trabecular meshwork may still be partially functional. As the disease progresses, synechial angle closure develops and the IOP becomes less responsive to medical IOP-lowering therapy; surgical IOP-lowering intervention is often needed at this stage.

3.4 Conjunctiva/Sclera and Cornea

Conjunctival hyperemia and ciliary flush may be seen in NVG, especially during acute elevations of IOP. Microcystic corneal edema may also be observed with acute IOP elevations. However, the cornea may be clear despite extremely elevated IOP, typically if the IOP increase has been gradual or chronic, and this may be associated with worse outcomes if it is an indication of long-term IOP elevation that has had a longer amount of time to cause severe glaucomatous optic neuropathy.

3.5 Anterior Chamber

Bleeding from NVI can lead to microhyphema or hyphema. Mild anterior chamber inflammation can also be observed. In advanced disease where the angle has become synechially closed, the anterior chamber may appear to be shallow due to the broad PAS.

3.6 Iris

Examination of the iris prior to dilation is critical to assess for NVI (rubeosis iridis). Neovascularization is usually first noted at the pupillary border. Whereas normal iris vessels usually lie in the stroma and are radial in orientation, neovessels appear on the iris surface and do not follow an organized growth pattern. Early, subtle neovascularization is best detected using the high-magnification setting on the slit lamp. Corectopia and ectropion uveae may be noted in advanced stages due to peripheral anterior synechiae and contraction of the fibrovascular membrane that forms over the iris. This membrane may also give a smooth, glistening appearance to the iris. NVG can also lead to posterior synechiae or an inflammatory membrane at the pupil margin; if present for 360°, posterior synechiae can even lead to pupillary block and iris bombe configuration.

3.7 Gonioscopy

Gonioscopy is critical in the assessment of NVG and should be performed prior to dilation. Although NVA usually develops after NVI, in some cases NVA can be seen without any NVI at the pupillary border [15]. In the Central Vein Occlusion Study (CVOS), for example, 10% of eyes with nonischemic CRVO and 6% of eyes with ischemic CRVO developed NVA without apparent NVI [16]. It is therefore critical to perform gonioscopy in patients with NVG or those who are at risk for it due to underlying retinal disease such as PDR and CRVO, even when no NVI is noted. Gonioscopy is crucial even in the absence of elevated IOP, as it may help detect NVA that warrants more aggressive treatment of the underlying retinopathy.

In early stages of NVG, neovessels appear over the angle structures but the angle still appears open. As the disease progresses, peripheral anterior synechiae develop and lead to synechial angle closure. Indentation gonioscopy may reveal that an angle that appeared to be completely synechially closed may in fact be open in some areas with indentation, revealing NVA adjacent to areas of PAS.

3.8 Lens

Examining the lens status can help with treatment planning. The presence of a visually significant cataract could be a sign that combined cataract and glaucoma surgery would be beneficial. In eyes with history of intravitreal injection, assessing for inadvertent needle violation of the lens capsule can prevent unanticipated intraoperative events. If the eye is pseudophakic, noting whether the intraocular lens is in the capsular bag, sulcus, or anterior chamber may also assist with surgical planning.

3.9 Dilated Fundus Examination

In some cases, vitreous hemorrhage may obscure the view of fundus details, and an ultrasound examination may be helpful to assess for retinal breaks, retinal detachment, or posterior pole masses. If a view is possible, glaucomatous changes of the optic nerve may be noted on dilated fundus examination, including increased cup-to-disc ratio, focal notching, disc hemorrhage, or atrophy of the retinal nerve fiber layer. However, elevated IOP may not have been present with enough severity or duration to cause any signs of glaucomatous structural change. It is critical to examine the optic nerve in both eyes to assess for possible asymmetry. Glaucomatous optic nerve damage in the other eye of a patient with NVG secondary to CRVO in the eye in question may suggest that the CRVO was a result of uncontrolled primary open angle glaucoma. The optic nerve exam may also reveal pallor and fine vessels on the nerve head consistent with neovascularization of the disc. These changes may be driven by the underlying ischemic retinal disease or panretinal photocoagulation that was performed to treat PDR or CRVO.

A thorough dilated fundus examination also enables identification of possible underlying etiologies for NVG, including PDR (neovascularization of the disc or neovascularization elsewhere), old CRVO (optociliary shunt vessels, vessel sheathing), or ocular ischemic syndrome (mid-peripheral retinal hemorrhages). Presence of tractional retinal detachment in PDR or other disease that could require silicone oil for repair may impact surgical planning, such as placement of an aqueous shunt in an inferior rather than superior quadrant.

4 Ancillary Testing

While NVG is primarily a clinical diagnosis, ancillary testing can help assess the degree of glaucoma damage and identify underlying etiologies. Important tests that may be performed in the outpatient clinic setting are highlighted below.

4.1 Anterior Segment Photography

Anterior segment photographs prior to dilation may aid in the detection and documentation of NVI and could be particularly helpful in retina clinics where patients may often only be examined by the physician after dilation. Automated gonioscopy has the potential to circumferentially document the angle status, though it is not a perfect substitute for dynamic gonioscopy by a skilled examiner.

4.2 Visual Field Testing

Visual field testing using standard automated perimetry is a cornerstone of glaucoma diagnosis, assessment of disease severity, and monitoring for progression [17–19]. However, corneal edema, macular edema, macular ischemia, vitreous hemorrhage, or underlying retinal disease may limit the utility of visual field testing. Modifications such as using size V stimulus may improve the chances that visual field testing will provide useful information. Distinguishing whether field loss is due to glaucoma or other causes can be challenging. Glaucomatous field defects respect the horizontal meridian and classically present as a nasal step, arcuate scotoma, or with generalized depression in advanced disease. It is important to note that visual field loss in NVG patients can also be due to underlying retinal disease or its treatment (e.g., panretinal photocoagulation) [20].

4.3 Optical Coherence Tomography (OCT)

OCT provides high-speed, high-resolution imaging of the retinal nerve fiber layer (RNFL) and ganglion cell layer, which may be damaged before visual field defects are noted in glaucoma [21, 22]. It is critical to obtain a baseline OCT and assess for change over time. Of note, the presence of macular edema or other retinal pathology can affect thickness measurements and must be taken into account when interpreting data [23]. In particular, at initial presentation of NVG, disc edema may cause RNFL measurements to be artificially thickened, and macular edema may make ganglion cell layer segmentation challenging. As the inflammation and edema resolve, repeated OCT scans may indicate RNFL thinning, but this may be from resolution of edema instead of true glaucomatous progression.

Optical coherence tomography angiography (OCT-A) has potential to aid in detection of NVI before it is visible clinically [24, 25]. OCT-A relies on detecting changes between rapidly repeated OCT scans of the same area, highlighting vascular areas where moving red blood cells will vary in appearance between images. This noninvasive technology does not require intravascular dyes, but it is not as widely available as standard OCT.

4.4 Fluorescein Angiography

Fluorescein angiography (FA) is useful in imaging the retinal and choroidal vasculature and helps in the diagnosis of pathologic processes of the retina. It can be helpful for identifying an underlying etiology for NVG. In patients with PDR, FA leakage may be noted from the disc due to NVD or elsewhere in the retina due to NVE. In CRVO, perivenular hypoautofluorescence is seen due to autofluorescence blockage from hemorrhages and inner retinal edema [26]. Iris angiography is not widely utilized clinically, but it may be helpful

in the detection of subtle NVI before it becomes evident on slit-lamp biomicroscopy [27].

4.5 B-Scan Ultrasound

If no posterior view is possible on exam, a B-scan ultrasound should be performed to evaluate for posterior pathology, including vitreous hemorrhage, mass, or retinal detachment that may require additional treatment by a retina specialist. A suspicious mass may require additional neoplastic workup and would suggest that cyclophotocoagulation would be more appropriate than an aqueous shunt which could risk extraocular tumor spread. Retinal detachment may alter surgical urgency, and it is important to consider whether gas or silicone oil will be used.

4.6 Systemic Workup

Laboratory and radiology workup may be needed to identify an underlying systemic etiology for the development of NVG. This may include a blood glucose or hemoglobin A1c to evaluate for diabetes; a hypercoagulable workup in young patients with CRVO and no vascular risk factors; or a carotid doppler ultrasound to evaluate for carotid occlusive disease and ocular ischemic syndrome. This workup may be coordinated with the patient's primary care provider or performed in the emergency room depending on the clinical urgency.

5 Treatment

Once a clinical diagnosis of NVG has been made, prompt treatment is critical. Treatment of NVG will be covered in detail in other chapters, but in brief, the cornerstones of treatment involve controlling IOP with medications and/or surgery, as well as treating the underlying retinal disease, typically with a combination of intravitreal injections and panretinal photocoagulation.

6   Conclusion

Careful history taking, examination, and ancillary testing are critical in the clinical diagnosis of NVG. As many patients with NVG are asymptomatic, especially in the early stages, it is important to have a high suspicion for NVG in patients with predisposing conditions such as PDR and CRVO and to perform appropriate examination including gonioscopy. As the disease progresses, previously asymptomatic patients may develop severe pain and/or decreased vision which may prompt them to seek urgent medical attention in an emergency room setting, which will be discussed in detail in the next chapter.

References

1. Tolentino MJ, et al. Vascular endothelial growth factor is sufficient to produce iris neovascularization and neovascular glaucoma in a nonhuman primate. Arch Ophthalmol. 1996;114:964–70. https://doi.org/10.1001/archopht.1996.01100140172010.
2. Vancea PP, Abu-Taleb A. [Current trends in neovascular glaucoma treatment]. Rev Med Chir Soc Med Nat Iasi. 2005;109:264–8.
3. Hayreh SS, Zimmerman MB. Ocular neovascularization associated with central and hemicentral retinal vein occlusion. Retina. 2012;32:1553–65. https://doi.org/10.1097/IAE.0b013e318246912c.
4. Brown GC, Magargal LE, Schachat A, Shah H. Neovascular glaucoma. Etiologic considerations. Ophthalmology. 1984;91:315–20. https://doi.org/10.1016/s0161-6420(84)34293-2.
5. Nawaiseh I, et al. The impact of growth patterns of retinoblastoma (endophytic, exophytic, and mixed patterns). Turk Patoloji Derg. 2015;31:45–50. https://doi.org/10.5146/tjpath.2014.01278.
6. Mahdjoubi A, et al. Intravitreal bevacizumab for neovascular glaucoma in uveal melanoma treated by proton beam therapy. Graefes Arch Clin Exp Ophthalmol. 2018;256:411–20. https://doi.org/10.1007/s00417-017-3834-3.
7. Ali MJ, Honavar SG, Vemuganti GK. Ciliary body medulloepithelioma in an adult. Surv Ophthalmol. 2013;58:266–72. https://doi.org/10.1016/j.survophthal.2012.08.006.
8. Nakamura Y, Takeda N, Mochizuki M. A case of vasoproliferative retinal tumor complicated by neovascular glaucoma. Retin Cases Brief Rep. 2013;7:338–42. https://doi.org/10.1097/ICB.0b013e3182598eea.
9. Terelak-Borys B, Skonieczna K, Grabska-Liberek I. Ocular ischemic syndrome—a systematic review. Med Sci Monit. 2012;18:RA138–44. https://doi.org/10.12659/msm.883260.
10. Zhang J, et al. Glaucoma secondary to systemic lupus erythematosus. Chin Med J. 2014;127:3428–31.
11. Rao A, Padhy D. The child with spontaneous recurrent bleeding in the eye. BMJ Case Rep. 2014;2014:bcr2014203925. https://doi.org/10.1136/bcr-2014-203925.
12. Yang CH, Qureshi AA, Churchill WH, Saavedra AP. Long-term plasmapheresis in conjunction with thalidomide and dexamethasone for the treatment of cutaneous ulcers and neovascular glaucoma in recalcitrant type I cryoglobulinemia. JAMA Dermatol. 2014;150:426–8. https://doi.org/10.1001/jamadermatol.2013.8700.
13. Pichi F, et al. Neovascular glaucoma induced by peripheral retinal ischemia in neurofibromatosis type 1: management and imaging features. Case Rep Ophthalmol. 2013;4:69–73. https://doi.org/10.1159/000350956.
14. Servais GE, Thompson HS, Hayreh SS. Relative afferent pupillary defect in central retinal vein occlusion. Ophthalmology. 1986;93:301–3. https://doi.org/10.1016/s0161-6420(86)33751-5.
15. Blinder KJ, Friedman SM, Mames RN. Diabetic iris neovascularization. Am J Ophthalmol. 1995;120:393–5. https://doi.org/10.1016/s0002-9394(14)72173-7.
16. Baseline and early natural history report. The Central Vein Occlusion Study. Arch Ophthalmol. 1993;111:1087–95. https://doi.org/10.1001/archopht.1993.01090080083022.
17. Nelson-Quigg JM, Twelker JD, Johnson CA. Response properties of normal observers and patients during automated perimetry. Arch Ophthalmol. 1989;107:1612–5. https://doi.org/10.1001/archopht.1989.01070020690029.
18. Advanced Glaucoma Intervention Study. 2. Visual field test scoring and reliability. Ophthalmology. 1994;101:1445–55.
19. Chauhan BC, et al. Rates of glaucomatous visual field change in a large clinical population. Invest Ophthalmol Vis Sci. 2014;55:4135–43. https://doi.org/10.1167/iovs.14-14643.
20. Maguire MG, et al. Visual field changes over 5 years in patients treated with panretinal photocoagulation or ranibizumab for proliferative diabetic retinopathy. JAMA Ophthalmol. 2020;138:285–93. https://doi.org/10.1001/jamaophthalmol.2019.5939.
21. Huang D, et al. Optical coherence tomography. Science. 1991;254:1178–81. https://doi.org/10.1126/science.1957169.
22. Quigley HA, Miller NR, George T. Clinical evaluation of nerve fiber layer atrophy as an indicator of glaucomatous optic nerve damage. Arch Ophthalmol. 1980;98:1564–71. https://doi.org/10.1001/archopht.1980.01020040416003.
23. Hwang DJ, Lee EJ, Lee SY, Park KH, Woo SJ. Effect of diabetic macular edema on peripapillary retinal nerve fiber layer thickness profiles. Invest Ophthalmol Vis Sci. 2014;55:4213–9. https://doi.org/10.1167/iovs.13-13776.
24. Roberts PK, Goldstein DA, Fawzi AA. Anterior segment optical coherence tomography angiography

for identification of iris vasculature and staging of iris neovascularization: a pilot study. Curr Eye Res. 2017;42:1136–42. https://doi.org/10.1080/02713683. 2017.1293113.

25. Shiozaki D, et al. Observation of treated iris neo-vascularization by swept-source-based en-face anterior-segment optical coherence tomography angiography. Sci Rep. 2019;9:10262. https://doi. org/10.1038/s41598-019-46514-z.

26. Pichi F, et al. Perivenular whitening in central vein occlusion described by fundus autofluorescence and spectral domain optical coherence tomography. Retina. 2012;32:1438–9. https://doi.org/10.1097/ IAE.0b013e31825dd2a7.

27. Sanborn GE, Symes DJ, Magargal LE. Fundus-iris fluorescein angiography: evaluation of its use in the diagnosis of rubeosis iridis. Ann Ophthalmol. 1986;18:52–8.

Clinical Diagnosis of Neovascular Glaucoma in the Emergency Room

Christos N. Theophanous and Katy C. Liu

1 Disease Pathogenesis

In patients with neovascular glaucoma (NVG), an acute rise in intraocular pressure (IOP) often prompts a visit to the emergency room because patients experience severe pain and/or decreased vision. Acute IOP elevation in NVG is often due to neovascularization of the angle (NVA) which obstructs aqueous outflow through the trabecular meshwork; as the disease progresses, peripheral anterior synechiae can develop and cause synechial angle closure [1]. Acute IOP elevation in NVG can also occur due to hyphema secondary to neovascularization of the iris (NVI) in the absence of NVA [2]. Patients with NVG may also present to the emergency room with visual symptoms related to underlying retinal neovascularization such as macular edema or vitreous hemorrhage.

C. N. Theophanous
Department of Ophthalmology and Visual Science, University of Chicago, Chicago, IL, USA

K. C. Liu (✉)
Department of Ophthalmology, Duke University, Durham, NC, USA
e-mail: katy.liu@duke.edu

2 Clinical Presentation

The acute onset of symptoms in NVG can be a manifestation of previously undiagnosed disease or varying stages of the disease course. Common presenting symptoms include blurry vision, eye pain, eye redness, tearing, photophobia, or ocular irritation [3]. Ocular symptoms may also be associated with headache, nausea, and vomiting. In some cases, the presenting symptoms at different stages of NVG can be indistinguishable. For instance, a patient presenting with blurry vision may have decreased vision due to microcystic corneal edema in the setting of acute IOP elevation, obscuration from hyphema or vitreous hemorrhage, macular edema secondary to underlying retinal pathology, or acute ischemia from a retinal vessel occlusion. Blurry vision may also be due to glaucomatous optic neuropathy in later stages of NVG. In cases with more indolent and gradual IOP elevation, the patient may not complain of eye redness, pain or photophobia, but rather, presentation to the emergency room may be preceded by slow, painless vision loss.

3 Patient History

Given the variety of possible presenting symptoms and the spectrum of underlying causes for NVG, it is critical to obtain a detailed history with the following key elements:

1. *Elicit the Nature of Symptoms.* A careful history should include characterization of symptom quality, onset, duration, and associated signs or symptoms. Pertinent history-taking can suggest symptom etiology or the extent of disease. For example, eye pain characterized as deep, aching pain with or without headaches, nausea and vomiting, or halos around lights is more likely related to acute IOP elevation, whereas ocular irritation or foreign body sensation is more likely secondary to microcystic corneal edema. If eye pain or redness is present, it is useful to elicit whether the symptoms developed suddenly or gradually, which can suggest rapid versus gradual IOP elevation, respectively. If presenting symptoms are associated with preceding transient visual loss, i.e., amaurosis fugax, the history may indicate ocular ischemic syndrome (OIS) as an underlying etiology [4]. It is also important to ask about symptoms in the fellow eye. Since visual outcomes can be poor in many cases of NVG, identification of early or subtle changes in the fellow eye can facilitate closer monitoring and early intervention.

2. *Elicit the Timing of Symptoms.* The temporal relationship between symptoms can suggest underlying causes for NVG. For instance, sudden vision loss months before presentation could suggest NVG secondary to a central retinal vein occlusion (CRVO), whereas more recent vision loss weeks prior to presentation could favor NVG due to an underlying central retinal artery occlusion (CRAO) [5]. In patients with proliferative diabetic retinopathy (PDR), the onset of NVG is usually associated with periods of uncontrolled hyperglycemia [3].

3. *Elicit a Thorough Medical History.* Vasculopathic or ischemic systemic risk factors should raise concern for NVG. In particular, it is important to inquire about hypertension, hyperlipidemia, coronary artery disease, diabetes mellitus, history of cerebrovascular accident, coagulopathies, autoimmune conditions, vasculitis, and carotid occlusive disease. The degree of control of these medical conditions can correlate with onset or worsening of NVG. For instance, poor glycemic control, uncontrolled hypertension, or recent vasculitis flares can lead to retinal ischemia and predispose to new onset or worsening NVG. Oncologic history should also be solicited as the presence of tumors or a history of head and neck radiation are risk factors for NVG. For surgical planning purposes, it is also helpful to inquire about use of aspirin or anticoagulant medications.

4. *Elicit a Complete Ocular History.* Given the variety of underlying ischemic etiologies that can result in NVG, known history of PDR, CRAO, CRVO, OIS, or other less common ischemic conditions should raise concern for NVG [6]. If the patient cannot recall specific ocular diagnoses, a history of retinal laser or intravitreal injections (i.e., anti-vascular endothelial growth factor (anti-VEGF) injections) may indicate prior treatments for retinal ischemia. A history of vitrectomy surgery should be elicited, as NVG can result from chronic retinal detachment, and eyes with PDR may have previously undergone pars plana vitrectomy. It is also helpful to inquire about a history of glaucoma or the use of IOP-lowering medications.

4 Physical Examination

The diagnosis of neovascular glaucoma can usually be confirmed by a careful physical examination. The following clinical signs are useful in the diagnosis of NVG:

1. *Vitals and Medical Examination.* Patients seen in the emergency room have generally undergone a full medical examination prior to consultation. Vitals should be reviewed with attention to elevated blood pressure indicating underlying hypertension. Laboratory values such as blood glucose and hemoglobin A1c (HbA1c) can be diagnostic for diabetes and the degree of control. A comprehensive physical examination can elicit signs of vasculopathy. For patients with suspected OIS, auscultation for carotid bruits

should be specifically performed. Notably, the patient's medical status is important for treatment planning; if the patient is being treated for more emergent or life-threatening conditions (e.g., hypertensive emergency or electrolyte imbalance from missed dialysis), or if the patient's condition prohibits anesthesia clearance for surgery, the glaucoma management may need to be modified accordingly.

2. *Visual Acuity and Pupil Exam.* Patients with NVG often present with poor visual acuity. A baseline visual acuity is useful, but there can be limitations to acquiring an accurate visual acuity assessment in the emergency room including lack of access to a Snellen chart, appropriate lighting, spectacles if checking near vision, and limited patient cooperation. Nonetheless, even an estimate of visual acuity can help guide treatment planning. For instance, very poor baseline vision, especially no light perception vision, may push treatment toward less invasive options such as transscleral cyclophotocoagulation over an incisional glaucoma surgery. Next, a careful pupillary exam should be performed prior to dilation to assess for pupillary response. The affected pupil can be poorly reactive in NVG, and it is also important to check for the presence of a relative afferent pupillary defect (RAPD). Notably, a RAPD may indicate a glaucomatous optic neuropathy, but a RAPD can also be present in other conditions such as an ischemic CRVO. In cases where the view to the pupil is obstructed, such as with significant hyphema or microcystic edema, assessment of RAPD can be performed by reverse testing of the unaffected eye.

3. *Intraocular Pressure.* Measuring IOP in the affected and contralateral eye is critical in the evaluation of NVG in the emergency room. IOP can stratify the acuity of the clinical presentation and the extent of disease. Of note, IOP is not always elevated in the affected eye; higher IOP in the contralateral eye can be suggestive of NVG secondary to OIS. In the emergency room setting, Goldmann

applanation tonometry may not be available or logistically feasible. Portable handheld tonometers such as a Tono-Pen® (Reichert, Depew, NY) or an iCare (iCare USA, Raleigh, NC) may be practical and are generally sufficient for IOP measurement in the emergency room setting.

4. *Confrontational Visual Fields.* Assessment of visual fields in the emergency room is important, as the patient may not appreciate monocular field changes in the affected eye. Retinal ischemia or advanced glaucoma can impact the visual field. Field defects can be suggestive of branch or hemiretinal vessel occlusion, and peripheral field loss may indicate advanced glaucoma. Notably, accurate visual field assessment in the acute setting may be limited by a variety of factors such as microcystic edema of the cornea, dense hyphema, or vitreous hemorrhage. In cases with microcystic edema, it is prudent to delay or repeat confrontational visual field evaluation after the IOP has been lowered.

5. *Conjunctival Examination.* Conjunctival hyperemia and ciliary flush can be observed in NVG patients, especially those with an acute rise in IOP. The conjunctiva should also be examined for evidence of prior glaucoma surgeries (i.e., trabeculectomies, aqueous shunts, or other implants such as XEN® Gel Stents (Allergan, Dublin, Ireland) or Ex-PRESS Shunts (Alcon Laboratories Inc., Fort Worth, TX)) which may inform patient's prior ocular history and guide surgical management decisions.

6. *Corneal Examination.* Corneal changes such as microcystic edema can be an indication of rapid IOP elevation and blur the view for a detailed ocular examination. If microcystic edema is present in the setting of high IOP, initial topical treatment with beta-adrenergic antagonists, carbonic anhydrase inhibitors, and alpha-2 agonists can help to reduce edema and improve the view. Of note, prostaglandin analogs are often avoided to prevent further breakdown of the blood-aqueous barrier and worsening inflammation. Similarly, anticholinergics are proinflamma-

tory which can worsen peripheral anterior synechiae formation and are generally contraindicated [7]. If microcystic edema limits the initial exam, an updated examination after resolution of the edema can reveal subtle and previously concealed anterior and posterior segment exam findings.

7. *Anterior Chamber Examination.* A hyphema or microhyphema may suggest the presence of anterior segment neovascularization. Suspicion for underlying NVI and NVA should be particularly high in cases of seemingly spontaneous hyphema in the absence of trauma or other predisposing factors such as uveitis-glaucoma-hyphema syndrome in a pseudophakic eye. Mild anterior chamber reaction may be present in some cases.

8. *Iris Examination.* Neovascularization of the iris, or rubeosis, is a hallmark feature of NVG, though it is possible to have NVA and elevated IOP without NVI. Fine blood vessels can be seen on the surface of the iris and typically grow in a meandering pattern, extending from the pupillary margin. In some cases of acutely high IOP, NVI may appear less visible until the IOP is lowered and there is less resistance to vessel filling. In chronic NVG, ectropion uveae can be present due to contraction of the fibrovascular membrane. In cases of chronic, mature NVI, iris vessels may persist even after treatment for neovascularization, but typically appear less engorged than before. Regressed NVI can appear as either an absence of previously noted vessels, white empty-appearing ghost vessels on the iris surface, or an avascular fibrous membrane. Importantly, the fellow eye should be carefully examined for active or regressed NVI.

9. *Gonioscopy and Iridocorneal Angle Examination.* Assessment of the angle by gonioscopy should ideally be performed prior to dilation. Gonioscopic findings in NVG include neovascularization of the angle (NVA), peripheral anterior synechiae, and/or small-layered hyphema in the inferior angle

that may not be large enough to observe on slit-lamp examination without the gonioprism. Usually, NVA develops later than NVI, although NVA can be present when NVI is not seen. Notably, if the patient is receiving anti-VEGF injections, active neovascularization may not be present. It is also critical to evaluate angle structures to determine the extent of angle closure. NVA can progress to peripheral anterior synechiae formation which, in later stages of the disease, can lead to synechial angle closure. It is critical to perform compression gonioscopy in suspected NVG; in angles that initially appear closed without visible NVA, indentation can reveal NVA in the deepened angle, confirming the diagnosis of NVG. The absence of angle structures that does not deepen with significant compression indicate a synechially closed angle.

The ability to perform gonioscopy may be limited in the emergency room setting due to a lack of available equipment or a poor view to the angle. Examination of the fellow eye is important to assess for asymmetric findings. If microcystic edema impairs the view to perform gonioscopy, a repeat exam following IOP reduction is recommended. Hypertonic saline drops may also provide enough temporary improvement in corneal edema to allow for a sufficient gonioscopic exam.

10. *Funduscopic Examination.* A careful funduscopic exam can reveal signs of the underlying etiology for the NVG. Pertinent exam findings include retinal hemorrhages, neovascularization of the disc or elsewhere, cystoid macular edema, vessel abnormalities (e.g., attenuation, tortuosity, dilation), emboli, cotton wool spots, or vitreous hemorrhage. Examination of the optic nerve may show glaucomatous cupping depending on the duration and degree of IOP elevation. Evaluation of the degree of optic nerve head cupping may be confounded by a variety of factors in NVG patients. In the acute setting, disc edema may mask the degree of cupping.

The neuroretinal rim may be difficult to identify with disc neovascularization that can obscure its contours, or by the presence of optic nerve pallor from an ischemic-underlying etiology. Visualization of the nerve may also be obscured during the initial examination by microcystic edema, hyphema, or vitreous hemorrhage. Dilated funduscopic examination of both eyes should be performed, as comparing the two eyes can aid in diagnosis of NVG in the affected eye as well as prognosis for developing NVG in the fellow eye. Importantly, patients may have NVG bilaterally but only complain of symptoms in the worse-seeing eye. In those cases, close monitoring and/or early treatment of the better-seeing eye will be critical in terms of the patient's long-term visual function.

5 Additional Testing

Further testing may be helpful if findings remain inconclusive, ophthalmic examination is limited, or suspected etiologies warrant additional workup. If there is limited view of the fundus, B-scan ultrasonography should be used to evaluate for vitreoretinal abnormalities such as vitreous hemorrhage or retinal detachments. If a computed tomography (CT) scan was ordered as diagnostic workup for a coexisting complaint (e.g., headache), neuroimaging may show vitreous opacities or gross retinal pathology. The resources of the emergency department may be particularly beneficial when workup or testing can be performed more quickly than in an outpatient setting. For instance, doppler ultrasound should be ordered if findings suggest OIS and underlying carotid occlusive disease. Laboratory tests can also be performed more easily in the emergency department. Depending on the clinical context, pertinent diagnostic laboratory tests can include blood glucose, HbA1c, complete blood count (CBC), erythrocyte sedimentation rate (ESR), C-reactive protein (CRP), coagulation factors, or autoimmune markers.

6 Treatment and Follow-Up

After the initial diagnostic workup for NVG is complete, a treatment and follow-up plan should be formulated. Immediate interventions to be performed in the emergency department depend on a variety of factors including specialist availability, severity of the patient's glaucoma, institutional practice patterns, and the patient's medical comorbidities, among others. Broadly, however, attempts should be made to lower IOP before the patient is discharged from the emergency department. Immediate IOP lowering generally consists of repeated rounds of topical IOP-lowering medications and oral or intravenous agents such as acetazolamide or mannitol. In refractory cases, anterior chamber paracentesis could be considered while weighing the risk of causing or worsening a hyphema. If possible, anti-VEGF intravitreal injections can be administered in the emergency department, although this capability will depend on the hospital level of care, availability of retina service coverage, and other factors. Patient factors such as medication adherence, lack of transportation, and other barriers to follow-up, and insurance status should also be taken into consideration in the treatment plan. For instance, performing surgical intervention, intravitreal injections, or panretinal photocoagulation treatment during the emergency department visit might be warranted for patients with barriers to timely outpatient follow-up. Once the patient is stabilized, close outpatient follow-up should be made with the appropriate glaucoma and retina specialists for further workup and management. The specific outpatient treatment options are discussed more thoroughly in a different chapter.

7 Conclusions

NVG patients often present to the emergency room with significant symptoms and visual changes. Careful history taking, review of medical records, and examination of both the affected and fellow eyes are critical to diagnosis of NVG and its underlying condition as well as determination of a suitable treatment plan. Both resource limitations in the emergency room and the potential presence of other active health issues may make evaluation more challenging than in the outpatient setting. Strategies should be employed to acquire the best assessment of the affected and fellow eyes as possible. Emergency room treatment should seek to quickly reduce the IOP, provide initial treatment for the underlying disease process, as reasonable, and a follow-up plan should be developed with attention to patient factors and circumstances.

References

1. Yang H, Yu X, Sun X. Neovascular glaucoma: handling in the future. Taiwan J Ophthalmol. 2018;8(2):60–6.
2. Hayreh SS. Neovascular glaucoma. Prog Retin Eye Res. 2007;26(5):470–85.
3. Rodrigues GB, Abe RY, Zangalli C, Sodre SL, Donini FA, Costa DC, Leite A, Felix JP, Torigoe M, Diniz-Filho A, de Almeida HG. Neovascular glaucoma: a review. Int J Retina Vitreous. 2016;14(2):26.
4. Mizener JB, Podhajsky P, Hayreh SS. Ocular ischemic syndrome. Ophthalmology. 1997;104(5):859–64.
5. Duker JS, Sivalingam A, Brown GC, Reber R. A prospective study of acute central retinal artery obstruction. The incidence of secondary ocular neovascularization. Arch Ophthalmol. 1991;109(3):339–42.
6. Shazly TA, Latina MA. Neovascular glaucoma: etiology, diagnosis and prognosis. Semin Ophthalmol. 2009;24(2):113–21.
7. Havens SJ, Gulati V. Neovascular glaucoma. Dev Ophthalmol. 2016;55:196–204.

Neovascular Glaucoma in Proliferative Diabetic Retinopathy

Jing Shan, Chu Jian Ma, and Catherine Q. Sun

1 Introduction

Neovascular glaucoma (NVG) most commonly occurs in the setting of retinal ischemia after development of proliferative diabetic retinopathy (PDR) [1]. Management of elevated intraocular pressure (IOP) secondary to NVG usually requires IOP-lowering medications and often also requires IOP-lowering surgery. Management of the underlying PDR usually requires a combination of antivascular endothelial growth factor (VEGF) injections and panretinal photocoagulation (PRP). Despite a multifaceted therapeutic approach that includes temporizing and permanent measures, the prognosis is often poor [2]. The advancements in diabetes and retinal treatment in the last few decades have increased therapeutic options for patients at risk of PDR and subsequent NVG. However, the detection and management of NVG still have substantial room for improvement.

J. Shan · C. J. Ma
Department of Ophthalmology, University of California, San Francisco, CA, USA

C. Q. Sun (✉)
Department of Ophthalmology, University of California, San Francisco, CA, USA

Frances I. Proctor Foundation, University of California, San Francisco, CA, USA
e-mail: catherine.sun@ucsf.edu

2 Epidemiology

2.1 Neovascular Glaucoma

NVG occurs in a small percentage of patients with diabetic retinopathy. In the 2016 Intelligent Research in Sight (IRIS®) Registry, the prevalence of NVG in the dataset was 0.23 per 100 patients, which is estimated to be 3% of all glaucoma patients in the dataset (excluding glaucoma suspects) [3]. Studies have found that among PDR patients, those with NVG tend to be younger (50.8 years vs. 56.1 years), have shorter duration of diabetes (9.2 years vs. 13.7 years) and higher hemoglobin A1c (HbA1c) (8.3% vs. 7.5%) than PDR patients without NVG [4]. Few studies have focused on the epidemiology of NVG, but there is more robust literature on the epidemiology and risk factors of diabetic retinopathy.

2.2 Proliferative Diabetic Retinopathy

In the United States (US) and globally, diabetes is a growing concern, affecting about 10% of Americans and 4% of the world's population [5]. The prevalence of diabetes mellitus (DM) in the US is expected to increase by 54% to more than 55 million Americans from 2015 to 2030, and globally from 463 million adults in 2019 to 578 million adults in 2030, which will have an enormous health and socioeconomic impact worldwide [6, 7].

PDR occurs in 7% of patients with DM globally [5]. In the US, the number of patients with vision threatening diabetic retinopathy, which includes PDR and diabetic macular edema, are expected to increase from 1.2 million in 2005 to 3.4 million in 2050 [8]. The prevalence of PDR is higher in those with type 1 DM (32%), compared to those with type 2 DM (3%) [9]. Other notable differences include a younger age of PDR onset for type 1 DM patients; studies have reported the mean age of onset of PDR to be between 34.9 and 38.0 years for type 1 DM patients and between 56.8 and 65.3 years for type 2 DM patients [10–14]. The difference in age of onset of PDR is likely related to the duration of the underlying diabetes, which is a major risk factor for development of diabetic retinopathy. The Los Angeles Latino Eye Study found that 18% of participants with type 1 or 2 DM for more than 15 years had PDR [15]. Similarly, the Wisconsin Epidemiologic Study of Diabetic Retinopathy found that PDR develops in 2% of type 2 DM patients with diabetes duration of less than 5 years and in 25% of type 2 DM patients with diabetes duration of 25 years or more [16]. Table 1 summarizes the pivotal studies relevant to diabetic retinopathy.

Table 1 Pivotal diabetic retinopathy studies

Study name	Interval	Study design	Patient population	Intervention	Study conclusions (relevant to PDR)
Systemic diabetes mellitus studies					
United Kingdom Prospective Diabetes Study (UKPDS) [77, 78]	1977–1991	RCT	Newly diagnosed type 2 DM *N = 5102 patients enrolled*	Intensive (medication) vs. conventional (diet) glycemic control	• Intensive therapy arm had mean HbA1c of 7.0% (compared to 7.9% in conventional) and reduction in microvascular complications (DR and nephropathy) but not macrovascular disease • Intensive therapy arm had 25% reduction in need for PRP
Wisconsin Epidemiologic Study of Diabetic Retinopathy [16, 79, 80]	1980–2007	Population-based cohort study	Diabetic patients in southern Wisconsin *N = 2990 patients sampled at baseline*	Observation	Incidence and progression of DR, and progression to PDR were highest in the group diagnosed before age 30. • DR occurred in type 1 DM patients 3–5 years after diagnosis and almost all patients were affected by 25 years (97%) • 25-year cumulative rate of progression to PDR was 42% in type 1 DM • Strongest relationship to DR progression was worse glycemic control

Table 1 (continued)

Study name	Interval	Study design	Patient population	Intervention	Study conclusions (relevant to PDR)
Diabetes Control and Complications Trial (DCCT) [81–83]	1984–1993	RCT	Type 1 DM *N = 1441 patients enrolled*	Intensive vs. conventional glycemic control	• For every 10% decrease in HbA1c, there was 43% decrease in risk of DR progression in intensive group and 45% in conventional group • Intensive control reduced risk of developing DR by 76% and development of PDR or severe NPDR by 47% • Intensive control increased risk of severe hypoglycemia by 2- to three-fold
Epidemiology of Diabetes Interventions and Complications Trial (EDIC) [84, 85]	1994–2013	Prospective cohort study	All participants of DCCT *N = 1375 patients participated*	All initiated intensive glycemic control	Former intensive therapy had persistent beneficial effect with reduced risk of DR progression, PDR, macular edema, need for PRP compared to former conventional control group from DCCT
Los Angeles Latino Eye Study [86, 87]	2000–2008	Population-based cohort study	Adult Latinos (≥40 years) in Los Angeles County *N = 6357 patients participated at baseline*	Observation	Latinos had higher incidence and progression of DR compared to non-Hispanic whites • 4-year incidence of DR: 34% • Progression of NPDR to PDR: 5.3% • Progression of NPDR to high-risk PDR: 1.9%
Action to Control Cardiovascular Risk in Diabetes (ACCORD) [88, 89]	2001–2009	RCT	Type 2 DM and high risk of cardiovascular disease *N = 10,251 patients enrolled*	Intensive (goal HbA1c <6%) vs. standard (goal HbA1c 7–7.9%) glycemic control	• Median HbA1c was 6.4% in intensive and 7.5% in standard therapy group • Intensive therapy had increased mortality (22% higher rate) and did not significantly reduce major cardiovascular events • Hypoglycemia and weight gain occurred more frequently in intensive therapy group

(continued)

Table 1 (continued)

Study name	Interval	Study design	Patient population	Intervention	Study conclusions (relevant to PDR)
Proliferative diabetic retinopathy treatment studies					
Diabetic Retinopathy Study (DRS) [90, 91]	1971–1979	RCT	1. Unilateral PDR or bilateral severe NPDR 2. VA 20/100 or better in each eye *N = 1758 patients enrolled*	Scatter laser photocoagulation (argon or xenon arc)	PRP reduced the risk of severe vision loss (worse than 5/200) by 50–60% in patients with high-risk PDR: • NVD ≥ 1/4–1/3 of disc area • Any NVD with VH • NVE ≥ 1/2 of disc area with VH PRP recommended for NVI
Early Treatment Diabetic Retinopathy Study (ETDRS) [92]	1985–1990	RCT	1. Bilateral NPDR or early PDR 2. VA 20/200 or better in each eye *N = 3711 patients enrolled*	1. PRP (argon) • Early full scatter vs. early mild scatter vs. delayed PRP. • Eyes with macular edema: Immediate vs. delayed focal PRP. 2. Aspirin 650 mg/ day or placebo	• Early PRP reduced the risk of development of high-risk PDR but had minimal effect on severe vision loss • Recommended that immediate PRP be reserved for eyes approaching high-risk PDR or severe bilateral NPDR, especially those with type 2 DM • Adverse effects of moderate vision loss and visual field loss occurred more after full scatter photocoagulation
Diabetic Retinopathy Vitrectomy Study (DRVS) [93–96]	1976–1983	*Three studies*: 1. Observational 2. RCT 3. RCT	1. Severe PDR from DM *N = 744 eyes* 2. Severe PDR with VA 20/400 or better *N = 370 eyes* 3. PDR with severe VH present for <6 months and VA 5/200 to light perception *N = 616 eyes*	1. Natural history 2 & 3. Early vs. delayed (1 year) vitrectomy	Early vitrectomy was beneficial for: • Eyes with useful vision (VA 20/400 or better) and advanced, active PDR that had received PRP • Type 1 over type 2 DM likely due to more severe neovascularization and fibrous proliferations in type 1 • Severe VH with VA 5/200 or worse for >1 month, especially if fellow eye had poor vision
DRCR.net Protocol N [97]	2010–2012	RCT	VH from PDR in type 1 or 2 DM patients *N = 261 patients enrolled*	Intravitreal ranibizumab vs. saline	• At 16 weeks, similar rates of vitrectomy in the saline (17%) vs. ranibizumab (12%) group • Faster VH clearing and fewer recurrent VH with ranibizumab • No increased risk of RD with ranibizumab

Table 1 (continued)

Study name	Interval	Study design	Patient population	Intervention	Study conclusions (relevant to PDR)
DRCR.net Protocol S [44, 45]	2012–2018	RCT	Newly diagnosed PDR *N = 394 eyes enrolled*	Intravitreal ranibizumab vs. prompt PRP	• At 2 and 5 years, ranibizumab was noninferior to PRP for VA • Ranibizumab group had better average VA, less peripheral field loss, reduced rates of DME, and fewer vitrectomies • Very low rates of NVG or NVI in both groups • Significant loss to follow-up: <65% in each group completed 5-year visit

PDR, proliferative diabetic retinopathy; RCT, randomized controlled trial; N, number; DM, diabetes mellitus; HbA1c, hemoglobin A1c; PRP, panretinal photocoagulation; DR, diabetic retinopathy; NPDR, nonproliferative diabetic retinopathy; VA, visual acuity; NVD, neovascularization of the disc; VH, vitreous hemorrhage; NVE, neovascularization elsewhere; NVI, neovascularization of the iris; RD, retinal detachment; DME, diabetic macular edema; NVG, neovascular glaucoma

3 Mechanism

NVG occurs secondary to posterior segment ischemia, which stimulates the growth of new blood vessels via a complex interaction of angiogenic factors. VEGF is a strong mitogen for vascular endothelial cells and plays a major role in mediating intraocular neovascularization in patients with ischemic disease [17]. Significantly higher levels of VEGF are found in ocular fluids of patients with PDR compared to controls [17].

Anterior segment neovascularization first occurs with endothelial budding at the capillary level of iris vessels [18]. The new vasculature lacks a muscular layer and ruptures easily [19]. A clinically transparent fibrovascular membrane containing proliferating myofibroblasts can develop on the surface of the iris and/or iridocorneal angle; such an invasion of the angle initially impedes aqueous humor outflow in an open-angle fashion but eventually, the fibrovascular membrane contracts to produce synechial angle closure with peripheral anterior synechiae (PAS) [20]. Glaucomatous optic neuropathy can result if the elevated IOP is not promptly controlled. The processes underlying NVG typically occur with severe stages of PDR, in which the drivers for neovascularization have been uninhibited during prolonged periods of poor diabetic control.

4 Diagnosis

NVG is diagnosed clinically through patient history and a complete ophthalmological examination. Patient history helps to determine the origin of ischemia and to establish an index of suspicion, which is important since exam findings can be subtle in the early stages of the disease.

4.1 History

An initial history should address duration of vision loss or pain, events surrounding the onset of acute symptoms, duration of diabetes, past glycemic control including most recent HbA1c, medications, past medical history (e.g., renal disease, systemic hypertension, pregnancy), and ocular history (e.g., trauma, ocular injections, laser, surgery).

Diabetic NVG usually occurs in the setting of poor glycemic control leading to PDR and neovascularization of the anterior segment. The United Kingdom Prospective Diabetes Study and the Diabetes Control and Complications Trial found strong correlations between HbA1c <7% and lower risk of diabetic retinopathy development and progression in both type 1 and type 2 DM patients [21–23]. Additionally, researchers have found disease duration to be a significant risk factor for developing diabetic retinopathy, independent of glycemic control [24–29]. After diabetic retinopathy is already present, glycemic control appears to be a more important risk factor than the duration of diabetes in predicting progression of retinopathy [19].

It is important to rule out other diagnoses that can lead to NVG if the suspicion for PDR is low. The onset of NVG associated with CRVO has historically been reported to be approximately 90 days after the CRVO but can range between 2 weeks and 2 years after the initial obstructive event and may be delayed if the patient is receiving anti-VEGF injections for macular edema. NVG after central retinal artery occlusion can occur as early as 2 weeks after artery occlusion [30]. A history of carotid artery occlusion ipsilateral to the NVG eye suggests ocular ischemic syndrome. Other etiologies of NVG will be discussed in detail in other chapters.

4.2   Exam

Patients should undergo a comprehensive ophthalmological exam including visual acuity (VA), IOP, pupillary assessment, gonioscopy prior to dilation, slit-lamp biomicroscopy, and dilated fundus exam. Multiple methods of IOP measurement should be performed if there is any concern for the accuracy of readings. If there is suspicion for macular edema, optical coherence tomography (OCT) can be performed. If the view to the fundus is obscured, ultrasound biomicroscopy should be performed to evaluate for any vitreous hemorrhage, vitreoretinal traction, or retinal detachment.

Signs supporting a diagnosis of NVG include elevated IOP with associated corneal edema and ciliary injection, NVI typically originating from the pupillary border, ectropion uveae resulting from contraction of a fibrovascular membrane overlying the iris, and/or neovascularization of the angle (NVA) with or without PAS. NVI typically precedes NVA though not always, thus it is important to perform gonioscopy even in the absence of NVI if there is clinical suspicion for NVG in a high-risk patient [19]. Gonioscopy is critical to assess the stage of NVG. Early in the disease process, the angle may appear open and normal. As the disease progresses, neovessels become visible in the angle and can eventually contract to form PAS and subsequent synechial angle closure. Careful examination of the iris should be performed prior to dilation since early NVI can appear very subtle. Early in the disease process, NVI will appear in isolated patches, most commonly at the pupil margin. These neovessels course in an irregular pattern over the surface of the iris, in contrast to the radial path of normal iris vessels. Early detection of NVA can be important in preventing the onset of angle closure.

The optic nerve exam can provide additional insight to the severity of glaucomatous optic neuropathy while the retinal exam can help establish the etiology of NVG. In a patient with diabetes, signs of posterior pole neovascularization, such as vitreous hemorrhage, neovascularization of the disc or elsewhere, are highly suggestive of PDR and increase suspicion for diabetic NVG. Due to the relatively symmetric nature of diabetic retinopathy, the presence of PDR in one eye increases the likelihood of PDR in the fellow eye. As such, both eyes should be dilated, and a thorough retinal exam should be performed. The presence of bilateral NVG should raise suspicion for PDR [31]. Alternatively, findings of a "blood and thunder" appearance in the fundus, along with a history of sudden painless vision loss approximately 90 days prior to the onset of NVG suggest CRVO as the underlying etiology. Findings of a cherry-red spot with retinal whitening, arterial attenuation, and disc pallor are suggestive of central retinal artery occlusion. Elevated IOP, mid-peripheral microaneurysms in the ipsilateral eye, and orbital pain are most suspicious for ocular ischemic syndrome.

4.3 Diagnostic Testing for Neovascularization of the Iris and Angle

Early detection of NVI may require the aid of diagnostic tests, which can involve iris or gonioscopic angiography or anterior-segment optical coherence tomography angiography (OCTA) [32, 33]. While these diagnostic tests have been described in the literature, they are not commonly used in practice since they are not readily available to all ophthalmologists, and additional evaluation of their efficacy and utility is needed.

Intravenously injected fluorescein or indocyanine green (ICG) can highlight neovessels, both in the fundus, iris, and angle. Studies have used iris fluorescein angiography (FA) to diagnose subclinical NVI before it became visible at the slit lamp [34, 35]. Iris FA was able to improve detection of NVI by 29.6% compared to slit-lamp examination alone when eyes with PDR and NVI or NVG (33 eyes) were compared to eyes with normal irises (100 eyes) [35]. Additionally, FA of the angle has been reported to identify more patients with NVA ($N = 56$) compared to gonioscopic exam alone ($N = 30$) out of a sample of 100 patients with DM [36]. However, NVI is most visible on FA in lightly pigmented irises since brown pigment masks fluorescence [37]. As such, ICG angiography has been demonstrated to be a potential diagnostic tool to assess iris perfusion and neovascularization since its fluorescence is not blocked by overlying pigment [38–40]. In comparison to FA, OCTA has the advantage of being a noninvasive diagnostic tool for the detection and management of vascular abnormalities. OCTA eliminates the need for intravascular dyes, which can cause mild to severe allergic reactions. OCTA allows visualization of the iris vasculature but will not show leakage from neovascularization, which can obscure vessels. In a pilot study of 50 patients, OCTA was able to image normal and pathologic iris vessels in healthy controls, patients at risk for NVI, and those with active and regressed NVI [32]. Abnormal NVI vessels were characterized by irregular orientation, tortuosity, smaller caliber capillaries, and more superficial location. Given the deeper location of normal iris vessels, NVI was more easily detected in darker-pigmented irises where normal vessels were obscured by pigment, compared to light irises which do not have a large amount of pigment obscuring normal iris vessels [32]. OCTA has also been used to successfully image NVI regression [33].

5 Management

The management of NVG remains difficult and requires close collaboration between the glaucoma and retina specialist. There are few studies with strong evidence to support therapy guidelines [1, 41]. Currently, the management of NVG aims to achieve two main goals:

1. Address the underlying disease responsible for neovascularization using therapies such as PRP, intravitreal injections of anti-VEGF agents, and systemic management to normalize blood sugar and blood pressure.
2. Control the IOP via topical and oral medications, lasers to decrease aqueous production by the ciliary body, and/or surgeries to increase aqueous outflow.

5.1 Treating the Underlying Proliferative Diabetic Retinopathy

Management of the underlying disease process is typically directed systemically and locally at the ischemic retina. HbA1c should be checked at least two times per year, with a general goal set at $\leq 7\%$ [42]. Blood pressure should be treated, although the benefits of intensive management of hypertension are inconclusive [42]. Patients should be encouraged to follow-up with their primary care provider or endocrinologist, and encouraged to be compliant with all aspects of their medical care.

In addition to systemic control of blood sugar and blood pressure, PRP and/or anti-VEGF injections are generally considered the treatment of choice when neovascularization is present. If the media is clear with good dilation of the iris, PRP can be performed at the time of initial presentation. Side effects of PRP include constriction of the peripheral visual field, impaired night vision, and worsening of diabetic macular edema, the last of which can sometimes be lessened with a pretreatment of intravitreal anti-VEGF injection [43]. If the view of the fundus is insufficient for PRP, then anti-VEGF agents are usually injected. Given the high IOP of NVG, it is often advisable to perform anterior chamber paracentesis at the time of injection.

Given the adverse effects of PRP, there has been interest in therapeutic alternatives. The Diabetic Retinopathy Clinical Research Network (DRCR.net) Protocol S study was a noninferiority study that compared the safety and effectiveness of prompt PRP versus serial anti-VEGF intravitreal injections (ranibizumab) with delayed PRP for PDR [44]. At 2-year and 5-year follow-up, mean VA letter improvement was similar in both groups [44, 45]. More patients in the PRP group developed diabetic macular edema and required vitrectomies [44]. At 2 years, there was no significant difference in NVG (2% vs. 3%) or NVI (1% vs. <1%) between the anti-VEGF and prompt PRP groups, respectively [44]. At 5 years, the percentage of eyes with NVG was still similar in both groups (anti-VEGF 3% vs. prompt PRP 4%) [45]. Other randomized controlled trials have similarly demonstrated that intravitreal anti-VEGF injections are a reasonable alternative therapy for PDR patients through 2 years [44, 46, 47].

The decision of whether to treat PDR with prompt PRP or serial anti-VEGF injections should be made with strong consideration of the patient's likelihood to follow-up and risk for rapid progression [19]. The therapeutic benefits of anti-VEGF injections are temporary and patients require frequent life-long injections. In those who do not adhere to follow-up, a retro-spective study using electronic health record data demonstrated worse visual outcomes with anti-VEGF injections compared to PRP, including higher rates of NVG [48]. In patients with NVG, one study suggested that both anti-VEGF and PRP should be given [49]. In this retrospective study, patients who received both PRP and anti-VEGF injections had fewer glaucoma surgeries than those who received anti-VEGF injections alone [49]. This may be due to the rapid onset of the antineovascular effect after anti-VEGF injection compared to PRP. Intravitreal bevacizumab resulted in complete neovascular regression in 83% of high-risk PDR eyes at 48 hours [50]. These eyes then had recurrence of neovascularization between 2 and 4 weeks after the initial injection [50]. In comparison, it can take weeks to months for neovascularization to regress after PRP [50, 51]. As such, it has been proposed that a combination treatment strategy of anti-VEGF and early PRP within 4 weeks of the anti-VEGF injection has a promising role for treating high-risk PDR [50, 52]. However, further research is needed in this area. *In patients with NVG secondary to PDR, we recommend initial prompt anti-VEGF injection with early PRP within 4 weeks of the anti-VEGF injection.*

Following anti-VEGF and/or PRP, neovessels in the angle that have been present for only a short time may fully regress, resulting in normalization of the IOP. However, some eyes may still require IOP-lowering eyedrops to control the IOP even after the NVA visibly regresses. In more severe cases, if extensive synechial angle closure has already developed, additional surgical interventions are often needed to adequately control the IOP.

5.2 Controlling Intraocular Pressure

5.2.1 Medical Management

The strategy for medical IOP-lowering in NVG secondary to PDR is similar to when the NVG is secondary to other etiologies. In the acute phase, topical beta blockers, alpha agonists, and carbonic anhydrase inhibitors (CAIs), along with oral CAIs are typically administered to rapidly lower IOP, barring contraindications. Prostaglandin analogs are generally considered to be less effective in acute NVG. Anticholinergic agents such as pilocarpine are generally contraindicated because they may increase inflammation, worsen synechial angle closure, and decrease uveoscleral outflow. Special attention should be paid if using oral CAI in patients with DM. Acetazolamide (Diamox) is cleared renally while methazolamide (Neptazane) is cleared renally and hepatically. Dose adjustments should be made for patients with renal compromise or who are on dialysis. These medications should be avoided in patients with creatinine clearance <10 mL/min or have severe hepatic impairment, especially liver cirrhosis [53]. They are contraindicated if patients have a sulfa allergy to a sulfonamide nonantibiotic drug or have a history of a severe allergic reaction to a sulfonamide antibiotic (e.g., anaphylaxis, Stevens-Johnson syndrome) [53]. IOP-lowering medications in the setting of NVG will be discussed in detail in a future chapter.

5.2.2 Laser and Surgical Management

There have been no randomized clinical trials enrolling only patients with NVG, and several small to medium-sized prospective and retrospective studies comparing the outcomes of laser cyclophotocoagulation (CPC), aqueous shunts or trabeculectomy include all etiologies of NVG. Table 2 summarizes the studies that compare surgical IOP-lowering treatments in the setting of NVG. The literature has been equivocal regarding NVG treatment outcomes. Studies have reported both better and comparable outcomes with aqueous shunt versus CPC [54–57]. Similarly, aqueous shunts have been shown to perform comparable and also worse than trabeculectomies [58–61]. Larger, longer-term randomized clinical trials are needed in this area to provide guidance for management.

Trabeculectomies have been relatively less successful in the setting of NVG despite modifications to improve its outcome, including the use of antimetabolites such as 5-fluorouracil (5FU)

or mitomycin C (MMC). Success rates as low as 28% have been reported at 5 years after trabeculectomy with 5FU for NVG treatment [62]. Other studies have reported 55% success rate at 35 months with postoperative 5FU administration and 54% success rate at 18 months with intraoperative MMC [63]. Younger patients under the age of 50 and patients with type 1 DM showed particularly poor prognoses [62]. It is worth mentioning that of the various etiologies of NVG from ischemic retinal disease, PDR demonstrated the most favorable prognosis in one study, with 77.6% of patients achieving an IOP of less than 21 mmHg at 24 months after trabeculectomy with MMC, versus only 41.4% in patients with retinal vein occlusion and 50% in patients with ocular ischemic syndrome [64]. Trabeculectomy in the setting of NVG will be discussed in detail in a future chapter.

While there are no large randomized clinical trials to serve as a basis for choosing aqueous shunts over trabeculectomy, aqueous shunts are generally considered the treatment of choice in the setting of NVG due to excessive conjunctival scarring and anterior segment neovascularization which can occlude the sclerostomy site of a trabeculectomy. Valved aqueous shunts (i.e., Ahmed) are often preferred over nonvalved aqueous shunts (i.e., Baerveldt, Molteno, Ahmed ClearPath) if immediate IOP lowering is needed, though success rates have been similar in the literature [65, 66]. Aqueous shunts have a wide range of reported success rates in the setting of NVG, ranging from 20% to 97% [41, 67]. The success rates of aqueous shunts were significantly lower in eyes with NVG: success rates at 5 years were 20.6% for patients with NVG compared to 81.8% other glaucoma diagnoses [68]. Worse preoperative VA and presence of a hypertensive phase in the postoperative period were risk factors for Ahmed valve failure in patients with NVG [69]. Patients with PDR had better prognoses than patients with CRVO after Molteno implantation, which is similar to the trend following trabeculectomy [70]. These findings suggest that studies investigating NVG outcomes should be stratified by underlying etiology to determine if there is truly a difference in out-

Table 2 Neovascular glaucoma comparative treatment studies

Cyclophotocoagulation versus aqueous shunt (tube)

Author (Year)	Study design	Intervention (N per group)	DM (%)	Prior PRP (%)	Mean IOP (mmHg) Pretreatment	Posttreatment	Complications	Success criteria	Study conclusions
Eid (1997) [54]	Retrospective	Nd:YAG TS-CPC (24 patients) vs. tube[a] (24 patients)	41.7% both groups	CPC 91.7%, Tube 70.8%	CPC 54.9 Tube 51.4	6 mo: CPC 25.7 (N = 23) Tube 18.9 (N = 21)	Phthisis: CPC 8%, tube 8%	• 6 ≤ IOP ≤25 ± Meds • No phthisis • No reoperation (CPC allowed) • No removal of tube • No enucleation	• IOP control was better with tube (66.7%) compared to CPC (37.5%) at mean follow-up (p = 0.04) • Success at 6 mo: CPC 79.2%, tube 87.5% • Success at 3 yr: CPC 28.8%, tube 56.7% • NLP at final visit: CPC 45.8%, tube 16.7%
Chalam (2002) [55]	Retrospective	Nd:YAG TS-CPC (30 patients) vs. Pars plana BGI 350 (18 patients)	CPC 60%, BGI 66.6%	CPC 10%, BGI 0%	CPC 53.8 BGI 62.8	6 mo: CPC 21 BGI 16.4	Hypotony: CPC 23.3%, BGI 5.6%	• 6 < IOP ≤21 ± Meds • No Phthisis • No NLP • No reoperation	• At 6 mo, IOP control was achieved in 76.6% of CPC and 94.4% of BGI (p = 0.13) • Success at 6 mo: CPC 76.7%, BGI 94.4% • NLP at 6 mo: CPC 23.3%, BGI 5.6%
Yildirim (2009) [56]	Prospective non-RCT	Diode TS-CPC[b] (33 patients) vs. AGV S2 (33 patients)	NA	NA	CPC 43.4 AGV 43.3	6 mo: CPC 17 AGV 19.7 24 mo: CPC 18.7 AGV 22.9	Hypotony: CPC 12%, AGV 3% Phthisis: CPC 0%, AGV 6% (All phthisical eyes had TRD)	• 5 < IOP < 21 ± Meds • No NLP • No reoperation	• Similar success rates at 12 and 24 mo between the groups • Success at 24 mo: CPC 63.6%, 59.3% AGV • No patients lost vision due to glaucoma surgery
Choy (2018) [57]	Prospective non-RCT	Diode TS-CPC[c] (8 eyes) vs. AGV S2 (12 eyes)	50% both groups	75% both groups	CPC 42.5 (6 eyes) AGV 41.5 (6 eyes)	Final visit: CPC 15.2 (28.5 mo, 6 eyes) AGV 14.7 (31.0 mo, 6 eyes)	Phthisis: CPC 0%, AGV 25%	• IOP ≤21 ± Meds • No hypotony-related maculopathy • No choroidal detachment	• Small study that showed similar rates of IOP control between groups • Success at final visit: CPC 85.8%, AGV 85.8% • NLP at final visit: CPC 12.5%, AGV 33.3%

Aqueous shunt (tube) versus trabeculectomy

Study	Design	Groups			Baseline IOP	Follow-up IOP	Complications	Success criteria	Outcomes
Engin (2011) [58]	Retrospective	AGV S2 (10 eyes) vs. Cyclectomy/Trab (C/T)d (25 eyes)	Main etiology	NA	AGV 50.2 C/T 52.7	*6 mo:* AGV 20.5 C/T 19.7 *12 mo:* AGV 21.5 C/T 21.2	*Hypotony:* AGV 20%, C/T 26% *Enucleation:* AGV 10%, C/T 0%	• $5 \leq IOP \leq 20$ • No meds	• Success rates trended higher for C/T at 1 yr (AGV 50% vs. C/T 72%, $p = 0.26$) • Vision preservation was similar in both groups at 1 yr one patient in AGV group developed NLP
Shen (2011) [59]	Retrospective	AGV (20 eyes) vs. Trab + MMC (20 eyes)	AGV 70%, Trab 65%	AGV 90%, Trab 85%	AGV 47.7 Trab 47.8	*Final visit:* AGV 13.7 (31 mo) Trab 16.5 (25 mo)	*Hypotony (at week 1):* AGV 0%, Trab 10% *SCH:* AGV 0%, Trab 10%	• $6 \leq IOP \leq 21$ ± Meds • No NLP • No reoperation • No removal of AGV	• VA, IOP, and success were similar between both groups • Success at 24 mo: AGV 60%, Trab 55% • NLP at final visit: AGV 20%, Trab 15%
Liu (2016) [60]	Prospective non-RCT	AGV FP7 (19 eyes) vs. Trab + MMC + IVR (18 eyes)	AGV 42.1%, Trab 33.3%	NA	AGV 49.8 Trab 57.1	*6 mo:* AGV 22.8 Trab 19.7	*Hypotony:* AGV 31.6%, Trab 0% *Enucleation:* AGV 10.5%, Trab 5.6%	• $6 \leq IOP \leq 21$ ± Meds • No NLP • No reoperation	• Trab + IVR had better success than AGV • Success at 6 mo: AGV 68.4%, Trab 94.4% • NLP at final visit: AGV 26.3%, Trab 22.2%. At baseline, 15.7% AGV and 16.6% Trab were NLP already
Sun (2017) [61]	Retrospective	AGV (23 patients) vs. Trab (22 patients) All received IVR + PRPe	55.6%	0%	AGV 44.9 Trab 43.5	*6 mo:* AGV 16.1 Trab 15.6 *12 mo:* AGV 15.1 Trab 15.9	No hypotony or phthisis	• $6 \leq IOP \leq 21$ ± Meds • No reoperation	• Similar IOP and success between AGV and Trab when combined with preop IVR and postop PRP • Success at 12 mo: AGV 82.6%, Trab 81.8%

(continued)

Table 2 (continued)

Author (Year)	Study design	Intervention (N per group)	DM (%)	Prior PRP (%)	Mean IOP (mmHg) Pretreatment	Posttreatment	Complications	Success criteria	Study conclusions
Aqueous shunt (tube)									
Yalvac (2007) [65]	Retrospective	AGV S2 *(38 eyes)* vs. Molteno single plate *(27 eyes)*	AGV 50%, MSP 55.6%	AGV 94.7%, MSP 92.6%	AGV 39.5 MSP 39.3	*6 mo:* AGV 17.8 MSP 20.9 *60 mo:* AGV 20.8 MSP 22.7	*Hypotony (0–3 mo):* AGV 3.5%, MSP 7.4% *SCH:* AGV 0%, MSP 3.7% *Phthisis:* AGV 7.9%, MSP 14.8%	• 5 < IOP <22 ± Meds • No NLP • No reoperation	• AGV had higher early success rate than MSP but both had poor long-term success • Success at 12 mo: AGV 63.2%, MSP 37% • Success at 60 mo: AGV 25.2%, MSP 29.6% • NLP at final visit: AGV 13%, MSP 22.2%
Shalaby (2020) [66]	Retrospective	AGV *(91 eyes)* vs. BGI 250 or 350 *(61 eyes)*	AGV 59.3% BGI 62.3%	AGV 76.9%, BGI 63.3%	AGV 41.4 BGI 39.3	*6 mo:* AGV 16.0 BGI 16.5	*Hypotony:* AGV 0%, BGI 1.6% *SCH:* AGV 4.4%, BGI 5.5%	• 5 ≤ IOP ≤21 ± Meds • No NLP • No reoperation • No removal of tube	• AGV and BGI had comparable outcomes with BGI eyes requiring fewer meds (1.5 vs. 2.5 meds respectively) • Success at 6 mo: AGV 21.6%, BGI 25.9% • NLP at final visit: AGV 18.7%, BGI 14.8%
Trabeculectomy versus ex-PRESS shunt									
Shinohara (2017) [98]	Retrospective	Trab + MMC *(39 eyes)* vs. Ex-PRESS (Ex) + MMC *(50 eyes)*	Trab 61.5%, Ex 88%	NA	Trab 35.1 Ex 33.4	*6 mo:* Trab 15.3 Ex 17.8	*Hypotony maculopathy:* Trab 2.6%, Ex 0%	• 5 ≤ IOP ≤21 ± Meds • No NLP • No reoperation	• Similar VA, IOP, and success rates between groups • Fewer early complications with Ex • Success at 6 mo: Trab 72.1%, Ex 78.0% • NLP at 6 mo: Trab 0%, Ex 2%

Study	Design	Intervention			Baseline IOP	Follow-up IOP	Complications	Success criteria	Results
Kawabata (2019) [99]	Retrospective	Trab + MMC (30 eyes) vs. Ex-PRESS + MMC (14 eyes)	Trab 80%, Ex 71.4%	All	Trab 35.4, Ex 37.4	NA	No hypotony, phthisis or SCH	• 4 ≤ IOP <21 • ± Meds • No reoperation	• At 1-yr follow-up, Trab was more effective but had more complications (i.e., hyphema, bleb leaks) than Ex • Success at 12 mo (including meds): Trab 69.3%, Ex 31.8% (p = 0.02)
Multiple modalities									
El-Saied (2021) [100]	Prospective non-RCT	1. Trab + MMC (10 eyes) 2. AGV (10 eyes) 3. Ex-PRESS + MMC (10 eyes) 4. Diode TS-CPC (10 eyes) All: IVB preop + PRP postop	100%	NA	Trab 29, AGV 29.5, Ex 27.8, CPC 30.3	*6 mo:* Trab 17.2, AGV 16.4, Ex 16.2, CPC 15.0 *12 mo:* Trab 17.0, AGV 16.2, Ex 13.8, CPC 13.0	*Hypotony:* Trab 0%, AGV 20%, Ex 10%, CPC 0%	• 6 < IOP ≤21 • IOP change ≥20% from baseline • ± Meds • No reoperation	• Similar effects on IOP at 1 yr between four interventions • Trab had highest incidence of intraoperative bleeding • Success at 12 mo: Trab 60%, AGV 40%, Ex 60%, CPC 60%

Studies included enrolled only cases with a diagnosis of neovascular glaucoma, had >5 cases per group and used surgical procedures or implants that are still in use today

N, number; DM, diabetes mellitus; PRP, panretinal photocoagulation; IOP, intraocular pressure; Tube, aqueous shunt; Nd:YAG, neodymium-doped yttrium aluminum garnet; TS-CPC, transscleral cyclophotocoagulation; Meds, medications; mo, months; NLP, no light perception; BGI, Baerveldt glaucoma implant; AGV, Ahmed glaucoma valve; TRD, tractional retinal detachment; RCT, randomized clinical trial; Trab, trabeculectomy; NA, not available; yr, year; MMC, mitomycin C; VA, visual acuity; SCH, suprachoroidal hemorrhage; IVR, intravitreal ranibizumab; MSP, Molteno single plate; IVB, intravitreal bevacizumab

[a] Aqueous shunts (tubes) were double-plated Molteno (N = 8), AGV (N = 8), BGI (N = 6), Schocket procedure (N = 2)

[b] CPC was performed using G-probe (Iridex, Mountain View, CA) with traditional CPC settings starting at 1500 mW and titrated to below audible "pop", 2-s duration for 16–20 applications over 270°

[c] CPC was performed using the G-probe with traditional CPC settings starting at 1750 mW with 2-s duration. Power was titrated down after two consecutive audible "pops" were heard and titrated up after two consecutive silent shots. CPC was repeated at >4-week intervals until IOP ≤21 or reached a maximum of 5 CPC treatments

[d] Cyclectomy/Trabeculectomy involved excision of ciliary body fragment of 2 × 4 mm. No antimetabolites were given

[e] All patients received intravitreal ranibizumab injection 7 days prior to glaucoma surgery and PRP 7 days after glaucoma surgery

[f] CPC was performed using the G-probe with laser settings of 1000–1500 mW titrated to avoid "pop" for 360° with eight shots per quadrant

comes in patients with NVG secondary to PDR compared to retinal vein occlusions, and to determine the best treatment strategy depending on the underlying etiology. Aqueous shunt surgery in the setting of NVG will be discussed in detail in a future chapter.

CPC decreases aqueous humor production through selective thermal coagulation of the ciliary body. Historically, CPC has been reserved for eyes with refractory glaucoma and poor visual potential. At 24 months, success rates of transscleral CPC and endocyclophotocoagulation have been reported to be 61.2% and 73.5%, respectively, in the setting of NVG [71, 72]. However, NVG patients are at increased risk for hypotony and phthisis bulbi after cyclodestructive procedures [56, 73–76]. To help reduce the risk of complications, newer cyclodestructive approaches have been introduced including micropulse transscleral CPC and transscleral CPC using a "slow coagulation" technique which increases the duration of laser and titrates laser energy to iris color to reduce damage to collateral tissue. Since CPC has traditionally been reserved for refractory glaucoma and eyes with poor visual potential, studies that directly compare CPC with trabeculectomy or aqueous shunts are prone to selection bias. Since transscleral CPC is typically a quick procedure, its utility and cost-effectiveness for select patients with poor visual potential and high risk of complications with incisional surgery need to be further studied. CPC in the setting of NVG will be discussed in detail in a future chapter.

6   Conclusions and Future Directions

NVG secondary to PDR is a challenging disease to manage and has historically been associated with poor visual prognosis. Despite the multitude of therapies aimed at regressing neovascularization and controlling IOP, the ultimate visual outcome in these eyes may be quite poor due to a combination of irreversible glaucomatous optic neuropathy and retinal ischemia or detachment related to the underlying PDR. The patient's preoperative visual acuity, degree of underlying retinal ischemia, and prior treatment with PRP have been shown to be strongest predictors of loss of light perception vision [66]. In this regard, prevention, early detection and early treatment of retinal ischemia, and subsequent anterior segment neovascularization are keys to improving visual outcomes in NVG secondary to PDR. To do so requires ophthalmologists to work synergistically across specialties and with patients to provide optimal NVG care.

The underlying disease processes for NVG typically develop over many years. Thus, there is a window of opportunity for improved outcome if there are better tools for earlier diagnosis, better systems in place to identify at-risk patients, and a systematic method for monitoring them closely. The use of OCTA imaging provides a noninvasive method to potentially detect subclinical NVI or NVA, but additional evaluation of its efficacy and utility are needed. Improved monitoring of at-risk patients requires the coordinated effort of multiple subspecialists, including retinal specialists, glaucoma specialists, primary care providers, endocrinologists, and potentially social workers. Electronic health records are a potential area where we can create decision support software or alerts to better monitor these patients without significantly increasing the burden on providers.

The field would benefit from more prospective studies that investigate NVG outcomes stratified by etiology and compare treatment options longterm. So far, this has been challenging because NVG is a relatively rare disease; identifying a large enough cohort of patients to power studies capable of providing clinically meaningful results is a lengthy, time-intensive process. The onset of electronic health records as well as large national databases, such as the American Academy of Ophthalmology's IRIS® Registry and the Sight Outcomes Research Collaborative (SOURCE) Ophthalmology Data Repository may allow us to better strive toward this worthy goal.

References

1. Hayreh SS. Neovascular glaucoma. Prog Retin Eye Res. 2007;26(5):470–85. https://doi.org/10.1016/j.preteyeres.2007.06.001.

2. Rodrigues GB, Abe RY, Zangalli C, Sodre SL, Donini FA, Costa DC, et al. Neovascular glaucoma: a review. Int J Retina Vitreous. 2016;2(1):26. https://doi.org/10.1186/s40942-016-0051-x.

3. Lee P, Wang CC, Adamis AP. Ocular neovascularization: an epidemiologic review. Surv Ophthalmol. 1998;43(3):245–69. https://doi.org/10.1016/s0039-6257(98)00035-6.

4. Takayama K, Someya H, Yokoyama H, Takamura Y, Morioka M, Sameshima S, et al. Risk factors of neovascular glaucoma after 25-gauge vitrectomy for proliferative diabetic retinopathy with vitreous hemorrhage: a retrospective multicenter study. Sci Rep. 2019;9(1):14858. https://doi.org/10.1038/s41598-019-51411-6.

5. Yau JWY, Rogers SL, Kawasaki R, Lamoureux EL, Kowalski JW, Bek T, et al. Global prevalence and major risk factors of diabetic retinopathy. Diabetes Care. 2012;35(3):556–64. https://doi.org/10.2337/dc11-1909.

6. Rowley WR, Bezold C, Arikan Y, Byrne E, Krohe S. Diabetes 2030: insights from yesterday, today, and future trends. Popul Health Manag. 2017;20(1):6–12. https://doi.org/10.1089/pop.2015.0181.

7. Saeedi P, Petersohn I, Salpea P, Malanda B, Karuranga S, Unwin N, et al. Global and regional diabetes prevalence estimates for 2019 and projections for 2030 and 2045: results from the international diabetes federation diabetes atlas, 9(th) edition. Diabetes Res Clin Pract. 2019;157:107843. https://doi.org/10.1016/j.diabres.2019.107843.

8. Saaddine JB, Honeycutt AA, Narayan KMV, Zhang X, Klein R, Boyle JP. Projection of diabetic retinopathy and other major eye diseases among people with diabetes mellitus: United States, 2005-2050. Arch Ophthalmol. 2008;126(12):1740–7. https://doi.org/10.1001/archopht.126.12.1740.

9. Weiss DI, Shaffer RN, Nehrenberg TR. Neovascular gluacoma complicating carotid-cavernous fistula. Arch Ophthalmol. 1963;69:304–7.

10. Thomas RL, Dunstan FD, Luzio SD, Chowdhury SR, North RV, Hale SL, et al. Prevalence of diabetic retinopathy within a national diabetic retinopathy screening service. Br J Ophthalmol. 2015;99(1):64–8. https://doi.org/10.1136/bjophthalmol-2013-304017.

11. Pedro R-A, Ramon S-A, Marc B-B, Juan F-B, Isabel M-M. Prevalence and relationship between diabetic retinopathy and nephropathy, and its risk factors in the North-east of Spain, a population-based study. Ophthalmic Epidemiol. 2010;17(4):251–65. https://doi.org/10.3109/09286586.2010.498661.

12. Knudsen LL, Lervang HH, Lundbye-Christensen S, Gorst-Rasmussen A. The North Jutland County diabetic retinopathy study: population characteristics. Br J Ophthalmol. 2006;90(11):1404–9. https://doi.org/10.1136/bjo.2006.093393.

13. Dedov I, Maslova O, Suntsov Y, Bolotskaia L, Milenkaia T, Besmertnaia L. Prevalence of diabetic retinopathy and cataract in adult patients with type 1 and type 2 diabetes in Russia. Rev Diabetic Stud. 2009;6(2):124–9. https://doi.org/10.1900/RDS.2009.6.124.

14. Thomas RL, Distiller L, Luzio SD, Chowdhury SR, Melville VJ, Kramer B, et al. Ethnic differences in the prevalence of diabetic retinopathy in persons with diabetes when first presenting at a diabetes clinic in South Africa. Diabetes Care. 2013;36(2):336–41. https://doi.org/10.2337/dc12-0683.

15. Varma R, Torres M, Peña F, Klein R, Azen SP. Prevalence of diabetic retinopathy in adult Latinos: the Los Angeles Latino eye study. Ophthalmology. 2004;111(7):1298–306. https://doi.org/10.1016/j.ophtha.2004.03.002.

16. Klein R, Klein BE, Moss SE, Davis MD, DeMets DL. The Wisconsin epidemiologic study of diabetic retinopathy. III. Prevalence and risk of diabetic retinopathy when age at diagnosis is 30 or more years. Arch Ophthalmol. 1984;102(4):527–32. https://doi.org/10.1001/archopht.1984.01040030405011.

17. Aiello LP, Avery RL, Arrigg PG, Keyt BA, Jampel HD, Shah ST, et al. Vascular endothelial growth factor in ocular fluid of patients with diabetic retinopathy and other retinal disorders. N Engl J Med. 1994;331(22):1480–7. https://doi.org/10.1056/NEJM199412013312203.

18. Havens SJ, Gulati V. Neovascular glaucoma developments in ophthalmology. 2016;55:196–204. https://doi.org/10.1159/000431196

19. Gartner S, Henkind P. Neovascularization of the iris (rubeosis iridis). Surv Ophthalmol. 1978;22(5):291–312. https://doi.org/10.1016/0039-6257(78)90175-3.

20. John T, Sassani JW, Eagle RC Jr. The myofibroblastic component of rubeosis iridis. Ophthalmology. 1983;90(6):721–8. https://doi.org/10.1016/s0161-6420(83)34520-6.

21. King P, Peacock I, Donnelly R. The UK prospective diabetes study (UKPDS): clinical and therapeutic implications for type 2 diabetes. Br J Clin Pharmacol. 1999;48(5):643–8. https://doi.org/10.1046/j.1365-2125.1999.00092.x.

22. Wong TY, Liew G, Tapp RJ, Schmidt MI, Wang JJ, Mitchell P, et al. Relation between fasting glucose and retinopathy for diagnosis of diabetes: three population-based cross-sectional studies. Lancet. 2008;371(9614):736–43. https://doi.org/10.1016/s0140-6736(08)60343-8.

23. Nathan DM, Genuth S, Lachin J, Cleary P, Crofford O, Davis M, et al. The effect of intensive treatment of diabetes on the development and progression of long-term complications in insulin-dependent diabetes mellitus. N Engl J Med. 1993;329(14):977–86. https://doi.org/10.1056/NEJM199309303291401.

24. Thomas RL, Dunstan F, Luzio SD, Roy Chowdury S, Hale SL, North RV, et al. Incidence of diabetic retinopathy in people with type 2 diabetes mellitus attending the diabetic retinopathy screening service for wales: retrospective analysis. BMJ. 2012;344. https://doi.org/10.1136/bmj.e874

25. Jones CD, Greenwood RH, Misra A, Bachmann MO. Incidence and progression of diabetic retinopathy during 17 years of a population-based screening program in England. Diabetes Care. 2012;35(3):592–6. https://doi.org/10.2337/dc11-0943.

26. Salinero-Fort MÁ, San Andrés-Rebollo FJ, de Burgos-Lunar C, Arrieta-Blanco FJ, Gómez-Campelo P. Four-year incidence of diabetic retinopathy in a Spanish cohort: the MADIABETES study. PLoS One. 2013;8(10):e76417-e. https://doi.org/10.1371/journal.pone.0076417

27. Xu J, Xu L, Wang YX, You QS, Jonas JB, Wei WB. Ten-year cumulative incidence of diabetic retinopathy. The Beijing Eye Study 2001/2011. PLoS One. 2014;9(10):e111320-e. https://doi.org/10.1371/journal.pone.0111320.

28. Kajiwara A, Miyagawa H, Saruwatari J, Kita A, Sakata M, Kawata Y, et al. Gender differences in the incidence and progression of diabetic retinopathy among Japanese patients with type 2 diabetes mellitus: a clinic-based retrospective longitudinal study. Diabetes Res Clin Pract. 2014;103(3):e7–10. https://doi.org/10.1016/j.diabres.2013.12.043.

29. Romero-Aroca P, Baget-Bernaldiz M, Fernandez-Ballart J, Plana-Gil N, Soler-Lluis N, Mendez-Marin I, et al. Ten-year incidence of diabetic retinopathy and macular edema. Risk factors in a sample of people with type 1 diabetes. Diabetes Res Clin Pract. 2011;94(1):126–32. https://doi.org/10.1016/j.diabres.2011.07.004.

30. Duker JS, Sivalingam A, Brown GC, Reber R. A prospective study of acute central retinal artery obstruction. The incidence of secondary ocular neovascularization. Arch Ophthalmol (Chicago, Ill: 1960). 1991;109(3):339–42. https://doi.org/10.1001/archopht.1991.01080030041034.

31. Ohrt V. The frequency of rubeosis iridis in diabetic patients. (0001-639X (Print)).

32. Roberts PK, Goldstein DA, Fawzi AA. Anterior segment optical coherence tomography angiography for identification of iris vasculature and staging of iris neovascularization: a pilot study. Curr Eye Res. 2017;42(8):1136–42. https://doi.org/10.1080/02713683.2017.1293113.

33. Shiozaki D, Sakimoto S, Shiraki A, Wakabayashi T, Fukushima Y, Oie Y, et al. Observation of treated iris neovascularization by swept-source-based en-face anterior-segment optical coherence tomography angiography. Sci Rep. 2019;9(1):10262. https://doi.org/10.1038/s41598-019-46514-z.

34. Mitsui Y, Matsubara M, Kanagawa M. Fluorescence iridocorneal photography. Br J Ophthalmol. 1969;53(8):505–12. https://doi.org/10.1136/bjo.53.8.505.

35. Li S, Wang Z, Li P, Dong Y. Application of iris fluorescein angiography combined with fundus fluorescein angiography in diabetic retinopathy with neovascular glaucoma. Zhonghua Shiyan Yanke Zazhi/Chin J Exp Ophthalmol. 2016;34:1112–5. https://doi.org/10.3760/cma.j.issn.2095-0160.2016.12.013.

36. Ohnishi Y, Ishibashi T Fau-Sagawa T, Sagawa T. Fluorescein gonioangiography in diabetic neovascularisation. (0721-832X (Print)).

37. Hayreh SS, Scott WE. Fluorescein iris angiography: I. Normal Pattern Arch Ophthalmol. 1978;96(8):1383–9. https://doi.org/10.1001/archopht.1978.03910060137009.

38. Chan TKJ, Rosenbaum AL, Rao R, Schwartz SD, Santiago P, Thayer D. Indocyanine green angiography of the anterior segment in patients undergoing strabismus surgery. Br J Ophthalmol. 2001;85(2):214. https://doi.org/10.1136/bjo.85.2.214.

39. Maruyama Y, Kishi S, Fau-Kamei Y, Kamei Y, Fau-Shimizu R, Shimizu R, Fau-Kimura Y, Kimura Y. Infrared angiography of the anterior ocular segment. (0039–6257 (Print)).

40. Ishibashi S, Tawara A Fau-Sohma R, Sohma R Fau-Kubota T, Kubota T, Fau-Toh N, Toh N. Angiographic changes in iris and iridocorneal angle neovascularization after intravitreal bevacizumab injection. (1538–3601 (Electronic)).

41. Sivak-Callcott JA, O'Day DM, Gass JD, Tsai JC. Evidence-based recommendations for the diagnosis and treatment of neovascular glaucoma. Ophthalmology. 2001;108(10):1767–76; quiz77, 800.

42. Standards of Medical Care in Diabetes-2019 abridged for primary care providers. Clin Diabetes. 2019;37(1):11–34. https://doi.org/10.2337/cd18-0105

43. Hamill E, Ali S, Weng C. An update in the management of proliferative diabetic retinopathy. Int Ophthalmol Clin. 2016;56:209–25. https://doi.org/10.1097/IIO.0000000000000136.

44. Gross JG, Glassman AR, Jampol LM, Inusah S, Aiello LP, Antoszyk AN, et al. Panretinal photocoagulation vs intravitreous ranibizumab for proliferative diabetic retinopathy: a randomized clinical trial. JAMA. 2015;314(20):2137–46. https://doi.org/10.1001/jama.2015.15217.

45. Gross JG, Glassman AR, Liu D, Sun JK, Antoszyk AN, Baker CW, et al. Five-year outcomes of panretinal photocoagulation vs intravitreous ranibizumab for proliferative diabetic retinopathy: a randomized clinical trial. JAMA Ophthalmol. 2018;136(10):1138–48. https://doi.org/10.1001/jamaophthalmol.2018.3255.

46. Figueira J, Fletcher E, Massin P, Silva R, Bandello F, Midena E, et al. Ranibizumab plus panretinal photocoagulation versus panretinal photocoagulation alone for high-risk proliferative diabetic retinopathy (PROTEUS study). Ophthalmology. 2018;125(5):691–700. https://doi.org/10.1016/j.ophtha.2017.12.008.

47. Sivaprasad S, Prevost AT, Vasconcelos JC, Riddell A, Murphy C, Kelly J, et al. Clinical efficacy of intravitreal aflibercept versus panretinal photocoagulation for best corrected visual acuity in patients with proliferative diabetic retinopathy at 52 weeks (CLARITY): a multicentre, single-blinded, randomised, controlled, phase 2b, non-inferiority trial. Lancet. 2017;389(10085):2193–203. https://doi.org/10.1016/s0140-6736(17)31193-5.

48. Obeid A, Su D, Patel SN, Uhr JH, Borkar D, Gao X, et al. Outcomes of eyes lost to follow-up with proliferative diabetic retinopathy that received panretinal photocoagulation versus intravitreal antivascular endothelial growth factor. Ophthalmology. 2019;126(3):407–13. https://doi.org/10.1016/j.ophtha.2018.07.027.

49. Olmos LC, Sayed MS, Moraczewski AL, Gedde SJ, Rosenfeld PJ, Shi W, et al. Long-term outcomes of neovascular glaucoma treated with and without intravitreal bevacizumab. Eye (Lond). 2016;30(3):463–72. https://doi.org/10.1038/eye.2015.259.

50. Shakarchi FI, Shakarchi AF, Al-Bayati SA. Timing of neovascular regression in eyes with high-risk proliferative diabetic retinopathy without macular edema treated initially with intravitreous bevacizumab. Clin Ophthalmol (Auckland, NZ). 2018;13:27–31. https://doi.org/10.2147/OPTH.S182420.

51. Vander JF, Duker Js Fau - Benson WE, Benson We Fau - Brown GC, Brown Gc Fau - McNamara JA, McNamara Ja Fau - Rosenstein RB, Rosenstein RB. Long-term stability and visual outcome after favorable initial response of proliferative diabetic retinopathy to panretinal photocoagulation. (0161–6420 (Print)).

52. American Academy of Ophthalmology Retina/Vitreous Panel. Preferred Practice Pattern®Guidelines. Diabetic retinopathy. San Francisco, CA: American Academy of Ophthalmology; 2017. Available at: www.aao.org/ppp

53. Chak G, Patel R, Allingham RR. Acetazolamide: considerations for systemic administration. EyeNet Magazine. 2015.

54. Eid TE, Katz LJ, Spaeth GL, Augsburger JJ. Tube-shunt surgery versus neodymium:YAG Cyclophotocoagulation in the management of neovascular glaucoma. Ophthalmology. 1997;104(10):1692–700. https://doi.org/10.1016/S0161-6420(97)30078-5.

55. Chalam KV, Gandham S, Gupta S, Tripathi BJ, Tripathi RC. Pars plana modified Baerveldt implant versus neodymium:YAG cyclophotocoagulation in the management of neovascular glaucoma. Ophthalmic Surg Lasers. 2002;33(5):383–93.

56. Yildirim N, Yalvac IS, Sahin A, Ozer A, Bozca T. A comparative study between diode laser cyclophotocoagulation and the Ahmed glaucoma valve implant in neovascular glaucoma: a long-term follow-up. J Glaucoma. 2009;18(3)

57. Choy BNK, Lai JSM, Yeung JCC, Chan JCH. Randomized comparative trial of diode laser transscleral cyclophotocoagulation versus Ahmed glaucoma valve for neovascular glaucoma in Chinese - a pilot study. Clin Ophthalmol. 2018;12:2545–52. https://doi.org/10.2147/opth.S188999.

58. Engin KN, Yılmazlı C, Engin G, Bilgiç L. Results of combined cyclectomy/trabeculectomy procedure compared with Ahmed glaucoma valve implant in neovascular glaucoma cases. ISRN Ophthalmol. 2011;2011:680827. https://doi.org/10.5402/2011/680827

59. Shen CC, Salim S, Du H, Netland PA. Trabeculectomy versus Ahmed glaucoma valve implantation in neovascular glaucoma. Clin Ophthalmol. 2011;5:281–6. https://doi.org/10.2147/opth.S16976.

60. Liu L, Xu Y, Huang Z, Wang X. Intravitreal ranibizumab injection combined trabeculectomy versus Ahmed valve surgery in the treatment of neovascular glaucoma: assessment of efficacy and complications. BMC Ophthalmol. 2016;16:65. https://doi.org/10.1186/s12886-016-0248-7.

61. Sun JT, Liang HJ, An M, Wang DB. Efficacy and safety of intravitreal ranibizumab with panretinal photocoagulation followed by trabeculectomy compared with Ahmed glaucoma valve implantation in neovascular glaucoma. Int J Ophthalmol. 2017;10(3):400–5. https://doi.org/10.18240/ijo.2017.03.12.

62. Tsai JC, Feuer WJ, Parrish RK 2nd, Grajewski AL. 5-fluorouracil filtering surgery and neovascular glaucoma. Long-term follow-up of the original pilot study. Ophthalmology. 1995;102(6):883–7. https://doi.org/10.1016/s0161-6420(95)30938-4.

63. Sisto D, Vetrugno M, Trabucco T, Cantatore F, Ruggeri G, Sborgia C. The role of antimetabolites in filtration surgery for neovascular glaucoma: intermediate-term follow-up. Acta Ophthalmol Scand. 2007;85(3):267–71. https://doi.org/10.1111/j.1600-0420.2006.00810.x.

64. Nakano S, Nakamuro T, Yokoyama K, Kiyosaki K, Kubota T. Prognostic factor analysis of intraocular pressure with neovascular glaucoma. J Ophthalmol. 2016;2016:1205895. https://doi.org/10.1155/2016/1205895

65. Yalvac IS, Eksioglu U, Satana B, Duman S. Long-term results of Ahmed glaucoma valve and Molteno implant in neovascular glaucoma. Eye. 2007;21(1):65–70. https://doi.org/10.1038/sj.eye.6702125.

66. Shalaby WS, Myers JS, Razeghinejad R, Katz LJ, Pro M, Dale E, et al. Outcomes of valved and nonvalved tube shunts in neovascular glaucoma. Ophthalmol Glaucoma. 2020. https://doi.org/10.1016/j.ogla.2020.09.010

67. Assaad MH, Baerveldt G, Rockwood EJ. Glaucoma drainage devices: pros and cons. Curr Opin Ophthalmol. 1999;10(2):147–53. https://doi.org/10.1097/00055735-199904000-00012.

68. Netland PA, Ishida K, Boyle JW. The Ahmed glaucoma valve in patients with and without neovascular glaucoma. J Glaucoma. 2010;19(9):581–6. https://doi.org/10.1097/IJG.0b013e3181ca7f7f.

69. Hernandez-Oteyza A, Lazcano-Gómez G, Jimenez-Roman J, Hernández GC. Surgical outcome of Ahmed valve implantation in Mexican patients with neovascular glaucoma. J Curr Glaucoma Pract DVD. 2014;8:86–90. https://doi.org/10.5005/jp-journals-10008-1168.

70. Mermoud A, Salmon JF, Alexander P, Straker C, Murray AD. Molteno tube implantation for neovascular glaucoma. Long-term results and factors influencing the outcome. Ophthalmology. 1993;100(6):897–902.

71. Lima FE, Magacho L, Carvalho DM, Susanna R Jr, Avila MP. A prospective, comparative study between endoscopic cyclophotocoagulation and the Ahmed drainage implant in refractory glaucoma. J Glaucoma. 2004;13(3):233–7.

72. Feldman RM, el-Harazi SM, LoRusso FJ, McCash C, Lloyd WC 3rd, Warner PA. Histopathologic findings following contact transscleral semiconductor diode laser cyclophotocoagulation in a human eye. J Glaucoma. 1997;6(2):139–40.

73. Iliev ME, Gerber S. Long-term outcome of transscleral diode laser cyclophotocoagulation in refractory glaucoma. Br J Ophthalmol. 2007;91(12):1631–5. https://doi.org/10.1136/bjo.2007.116533.

74. Murphy CC, Burnett CAM, Spry PGD, Broadway DC, Diamond JP. A two centre study of the dose-response relation for transscleral diode laser cyclophotocoagulation in refractory glaucoma. Br J Ophthalmol. 2003;87(10):1252–7. https://doi.org/10.1136/bjo.87.10.1252.

75. Ramli N, Htoon HM, Ho CL, Aung T, Perera S. Risk factors for hypotony after transscleral diode cyclophotocoagulation. J Glaucoma. 2012;21(3):169–73. https://doi.org/10.1097/IJG.0b013e318207091a.

76. Oguri A, Takahashi E, Tomita G, Yamamoto T, Jikihara S, Kitazawa Y. Transscleral cyclophotocoagulation with the diode laser for neovascular glaucoma. Ophthalmic Surg Lasers. 1998;29(9):722–7.

77. UK prospective diabetes study (UKPDS). VIII. Study design, progress and performance. Diabetologia. 1991;34(12):877–90.

78. Intensive blood-glucose control with sulphonylureas or insulin compared with conventional treatment and risk of complications in patients with type 2 diabetes (UKPDS 33). UK prospective diabetes study (UKPDS) Group. Lancet 1998;352(9131):837–853.

79. Klein R, Knudtson MD, Lee KE, Gangnon R, Klein BE. The Wisconsin epidemiologic study of diabetic retinopathy: XXII the twenty-five-year progression of retinopathy in persons with type 1 diabetes. Ophthalmology. 2008;115(11):1859–68. https://doi.org/10.1016/j.ophtha.2008.08.023.

80. Klein R, Klein BEK, Moss SE, Davis MD, DeMets DL. The Wisconsin epidemiologic study of diabetic retinopathy: IX. Four-year incidence and progression of diabetic retinopathy when age at diagnosis is less than 30 years. Arch Ophthalmol. 1989;107(2):237–43. https://doi.org/10.1001/archopht.1989.01070010243030.

81. The diabetes control and complications trial (DCCT): design and methodologic considerations for the feasibility phase. Diabetes. 1986;35(5):530–45. https://doi.org/10.2337/diab.35.5.530

82. The effect of intensive treatment of diabetes on the development and progression of long-term complications in insulin-dependent diabetes mellitus. N Engl J Med. 1993;329(14):977–86. https://doi.org/10.1056/nejm199309303291401

83. The relationship of glycemic exposure (HbA1c) to the risk of development and progression of retinopathy in the diabetes control and complications trial. Diabetes. 1995;44(8):968–83.

84. Epidemiology of diabetes interventions and complications (EDIC). Design, implementation, and preliminary results of a long-term follow-up of the diabetes control and complications trial cohort. Diabetes Care. 1999;22(1):99–111. https://doi.org/10.2337/diacare.22.1.99

85. Effect of intensive diabetes therapy on the progression of diabetic retinopathy in patients with type 1 diabetes: 18 years of follow-up in the DCCT/EDIC. Diabetes. 2015;64(2):631–42. https://doi.org/10.2337/db14-0930

86. Varma R, Paz SH, Azen SP, Klein R, Globe D, Torres M, et al. The Los Angeles Latino eye study: design, methods, and baseline data. Ophthalmology. 2004;111(6):1121–31. https://doi.org/10.1016/j.ophtha.2004.02.001.

87. Varma R, Choudhury F, Klein R, Chung J, Torres M, Azen SP. Four-year incidence and progression of diabetic retinopathy and macular edema: the Los Angeles Latino eye study. Am J Ophthalmol. 2010;149(5):752–61.e3. https://doi.org/10.1016/j.ajo.2009.11.014.

88. Buse JB. Action to control cardiovascular risk in diabetes (ACCORD) trial: design and methods. Am J Cardiol. 2007;99(Suppl 12):S21–S33. https://doi.org/10.1016/j.amjcard.2007.03.003.

89. Effects of intensive glucose lowering in type 2 diabetes. N Engl J Med. 2008;358(24):2545–59. https://doi.org/10.1056/NEJMoa0802743

90. Photocoagulation treatment of proliferative diabetic retinopathy: the second report of diabetic retinopathy study findings. Ophthalmology. 1978;85(1):82–106. https://doi.org/10.1016/s0161-6420(78)35693-1

91. Preliminary report on effects of photocoagulation therapy. The diabetic retinopathy study research group. Am J Ophthalmol. 1976;81(4):383–96. https://doi.org/10.1016/0002-9394(76)90292-0.

92. Early treatment diabetic retinopathy study design and baseline patient characteristics. ETDRS report number 7. Ophthalmology. 1991;98(5 Suppl):741–56. https://doi.org/10.1016/s0161-6420(13)38009-9.

93. Two-year course of visual acuity in severe proliferative diabetic retinopathy with conventional management: diabetic retinopathy Vitrectomy study (DRVS) report #1. Ophthalmology. 1985;92(4):492–502. https://doi.org/10.1016/S0161-6420(85)34002-2

94. Early vitrectomy for severe proliferative diabetic retinopathy in eyes with useful vision. Results of a randomized trial--Diabetic Retinopathy Vitrectomy Study Report 3. The Diabetic Retinopathy Vitrectomy Study Research Group. Ophthalmology. 1988;95(10):1307–20. https://doi.org/10.1016/s0161-6420(88)33015-0

95. Early vitrectomy for severe vitreous hemorrhage in diabetic retinopathy: four-year results of a randomized trial: diabetic retinopathy study report 5. Arch Ophthalmol. 1990;108(7):958–64. https://doi.org/10.1001/archopht.1990.01070090060040

96. Early vitrectomy for severe vitreous hemorrhage in diabetic retinopathy: two-year results of a randomized trial diabetic retinopathy Vitrectomy study report 2 the diabetic retinopathy vitrectomy study research group. Arch Ophthalmol. 1985;103(11):1644–52. https://doi.org/10.1001/archopht.1985.01050110038020

97. Diabetic Retinopathy Clinical Research N. Randomized clinical trial evaluating intravitreal ranibizumab or saline for vitreous hemorrhage from proliferative diabetic retinopathy. JAMA Ophthalmol. 2013;131(3):283–93. https://doi.org/10.1001/jamaophthalmol.2013.2015.

98. Shinohara Y, Akiyama H, Magori M, Kishi S. Short-term outcomes after EX-PRESS implantation versus trabeculectomy alone in patients with neovascular glaucoma. Clin Ophthalmol. 2017;11:2207–13. https://doi.org/10.2147/opth.S151200.

99. Kawabata K, Shobayashi K, Iwao K, Takahashi E, Tanihara H, Inoue T. Efficacy and safety of ex-PRESS® mini shunt surgery versus trabeculectomy for neovascular glaucoma: a retrospective comparative study. BMC Ophthalmol. 2019;19(1):75. https://doi.org/10.1186/s12886-019-1083-4.

100. El-Saied HMA, Abdelhakim M. Various modalities for management of secondary angle closure neovascular glaucoma in diabetic eyes: 1-year comparative study. Int Ophthalmol. 2021; https://doi.org/10.1007/s10792-020-01673-1.

Neovascular Glaucoma in Retinal Vein Occlusions

Nicholas A. Johnson and Atalie C. Thompson

1 Introduction

A retinal vein occlusion (RVO) is defined as an obstruction of the retinal venous system due to thrombosis, compression, or vascular disease [1]. Occlusions are primarily classified based on their location within the venous system which yields three fundamental types of RVOs: central retinal vein occlusion (CRVO), hemiretinal vein occlusions (HRVO), and branch retinal vein occlusion (BRVO). CRVOs are occlusions that occur within the central retinal vein, usually within or posterior to the optic nerve head. HRVOs are occlusions of either the superior or inferior branches of the central retinal vein bifurcation and therefore affect half of the retina. Finally, BRVOs are occlusions of distal veins stemming from the central retinal vein and are typically the result of venous compression by a crossing artery (Fig. 1).

Atherosclerotic risk factors are associated with all types of RVO, but each subtype is associated with its own unique risk factors. Systemic hypertension has been shown to be associated with both CRVOs and BRVOs [2–4]. However, CRVOs have also been shown to be associated with glaucoma, sleep apnea, homocystinuria, and thrombophilia in young patients [2, 5–8]. Meanwhile, BRVOs have been shown to be associated with arteriosclerosis, diabetes, obesity, and thrombophilia [3, 9].

Retinal vein occlusions may be ischemic or nonischemic in nature. While nonischemic manifestations pose little risk for neovascular complications, it is well known that conditions which induce hypoxia increase the risk of neovascular complications [10–13].

N. A. Johnson
Duke University School of Medicine,
Durham, NC, USA

A. C. Thompson (✉)
Duke University School of Medicine,
Durham, NC, USA

Department of Ophthalmology, Atrium - Wake Forest
Baptist Health, Winston Salem, NC, USA
e-mail: atalie.thompson@duke.edu

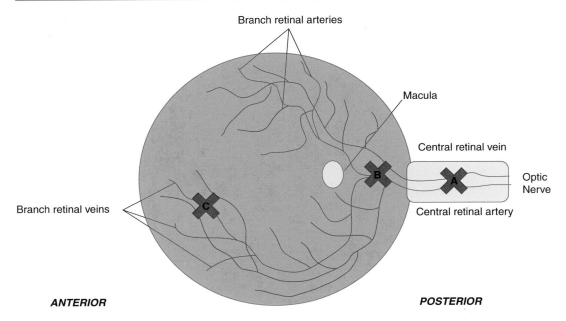

Fig. 1 Types of retinal vein occlusions. "*X*" marks the relative locations of (**a**) Central retinal vein occlusion (CRVO), (**b**) Hemi-retinal vein occlusion (HRVO), (**c**) Branch retinal vein occlusion (BRVO)

2 Pathogenesis of Neovascularization

Neovascular glaucoma (NVG) is a type of secondary glaucoma characterized by elevated intraocular pressure (IOP) due to the neovascularization of the iridocorneal angle [14]. Ischemic retinal diseases such as diabetic retinopathy and retinal vein occlusions, which promote abnormal angiogenesis and blood vessel collateralization, are therefore the most common causes for the development of NVG [13].

In 1948, Michaelson described the presence of vascular proliferative factors in the retina which may play significant roles in the pathogenesis of retinal diseases [15]. Endothelial vascular cells respond to proangiogenic factors such as vascular endothelial growth factor (VEGF), fibroblast growth factor (FGF), platelet-derived growth factor (PDGF), and others, which are released in response to tissue hypoxia [14]. Hypoxia-induced angiogenesis then begins from existing vasculature. Endothelial cells undergo proliferation, migration, and morphogenesis to form new vasculature [16]. Stabilization of this newly formed

vasculature occurs through the formation of a transparent fibrovascular membrane which reinforces new vessels. This membrane may obstruct aqueous flow through the trabecular meshwork, resulting in elevated IOP. As the disease progresses, myofibroblasts of the membrane contract, causing flattening and effacement of the iris, with subsequent development of ectropion uveae, peripheral anterior synechiae (PAS), and eventually secondary synechial angle closure [17].

Prior to the widespread use of anti-VEGF therapy, NVG was colloquially referred to as "100-day glaucoma" due to the notion that neovascularization following ischemia took approximately 3 months [12]. However, more recent studies conducted in the anti-VEGF era have reported that the onset of neovascularization may not be during the first 3 months if the eye is undergoing serial anti-VEGF injections (for example, for macular edema); in this setting, the onset of neovascularization can occur many months after the last anti-VEGF injection [2]. This delayed onset is an important factor to consider when evaluating patients undergoing serial injections.

2.1 Risk Factors for Neovascularization

Although it has been established that ischemic RVOs are associated with greater risk of NVG when compared to nonischemic variants [10–12, 18], there is ongoing debate as to the definitions of ischemic versus nonischemic occlusions. While many studies [19–22] have used imaging modalities such as fluorescein angiography to quantify degree of ischemia, Hayreh and colleagues studied multiple patient factors to investigate which would have the greatest risk of neovascular conversion [12]. Their group tested four functional tests (i.e., visual acuity, Goldmann visual fields, relative afferent pupillary defect (RAPD), and electroretinography (ERG)) against two morphological tests (i.e., ophthalmoscopy and fluorescein angiography). Their study, which was published in 1990, reported that the functional tests yielded greater predictive value than the morphological tests, with RAPD showing the greatest reliability [12].

Expanding on Hayreh's research, a recent study published in 2019 by Rong et al. examined the risk of neovascular complications in a population of patients with ischemic and nonischemic CRVO [2]. This analysis reported systemic hypertension as a novel association with the onset of NVG following CRVO. The authors proposed that this increased risk of NVG in patients with systemic hypertension may be due to retinovascular changes from hypertensive retinopathy, which may render the retinal vasculature less likely to adapt to acute ischemic events such as CRVO, thereby increasing the risk of neovascularization [11, 23, 24].

3 Diagnosis

3.1 Clinical Features

Patients with RVO may or may not present with decreased vision. If present, the decreased vision is painless due to the lack of trigeminal innervation of the retina [25–28]. The visual deficit is typically a scotoma with blurry or gray vision and may be accompanied by decreased visual acuity. The severity of the deficit is dependent on the degree of insult and the presence of complications such as macular ischemia, macular edema, or vitreous hemorrhage [29]. Therefore, it is not uncommon for patients with mild or macular-sparing occlusions to be asymptomatic. Patients with chronic prior RVO leading to neovascular complications may present acutely and symptomatically with a red, painful eye and severely decreased acuity secondary to the elevated IOP [14].

3.2 Diagnostic Testing

In patients with suspected RVO, a careful medical investigation for underlying systemic risk factors should be performed. Systemic conditions such as hypertension and diabetes are risk factors for RVO, and should be addressed to prevent further complications [30]. Patients should undergo standard ophthalmic evaluation including IOP measurement, slit-lamp exam with undilated gonioscopy, dilated fundoscopic exam, and possible ancillary imaging. IOP may be initially low in the setting of ciliary body hyposecretion, while elevated IOP due to NVG is a later finding [1, 14].

Slit-lamp exam of patients with anterior segment neovascularization shows the presence of thin, tortuous capillaries on the surface of the iris often near the pupil margin (Fig. 2). It is important to differentiate abnormal neovessels from normal vessels. Characteristics of these neovessels include individual vascular trunks at the base of the iris which cross over the ciliary trunk and then branch. As vessels progress from the base of the iris and across the ciliary band, they may occlude the trabecular meshwork, which may or may not be seen as neovascularization of the angle (NVA) on gonioscopy. The fibrous lining of these vessels is transparent, so the IOP may become elevated even when the angle anatomy still appears grossly normal on gonioscopy [14, 31]. If the anterior segment neovessels rupture, there may be microhyphema or a layered hyphema in the inferior angle, which can sometimes be too small to see without gonioscopy.

Fig. 2 Neovascularization of the iris at the
pupillary margin

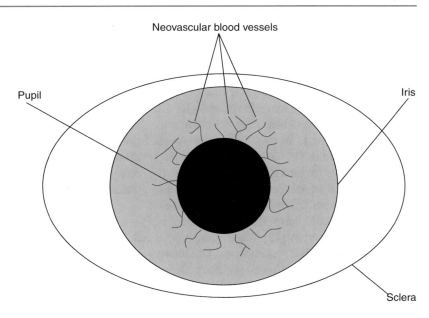

In patients with RVO, dilated fundoscopy is useful for the assessment of macular edema, neovascularization of the optic disc and/or retina, and glaucomatous changes to the optic nerve head. Vascular changes due to the occluded veins, such as the presence of hemorrhages, cotton wool spots, or dilated, tortuous veins may be seen in the acute setting. Other signs such as vascular whitening, atrophy, and development of collaterals indicate longstanding disease [32]. In determining risk factors for NVG conversion, a number of studies have reported no association between macular edema and risk of developing NVG [2, 6, 12].

While the diagnoses of both RVO and NVG are largely clinical, imaging can alert clinicians toward potential complications. Fluorescein angiography (FA) can help to determine the degree of retinal nonperfusion and detect subtle neovascularization. This imaging modality was utilized by the Central Vein Occlusion Study (CVOS) to differentiate ischemic versus nonischemic subtypes of CRVO [4]. This study defined <10 disc areas of capillary nonperfusion as nonischemic and ≥10 disc areas of nonperfusion as ischemic, a standard which has been utilized in other studies [4, 33–37]. In the CVOS study group, the risk of developing NVI and NVA increases with greater disc areas of nonperfusion

[4]. Recent studies suggest there may be added benefit in using improved imaging technologies such as wide-angle fundus fluorescein angiography (WA-FFA), which allows for a larger area of the retina to be imaged [19–22]. Ocular coherence tomography (OCT) can also be used for monitoring macular edema. Although current studies suggest that the presence of macular edema with an RVO is not a direct risk factor for NVG, tracking its progression may be useful for monitoring response to treatment. Additionally, eyes with macular edema are at lower risk of developing NVG if the eye is already undergoing serial anti-VEGF treatment for the macular edema. Therefore, although macular edema itself may not play a role in NVG development, treatment of macular edema with anti-VEGF can be considered protective against NVG development. The utility of optic nerve OCT in the management of NVG is limited, but there is evidence to suggest that it may be useful for staging disease severity [38].

More recently, angiography studies such as OCT with angiography (OCTA) and iris angiography have been proposed as tools for the early detection of neovascularization that cannot be appreciated on clinical examination. These tools can detect subclinical neovascularization of the retina and iris in patients with PDR and RVO

[39–41]. Although early detection may help prevent complications from untreated neovascularization, the clinical utility of these findings needs to be explored further. While these angiography tools have proven useful in the research setting, they are not currently routinely utilized by ophthalmologists for the purposes of clinical diagnosis and management.

4 Management and Treatment

Once diagnosis has been confirmed, serial examination with close follow-up should include IOP measurement, slit-lamp exam with undilated gonioscopy, and dilated fundoscopy [29]. Nonischemic CRVO with VA better than 20/40 at presentation has a more favorable prognosis; therefore, early treatment is not recommended and strict monitoring for the first 3 months and then every 2 months thereafter for the first year is advisable. Nonischemic CRVO with VA worse than or equal to 20/40 at presentation and ischemic CRVO have a less favorable prognosis; thus, early treatment with a similar strict follow-up protocol is recommended [30].

Treatment of NVG secondary to RVO consists of medical, surgical, and laser therapies. The goals of treatment are: (1) treatment of macular edema, more commonly with medications such as anti-VEGF or glucocorticoid injections than with macular focal or grid laser, (2) treatment of underlying retinal neovascularization with anti-VEGF therapy or panretinal photocoagulation (PRP), and (3) control of IOP using IOP-lowering eye drops or oral medications, or IOP-lowering surgery.

4.1 Anti-VEGF Medications

Intravitreal anti-VEGF injections are a mainstay for treatment of macular edema and NVG secondary to RVO due to its utility in both conditions. Anti-VEGF therapy has been shown to treat macular edema that arises secondary to both CRVO and BRVO [33, 42, 43]. The United States Food and Drug Administration (FDA) has approved intravitreal injection of ranibizumab and aflibercept for the treatment of macular edema associated with RVOs as both drugs have shown good long-term efficacy in multiple clinical trials [33, 44–47]. Bevacizumab is a less expensive anti-VEGF medication which has also shown favorable outcomes, though it is not FDA-approved for intravitreal use [48–52]. These anti-VEGF medications have also been shown to be useful for regressing anterior segment neovascularization and suppressing the underlying neovascular drive in patients with NVG [53–56].

While anti-VEGF therapies have been shown to improve visual outcomes in both NVG and RVO patients, these treatments are not without potential drawbacks. Direct risks of intravitreal injections include cataract formation, elevations in IOP, retinal detachment or tear, intraocular hemorrhage, and infection leading to endophthalmitis [57]. Furthermore, the Rubeosis Anti-VEGF trial (RAVE) demonstrated that while anti-VEGF is useful in the short-term, the long-term effects of these medications in preventing NVG progression may be limited. In a small sample of 20 patients, intravitreal ranibizumab injections were of clinical benefit to patients, but delayed rather than prevented neovascular progression [43]. Although anti-VEGF injections alone may delay rather than prevent progression to NVG, injections can provide a synergistic protective antineovascular effect when used in combination with PRP by preventing the conversion of iris and angle neovascularization to NVG.

Retinal laser photocoagulation can be used as an alternative treatment for macular edema secondary to BRVO in cases refractory to anti-VEGF injections or in those who cannot tolerate repeated injections. The Branch Vein Occlusion Study (BVOS) showed that macular grid laser photocoagulation improved visual acuity by at least two lines from baseline in patients with chronic macular edema (>3 months) secondary to BRVO and baseline visual acuity 20/40 or worse [58]. Notably, the Central Vein Occlusion Study (CVOS) found that neither prophylactic treatment with PRP nor macular grid laser photocoagulation yielded significant improvement in visual acuity in patients with ischemic and nonischemic variants of CRVO [4]. However, Hayreh has raised issues concerning limitations of the CVOS study, such as lack of visual field data [59]. In a previous study by Hayreh and colleagues, the use of PRP for ischemic CRVO resulted in significant worsening of peripheral visual field compared to eyes which did not receive laser therapy [60]. Although the authors of the CVOS study agreed with Hayreh's concerns, the results of the CVOS study are still the basis of the "gold standard" of treatment, which is to reserve the use of PRP until after neovascularization has developed.

Because PRP leads to regression of neovascularization in eyes that have not received prophylactic photocoagulation, it should be promptly initiated at the first sign of neovascularization. RVO patients should be closely monitored for neovascularization during follow-up, particularly in eyes with the following risk factors, as determined by the results of the CVOS study: increased retinal nonperfusion, prophylactic PRP treatment, VA worse than 20/200, duration less than 1 month, moderate or severe venous tortuosity, and significant retinal hemorrhage [61].

Imaging studies such as OCT/OCTA and iris angiography may also be helpful for confirming presence of macular edema and earlier detection of iris neovascularization [38, 39, 41]. Eyes demonstrating neovascularization with decreased vision, RAPD, or systemic hypertension are at increased risk for progressing to NVG, and may require more frequent follow-up [2]. However, the absence of these risk factors does not necessarily decrease the risk of NVG. Therefore, close follow-up every 2–4 weeks after PRP therapy is recommended to be certain that iris neovascularization is not progressing and that supplemental PRP is not needed [62].

4.2   Glucocorticoids

Although anti-VEGF therapy is the most common treatment for macular edema associated with RVO, intravitreal and subtenons injections of glucocorticoids can also be utilized, especially in refractory cases and in pseudophakic eyes.

Triamcinolone acetonide injection has been shown to effectively treat macular edema in patients with BRVO [63–68]. Subtenons steroid injections are commonly performed clinically and have been shown to be a safe and effective first-line treatment for macular edema [69, 70]. Intravitreal steroid injections are also commonly administered. A comparative study by Hayashi and Hayashi demonstrated that intravitreal steroid injection, which is the current standard route of administration, was more efficacious than repeated retrobulbar injections [71]. More recently, intravitreal sustained-release dexamethasone implants have also proven beneficial for patients with macular edema [72, 73]. One comparative study showed comparable efficacy between intravitreal dexamethasone implant versus intravitreal anti-VEGF injections [74].

A study by Oh and colleagues demonstrated that patients receiving early intravitreal steroid injections (within <3 months of BRVO) had better visual acuity and improved foveal thickness outcomes compared to patients receiving treatment >3 months after BRVO [75]. With regard to the use of triamcinolone for CRVO, the Standard Care versus Corticosteroid for Retinal Vein Occlusion (SCORE) study showed that triamcinolone injection was superior to observation for treating vision loss from macular edema secondary to CRVO [35]. However, side effects of intravitreal triamcinolone include cataract formation and IOP elevation which may occur in the first 1–3 months following injection [64, 66–68]. In the majority of patients, these IOP elevations can be readily controlled with IOP-lowering eyedrops, resulting in adequate IOP control by the 6–8-month follow-up period [67, 68, 76–78].

Sustained release dexamethasone implantation has also proven effective for treatment of macular edema associated with RVO [72, 79, 80]. A study by Haller et al. showed that dexamethasone implant both reduces risk of vision loss and improves speed and incidence of visual improvement [72]. Similarly, Ferrini and Ambresin found that intravitreal dexamethasone implantation significantly reduced the amount of macular edema as early as 1 day following treatment, with complete resolution by 1 month [79]. Intravitreal steroid implantation has also been shown to provide similar improvements in BCVA and central foveal thickness as intravitreal anti-VEGF injections [74]. One advantage of intravitreal steroid implantation treatment, however, is decreased need for repeated injections. Side effects of sustained-release steroid implants are similar to those of intravitreal steroid injection, including elevated IOP and cataract formation.

With regard to NVG management, topical corticosteroids may be helpful in reducing inflammation during the acute presentation, postoperative period, and/or when the NVG occurs due to underlying inflammatory disease [32, 81].

4.3   IOP-Lowering Medications

The strategy for medical IOP-lowering in NVG secondary to RVO is similar to when the NVG is secondary to other etiologies. Topical IOP-lowering eyedrops are the medications of choice to treat elevated IOP in patients with NVG. Aqueous humor suppressants such as beta blockers, alpha agonists, and carbonic anhydrase inhibitors (CAIs) have excellent efficacy and are well tolerated by patients. These agents work by suppressing aqueous production and possibly increasing uveoscleral outflow [59, 82]. Prostaglandin analogs may be effective for enhancing aqueous outflow but may worsen inflammation [54]. As a result, they are usually not considered first-line IOP-lowering therapy in the management of NVG. Anticholinergic agents, such as pilocarpine, are also avoided because they may increase inflammation, worsen secondary angle closure, and decrease uveoscleral outflow [54]. Although pilocarpine can be used to treat angle closure in the setting of primary angle closure from pupillary block or plateau iris syndrome, it can potentially worsen secondary angle closure due to lens-induced etiologies or aqueous misdirection by precipitating paradoxical shallowing of the anterior chamber [83]. Oral carbonic anhydrase inhibitors, such as acetazolamide, can be prescribed when topical treatment is not sufficient to lower IOP [84]. IOP-lowering medi-

cations in the setting of NVG will be discussed in detail in a different chapter.

4.4   IOP-Lowering Surgery

Eyes with NVG often require IOP-lowering surgery to achieve adequate IOP control, because medical IOP-lowering therapy may be insufficient especially in the setting of synechial angle closure. The surgical strategy for IOP-lowering is similar to when the NVG is secondary to other etiologies. Aqueous shunts are the most common surgical procedure of choice in NVG; trabeculectomy has a relatively higher failure rate in NVG because fibrovascular tissue in the anterior segment and/or external scarring and fibrosis of the conjunctiva can limit aqueous outflow [78]. Transscleral cyclophotocoagulation (CPC), a nonincisional laser procedure which lowers aqueous production, is another strategy for IOP-lowering in NVG refractory to medical IOP-lowering therapy [85–87]. CPC has historically been reserved for NVG eyes with poorer visual potential and has been shown to have comparable efficacy to aqueous shunt surgery [88, 89]. A distinct advantage of CPC is the easier learning curve and faster surgical time compared to traditional incisional procedures. With the advent of micropulse technology and modified laser settings, there may be a growing role for CPC in patients with NVG; further research is needed in this area. IOP-lowering surgeries in the setting of NVG will be discussed in detail in other chapters.

5   Conclusion

NVG is a particularly aggressive form of glaucoma that often arises secondary to ischemic retinal events such as RVO. Ischemic RVOs induce hypoxia-driven angiogenesis which leads to neovascularization of the angle that obstructs aqueous outflow. The diagnosis of RVO and its associated complications (i.e. macular edema, NVG, etc.) is largely clinical and requires thorough ophthalmic evaluation. Factors associated with increased risk of neovascularization and conversion to NVG have been established by previous studies [2, 61]. Certain imaging tools such as FA and OCT/OCTA may be useful for classifying disease progression and monitoring response to treatment. Treatment for NVG secondary to RVO is multifactorial and aimed at resolution of macular edema with anti-VEGF or glucocorticoids, prevention of neovascularization using anti-VEGF or PRP, and control of IOP using medications or surgery. Despite these treatment strategies, NVG secondary to RVO is often a difficult condition to manage, and complications are frequent. As such, it is important for clinicians to educate patients about potential treatment options while managing expectations with regard to visual prognosis.

References

1. Interim Guidelines for Management of Retinal Vein Occlusion [Internet]. [cited 2020 Nov 24]. Available from: https://www.rcophth.ac.uk/wp-content/uploads/2014/12/2010-SCI-095-RVO-Interim-Guidelines-Dec-2010-FINAL.pdf
2. Rong AJ, Swaminathan SS, Vanner EA, Parrish RK. Predictors of neovascular glaucoma in central retinal vein occlusion. Am J Ophthalmol. 2019;204:62–9.
3. Yen Y-C, Weng S-F, Chen H-A, Lin Y-S. Risk of retinal vein occlusion in patients with systemic lupus erythematosus: a population-based cohort study. Br J Ophthalmol. 2013;97(9):1192–6.
4. Natural history and clinical management of central retinal vein occlusion. The central vein occlusion study group. Arch Ophthalmol. 1997;115(4):486–91.
5. Fong AC, Schatz H. Central retinal vein occlusion in young adults. Surv Ophthalmol. 1993;37(6):393–417.
6. Glacet-Bernard A, Leroux les Jardins G, Lasry S, Coscas G, Soubrane G, Souied E, et al. Obstructive sleep apnea among patients with retinal vein occlusion. Arch Ophthalmol. 2010;128(12):1533–8.
7. Chou K-T, Huang C-C, Tsai D-C, Chen Y-M, Perng D-W, Shiao G-M, et al. Sleep apnea and risk of retinal vein occlusion: a nationwide population-based study of Taiwanese. Am J Ophthalmol. 2012;154(1):200–205.e1.
8. Lahey JM, Tunç M, Kearney J, Modlinski B, Koo H, Johnson RN, et al. Laboratory evaluation of hypercoagulable states in patients with central retinal vein occlusion who are less than 56 years of age. Ophthalmology. 2002;109(1):126–31.
9. Risk factors for branch retinal vein occlusion. The eye disease case-control study group. Am J Ophthalmol. 1993;116(3):286–96.
10. Quinlan PM, Elman MJ, Bhatt AK, Mardesich P, Enger C. The natural course of central retinal vein occlusion. Am J Ophthalmol. 1990;110(2):118–23.
11. Zegarra H, Gutman FA, Conforto J. The natural course of central retinal vein occlusion. Ophthalmology. 1979;86(11):1931–42.
12. Hayreh SS, Klugman MR, Beri M, Kimura AE, Podhajsky P. Differentiation of ischemic from nonischemic central retinal vein occlusion during the early acute phase. Graefes Arch Clin Exp Ophthalmol. 1990;228(3):201–17.
13. Haefliger IO, Zschauer A, Anderson DR. Relaxation of retinal pericyte contractile tone through the nitric oxide-cyclic guanosine monophosphate pathway. Invest Ophthalmol Vis Sci. 1994;35(3):991–7.
14. Barac IR, Pop MD, Gheorghe AI, Taban C. Neovascular secondary glaucoma, etiology and pathogenesis. Rom J Ophthalmol. 2015;59(1):24–8.
15. Michaelson I. The mode of development of the vascular system of the retina, with some observations on its significance for certain retinal diseases [Internet]. undefined. 1948 [cited 2020 Nov 24]. Available from: http://The-mode-of-development-of-the-vascular-system-of-Michaelson/69f11a4f0ce22a430e1c8483d437c529f1e6c287/
16. Adair TH, Montani J-P. Overview of angiogenesis [Internet]. Angiogenesis. Morgan & Claypool Life Sciences; 2010 [cited 2020 Nov 24]. Available from: https://www.ncbi.nlm.nih.gov/books/NBK53238/
17. John T, Sassani JW, Eagle RC. The myofibroblastic component of Rubeosis Iridis. Ophthalmology. 1983;90(6):721–8.
18. Laatikainen L, Kohner EM, Khoury D, Blach RK. Panretinal photocoagulation in central retinal vein occlusion: a randomised controlled clinical study. Br J Ophthalmol. 1977;61(12):741–53.
19. Yasuda Y, Hirano Y, Esaki Y, Tomiyasu T, Suzuki N, Yasukawa T, et al. Peripheral microvascular abnormalities detected by wide-field fluorescein angiography in eyes with branch retinal vein occlusion. Ophthalmic Res. 2019;61(2):107–14.
20. Thomas AS, Thomas MK, Finn AP, Fekrat S. Use of the ischemic index on widefield fluorescein angiography to characterize a central retinal vein occlusion as ischemic or nonischemic. Retina. 2019;39(6):1033–8.
21. Storch M, Bemme S, Rehak M, Hoerauf H, Feltgen N. Ultra-widefield angiography for retinal vein occlusion: how large is large enough? Ophthalmologe. 2018;115(6):499–504.
22. Böker A, Seibel I, Rübsam A, Joussen AM, Zeitz O. Peripheral ischemia in diabetic retinopathy and retinal vein occlusion: new insights with ultra-wide-angle fundus imaging and wide-angle fluorescein angiography. Klin Monatsbl Augenheilkd. 2018;235(9):974–9.

23. Sinclair SH, Gragoudas ES. Prognosis for rubeosis iridis following central retinal vein occlusion. Br J Ophthalmol. 1979;63(11):735–43.
24. Tso MO, Jampol LM. Pathophysiology of hypertensive retinopathy. Ophthalmology. 1982;89(10):1132–45.
25. Kiel JW. The ocular circulation [internet]. San Rafael (CA): Morgan & Claypool Life Sciences; 2010 [cited 2020 Dec 5]. (Integrated Systems Physiology: from Molecule to Function to Disease). Available from: http://www.ncbi.nlm.nih.gov/books/NBK53323/
26. Laties AM. Central retinal artery innervation. Absence of adrenergic innervation to the intraocular branches. Arch Ophthalmol. 1967;77(3):405–9.
27. Ye XD, Laties AM, Stone RA. Peptidergic innervation of the retinal vasculature and optic nerve head. Invest Ophthalmol Vis Sci. 1990;31(9):1731–7.
28. Ehinger B. Adrenergic nerves to the eye and to related structures in man and in the cynomolgus monkey (Macaca Irus). Invest Ophthalmol Vis Sci. 1966;5(1):42–52.
29. Ip M, Hendrick A. Retinal vein occlusion review. Asia Pac J Ophthalmol (Phila). 2018;7(1):40–5.
30. La Spina C, De Benedetto U, Parodi MB, Coscas G, Bandello F. Practical management of retinal vein occlusions. Ophthalmol Ther [Internet]. 2012 Dec [cited 2021 Jun 13];1(1). Available from: https://www.ncbi.nlm.nih.gov/pmc/articles/PMC4108135/
31. Green WR, Chan CC, Hutchins GM, Terry JM. Central retinal vein occlusion: a prospective histopathologic study of 29 eyes in 28 cases. Trans Am Ophthalmol Soc. 1981;79:371–422.
32. Comer G. Retinal vein occlusion [Internet]. [cited 2020 Dec 5]. Available from: https://eyewiki.aao.org/Retinal_Vein_Occlusion
33. Brown DM, Heier JS, Clark WL, Boyer DS, Vitti R, Berliner AJ, et al. Intravitreal aflibercept injection for macular edema secondary to central retinal vein occlusion: 1-year results from the phase 3 COPERNICUS study. Am J Ophthalmol. 2013;155(3):429–437.e7.
34. Holz FG, Roider J, Ogura Y, Korobelnik J-F, Simader C, Groetzbach G, et al. VEGF trap-eye for macular oedema secondary to central retinal vein occlusion: 6-month results of the phase III GALILEO study. Br J Ophthalmol. 2013;97(3):278–84.
35. Ip MS, Scott IU, VanVeldhuisen PC, Oden NL, Blodi BA, Fisher M, et al. A randomized trial comparing the efficacy and safety of intravitreal triamcinolone with observation to treat vision loss associated with macular edema secondary to central retinal vein occlusion: the standard care vs corticosteroid for retinal vein occlusion (SCORE) study report 5. Arch Ophthalmol. 2009;127(9):1101–14.
36. Parodi MB, Iacono P, Petruzzi G, Parravano M, Varano M, Bandello F. Dexamethasone implant for macular edema secondary to ischemic retinal vein occlusions. Retina. 2015;35(7):1387–92.
37. Ramezani A, Esfandiari H, Entezari M, Moradian S, Soheilian M, Dehsarvi B, et al. Three intravitreal bevacizumab versus two intravitreal triamcinolone injections in recent-onset branch retinal vein

occlusion. Graefes Arch Clin Exp Ophthalmol. 2012;250(8):1149–60.
38. Bellotti A, Labbé A, Fayol N, El Mahtoufi A, Baudouin C. OCT and neovascular glaucoma. J Fr Ophthalmol. 2007;30(6):586–91.
39. You QS, Guo Y, Wang J, Wei X, Camino A, Zang P, et al. Detection of clinically unsuspected retinal neovascularization with wide-field optical coherence tomography angiography. Retina. 2020;40(5):891–7.
40. Ishibashi S, Tawara A, Sohma R, Kubota T, Toh N. Angiographic changes in iris and iridocorneal angle neovascularization after intravitreal bevacizumab injection. Arch Ophthalmol. 2010;128(12):1539–45.
41. Vaz-Pereira S, Morais-Sarmento T, Esteves MR. Optical coherence tomography features of neovascularization in proliferative diabetic retinopathy: a systematic review. Int J Retina Vitreous. 2020;6:26.
42. Braithwaite T, Nanji AA, Greenberg PB. Anti-vascular endothelial growth factor for macular edema secondary to central retinal vein occlusion. Cochrane Database Syst Rev. 2010;10:CD007325.
43. Brown DM, Wykoff CC, Wong TP, Mariani AF, Croft DE, Schuetzle KL, et al. Ranibizumab in preproliferative (ischemic) central retinal vein occlusion: the rubeosis anti-VEGF (RAVE) trial. Retina. 2014;34(9):1728–35.
44. Brown DM, Campochiaro PA, Singh RP, Li Z, Gray S, Saroj N, et al. Ranibizumab for macular edema following central retinal vein occlusion: six-month primary end point results of a phase III study. Ophthalmology. 2010;117(6):1124–1133.e1.
45. Campochiaro PA, Brown DM, Awh CC, Lee SY, Gray S, Saroj N, et al. Sustained benefits from ranibizumab for macular edema following central retinal vein occlusion: twelve-month outcomes of a phase III study. Ophthalmology. 2011;118(10):2041–9.
46. Campochiaro PA, Clark WL, Boyer DS, Heier JS, Brown DM, Vitti R, et al. Intravitreal aflibercept for macular edema following branch retinal vein occlusion: the 24-week results of the VIBRANT study. Ophthalmology. 2015;122(3):538–44.
47. Heier JS, Clark WL, Boyer DS, Brown DM, Vitti R, Berliner AJ, et al. Intravitreal aflibercept injection for macular edema due to central retinal vein occlusion: two-year results from the COPERNICUS study. Ophthalmology. 2014;121(7):1414–1420.e1.
48. Hikichi T, Higuchi M, Matsushita T, Kosaka S, Matsushita R, Takami K, et al. Two-year outcomes of intravitreal bevacizumab therapy for macular oedema secondary to branch retinal vein occlusion. Br J Ophthalmol. 2014;98(2):195–9.
49. Prager F, Michels S, Kriechbaum K, Georgopoulos M, Funk M, Geitzenauer W, et al. Intravitreal bevacizumab (Avastin) for macular oedema secondary to retinal vein occlusion: 12-month results of a prospective clinical trial. Br J Ophthalmol. 2009;93(4):452–6.
50. Ehlers JP, Decroos FC, Fekrat S. Intravitreal bevacizumab for macular edema secondary to branch retinal vein occlusion. Retina. 2011;31(9):1856–62.

51. Donati S, Barosi P, Bianchi M, Al Oum M, Azzolini C. Combined intravitreal bevacizumab and grid laser photocoagulation for macular edema secondary to branch retinal vein occlusion. Eur J Ophthalmol. 2012;22(4):607–14.
52. Kreutzer TC, Alge CS, Wolf AH, Kook D, Burger J, Strauss R, et al. Intravitreal bevacizumab for the treatment of macular oedema secondary to branch retinal vein occlusion. Br J Ophthalmol. 2008;92(3):351–5.
53. Karpilova MA, Durzhinskaya MH. Anti-VEGF drugs in the treatment of neovascular glaucoma. Vestn Oftalmol. 2019;135(5. Vyp. 2):299–304.
54. Rodrigues GB, Abe RY, Zangalli C, Sodre SL, Donini FA, Costa DC, et al. Neovascular glaucoma: a review. Int J Retina Vitreous. 2016;2:26.
55. Sun Y, Liang Y, Zhou P, Wu H, Hou X, Ren Z, et al. Anti-VEGF treatment is the key strategy for neovascular glaucoma management in the short term. BMC Ophthalmol. 2016;16(1):150.
56. Simha A, Aziz K, Braganza A, Abraham L, Samuel P, Lindsley KB. Anti-vascular endothelial growth factor for neovascular glaucoma. Cochrane Database Syst Rev. 2020;2:CD007920.
57. Sampat KM, Garg SJ. Complications of intravitreal injections. Curr Opin Ophthalmol. 2010;21(3):178–83.
58. Branch Vein Occlusion Study Group. Argon laser photocoagulation for macular edema in branch vein occlusion. Am J Ophthalmol. 2018;196:xxx–xxxviii.
59. Hayreh SS. Neovascular glaucoma. Prog Retin Eye Res. 2007;26(5):470–85.
60. Hayreh SS, Klugman MR, Podhajsky P, Servais GE, Perkins ES. Argon laser panretinal photocoagulation in ischemic central retinal vein occlusion. A 10-year prospective study. Graefes Arch Clin Exp Ophthalmol. 1990;228(4):281–96.
61. The Central Vein Occlusion Study Group N report. A randomized clinical trial of early panretinal photocoagulation for ischemic central vein occlusion. Ophthalmology. 1995;102(10):1434–44.
62. Fekrat S, Finkelstein D. Current concepts in the management of central retinal vein occlusion. Curr Opin Ophthalmol. 1997;8(3):50–4.
63. Cekiç O, Chang S, Tseng JJ, Barile GR, Weissman H, Del Priore LV, et al. Intravitreal triamcinolone treatment for macular edema associated with central retinal vein occlusion and hemiretinal vein occlusion. Retina. 2005;25(7):846–50.
64. Lee H, Shah GK. Intravitreal triamcinolone as primary treatment of cystoid macular edema secondary to branch retinal vein occlusion. Retina 2005;25(5):551–5.
65. Ozkiris A, Evereklioglu C, Erkiliç K, Ilhan O. The efficacy of intravitreal triamcinolone acetonide on macular edema in branch retinal vein occlusion. Eur J Ophthalmol. 2005;15(1):96–101.
66. Jonas JB, Akkoyun I, Kamppeter B, Kreissig I, Degenring RF. Branch retinal vein occlusion treated by intravitreal triamcinolone acetonide. Eye (Lond). 2005;19(1):65–71.
67. Chen SDM, Sundaram V, Lochhead J, Patel CK. Intravitreal triamcinolone for the treatment of ischemic macular edema associated with branch retinal vein occlusion. Am J Ophthalmol. 2006;141(5):876–83.
68. Cheng K-C, Wu W-C. Intravitreal triamcinolone acetonide for patients with macular edema due to branch retinal vein occlusion. Kaohsiung J Med Sci. 2006;22(7):321–30.
69. Kola M, Hacioglu D, Turk A, Erdol H. The effectiveness and reliability of posterior sub-Tenon triamcinolone acetonide injection in branch retinal vein occlusion-related macular edema. Cutan Ocul Toxicol. 2016;35(3):185–9.
70. Gurram MM. Effect of posterior sub–Tenon triamcinolone in macular edema due to non–ischemic vein occlusions. J Clin Diagn Res. 2013;7(12):2821–4.
71. Hayashi K, Hayashi H. Intravitreal versus retrobulbar injections of triamcinolone for macular edema associated with branch retinal vein occlusion. Am J Ophthalmol. 2005;139(6):972–82.
72. Haller JA, Bandello F, Belfort R, Blumenkranz MS, Gillies M, Heier J, et al. Randomized, sham-controlled trial of dexamethasone intravitreal implant in patients with macular edema due to retinal vein occlusion. Ophthalmology. 2010;117(6):1134–1146.e3.
73. Kuppermann BD, Blumenkranz MS, Haller JA, Williams GA, Weinberg DV, Chou C, et al. Randomized controlled study of an intravitreous dexamethasone drug delivery system in patients with persistent macular edema. Arch Ophthalmol. 2007;125(3):309–17.
74. Kim M, Lee DH, Byeon SH, Koh HJ, Kim SS, Lee SC. Comparison of intravitreal bevacizumab and dexamethasone implant for the treatment of macula oedema associated with branch retinal vein occlusion. Br J Ophthalmol. 2015;99(9):1271–6.
75. Oh JY, Seo JH, Ahn JK, Heo JW, Chung H. Early versus late intravitreal triamcinolone acetonide for macular edema associated with branch retinal vein occlusion. Korean J Ophthalmol. 2007;21(1):18–20.
76. Wingate RJ, Beaumont PE. Intravitreal triamcinolone and elevated intraocular pressure. Aust N Z J Ophthalmol. 1999;27(6):431–2.
77. Martidis A, Duker JS, Greenberg PB, Rogers AH, Puliafito CA, Reichel E, et al. Intravitreal triamcinolone for refractory diabetic macular edema. Ophthalmology. 2002;109(5):920–7.
78. Bakri SJ, Beer PM. The effect of intravitreal triamcinolone acetonide on intraocular pressure. Ophthalmic Surg Lasers Imaging. 2003;34(5):386–90.
79. Ferrini W, Ambresin A. Intravitreal dexamethasone implant for the treatment of macular edema after retinal vein occlusion in a clinical setting. Klin Monatsbl Augenheilkd. 2013;230(4):423–6.
80. Bonfiglio V, Reibaldi M, Fallico M, Russo A, Pizzo A, Fichera S, et al. Widening use of dexamethasone implant for the treatment of macular edema. Drug Des Devel Ther. 2017;11:2359–72.

81. Rodgin SG. Neovascular glaucoma associated with uveitis. J Am Optom Assoc. 1987;58(6):499–503.
82. Sivak-Callcott JA, O'Day DM, Gass JD, Tsai JC. Evidence-based recommendations for the diagnosis and treatment of neovascular glaucoma. Ophthalmology. 2001;108(10):1767–76; quiz1777, 1800.
83. Ritch R. The pilocarpine paradox. J Glaucoma. 1996;5(4):225–7.
84. Centofanti M, Manni GL, Napoli D, Bucci MG. Comparative effects of intraocular pressure between systemic and topical carbonic anhydrase inhibitors: a clinical masked, cross-over study. Pharmacol Res. 1997;35(5):481–5.
85. Delgado MF, Dickens CJ, Iwach AG, Novack GD, Nychka DS, Wong PC, et al. Long-term results of noncontact neodymium:yttrium-aluminum-garnet cyclophotocoagulation in neovascular glaucoma. Ophthalmology. 2003;110(5):895–9.
86. Nabili S, Kirkness CM. Trans-scleral diode laser cyclophoto-coagulation in the treatment of diabetic neovascular glaucoma. Eye (Lond). 2004;18(4):352–6.
87. Oguri A, Takahashi E, Tomita G, Yamamoto T, Jikihara S, Kitazawa Y. Transscleral cyclophotocoagulation with the diode laser for neovascular glaucoma. Ophthalmic Surg Lasers. 1998;29(9):722–7.
88. Choy BNK, Lai JSM, Yeung JCC, Chan JCH. Randomized comparative trial of diode laser transscleral cyclophotocoagulation versus Ahmed glaucoma valve for neovascular glaucoma in Chinese – a pilot study. Clin Ophthalmol. 2018;12:2545–52.
89. Yildirim N, Yalvac IS, Sahin A, Ozer A, Bozca T. A comparative study between diode laser cyclophotocoagulation and the Ahmed glaucoma valve implant in neovascular glaucoma: a long-term follow-up. J Glaucoma. 2009;18(3):192–6.

Neovascular Glaucoma in Ocular Ischemic Syndrome

Zhuangjun Si and Seenu M. Hariprasad

1 Background

Ocular ischemic syndrome (OIS) is the third most common cause of neovascular glaucoma (NVG) after proliferative diabetic retinopathy (PDR) and retinal vein occlusions (RVO). The pathophysiology is related to hypoperfusion of the eye, usually from ipsilateral stenosis of the common carotid or internal carotid arteries. The most common etiology of this carotid stenosis is atherosclerotic plaque buildup. However, any disease process which limits arterial flow to the ophthalmic artery, central retinal artery, and/or ciliary arteries can potentially cause OIS. As such, cases of giant cell arteritis, aortic arch syndrome, carotid artery dissection, Moyamoya, and Takayasu arteritis have been linked with OIS [1–4]. Typically, at least 90% stenosis of the ipsilateral carotid system is needed to produce OIS [5], as it reduces central retinal artery perfusion by

Z. Si
Department of Ophthalmology and Visual Science, The University of Chicago Medicine and Biological Sciences, Chicago, IL, USA

Duke Ophthalmology, Duke University School of Medicine, Durham, NC, USA

S. M. Hariprasad (✉)
Department of Ophthalmology and Visual Science, The University of Chicago Medicine and Biological Sciences, Chicago, IL, USA
e-mail: sharipra@bsd.uchicago.edu

50% [6, 7]. In 10% of cases of OIS, there is 100% bilateral carotid artery obstruction [5]. Of note, not all patients with significant carotid artery stenosis have OIS, possibly due to the formation of collateral vessels. Similar to other causes of NVG, the underlying ischemic drive induces pathological neovascularization of the anterior segment that eventually obstructs aqueous outflow at the iridocorneal angle.

OIS has been reported to present at a mean age of 65 years with a range between the sixth to ninth decade of life, affecting males more frequently than females, and there is no evidence to suggest any racial predilection [1]. The incidence of OIS has not been extensively studied, but Sturrock and Mueller in Switzerland estimated 7.5 cases/million persons annually [1, 8]. This is likely a conservative estimate, as OIS is easily misdiagnosed as its symptoms and clinical findings are nonspecific. Published epidemiologic data are limited, but, based on a commonly cited study of 208 patients with NVG, approximately 13% was attributable to carotid insufficiency [9].

2 Clinical Presentation

More than 90% of patients with OIS experience some degree of vision loss in the affected eye(s), usually over a period of weeks to months [5]. Presenting visual acuity (VA) is typically bimodally distributed, with 43% of eyes with OIS presenting with 20/20 to 20/50 vision and another 37% of eyes with OIS presenting with vision counting fingers (CF) or worse. After 1 year, only 24% of eyes had vision in the 20/20 to 20/50 range while 58% of eyes had vision that was CF or worse [10]. Macular ischemia leads to prolonged light recovery ("bright light amaurosis") as vasculature is unable to meet retinal metabolic demands [1].

Additionally, 10% of OIS patients experience amaurosis fugax for seconds to minutes [5]. This phenomenon is thought to be from emboli occluding the central retinal artery or vasospasms [11]. However, amaurosis fugax alone does not necessarily imply the presence of OIS; one third of patients with amaurosis fugax may have ipsilateral carotid artery obstruction of more than 75% or, in very rare cases, ophthalmic artery stenosis [12].

"Ocular angina" or pain in the orbital region has been documented in 40% of cases of patients with OIS, even in the setting of normal IOP [1, 5]. As the term "ocular angina" suggests, this dull pain is thought to arise from ischemia to the globe.

In patients with significant unilateral carotid disease, prominent collateral vessels from the external carotid system on the contralateral side may be seen on the forehead. Mistaking these vessels for those seen in giant cell arteritis may be devastating, as a subsequent temporal artery biopsy can disrupt collateral blood flow to the brain [1].

In OIS, anterior segment signs include dilated episcleral vessels, anterior chamber cell and flare, poorly reactive pupils, cataract, iris atrophy, and neovascularization of the iris (NVI) with or without neovascularization of the angle (NVA). NVI is seen in approximately 66–87% of eyes at the time of OIS presentation [5, 13]. However, only half of these OIS eyes with NVI develop elevated IOP even when the angle is synechially closed on gonioscopy. This is presumably due to a concomitant decrease in ciliary body perfusion and reduction in aqueous production. Diffuse episcleral injection may be present following long-standing ipsilateral internal carotid artery occlusion due to enlarged collateral external carotid arteries supplying the ophthalmic artery via retrograde flow [14]. Anterior chamber flare is typically observed in eyes with NVI and anterior chamber cell is seen in one fifth of eyes with OIS [5].

Posterior segment findings may be very similar to other etiologies of NVG including PDR and RVOs, and thus, a definitive diagnosis of OIS is often made by retina specialists. The most common posterior segment finding is retinal artery narrowing with dilated retinal veins; tortuosity or beading are less common [1]. Retinal hemorrhages, especially in the mid periphery, are seen in 80% of patients with OIS (Fig. 1a). More severe findings include neovascularization of the optic nerve and retina (35% and 8%, respectively) [5]. On fluorescein angiography (FA),

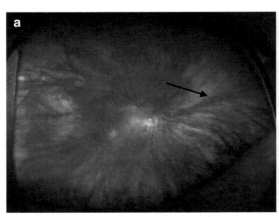
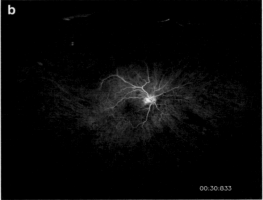
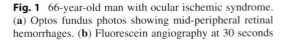

Fig. 1 66-year-old man with ocular ischemic syndrome. (**a**) Optos fundus photos showing mid-peripheral retinal hemorrhages. (**b**) Fluorescein angiography at 30 seconds of the same eye showing prolonged filling time and gradual peripheral nonperfusion

delayed or patchy choroidal filling (seen in 60% of OIS eyes) is the most specific finding while prolongation of the retinal arteriovenous transit time is most sensitive (seen in 95% of OIS eyes [1]) (Fig. 1b). However, the latter finding is often seen in central retinal artery occlusions (CRAO) and central retinal vein occlusions (CRVO) as well. Staining of both the large and small retinal vessels in later phases was seen in approximately 85% of eyes with OIS, which may be indicative of chronic hypoxic damage to endothelial cells [1, 5]. Gradual peripheral to mid-peripheral retinal nonperfusion may or may not be seen on FA (Fig. 1b) [5]. By comparison, in CRAO the FA typically does not show staining of vessels, and in CRVO, the FA typically shows staining of the veins with retinal artery sparing. Diabetic retinopathy can coexist with OIS and can be distinguished from OIS by the presence of hard exudates. Carotid artery stenosis does not appear to be protective against the development of diabetic retinopathy [15].

3 Systemic Associations and Management

Management of OIS is controversial due to the paucity of cases and lack of randomized prospective trials. In general, eyes with OIS have a poor visual prognosis. With NVI present, well over 90% of eye with OIS become legally blind within a year from either retinal pathology or glaucomatous optic neuropathy [10]. Treatment from an ophthalmic perspective consists of multiple components, including referral for management of comorbidities, controlling any anterior segment inflammation, ablation of ischemic retina, and management of elevated IOP or NVG.

One of the most important aspects of managing OIS is referring patients to their primary care provider for cardiovascular evaluation. The 5-year mortality for patients with OIS is 40% [16]. Two-thirds of these deaths are from cardiovascular disease; the second-leading cause is stroke. Systemic hypertension was present in 75% of OIS patients while diabetes mellitus was present in 56% [16]. Not surprisingly, nearly

20% of OIS patients had a history of peripheral vascular disease requiring a bypass. In a study of 32 patients with OIS, OIS was the first indicator for carotid artery workup in over two thirds of these patients [13]. Overall, for any patient with suspected OIS, a referral for cardiovascular workup is warranted due to the myriad of comorbidities and high mortality rate.

3.1 Revascularization of the Carotid Artery

Given the pathogenesis of OIS, it would seem that revascularization may be the most physiologic intervention. However, there are limited data on the effect of carotid endarterectomy (CEA) on OIS as cases are few and results are difficult to interpret due to the procedure's high complication rate and absence of a control group. Several investigators, including Cohn et al. and Geroulakos et al., have shown with Doppler imaging that flow velocities in the ophthalmic arteries improve after CEA [17, 18]. This was correlated with improved visual symptoms. However, these studies were small, and it is unclear if these hemodynamic changes lead to long-term visual benefits. Although there has been one documented case where a patient's symptoms, NVI, NVA, and retinal hemorrhages improved after uncomplicated CEA [19], other studies have been more equivocal. In a larger series of 52 patients with OIS undergoing CEA, 7% of eyes had improved vision and 60% of eyes had worse vision at postoperative year 1 [10]. However, CEA may reduce the risk of stroke in certain patients, and thus, the decision to proceed should be at the discretion of the vascular surgeon [20]. Occasionally, IOP spikes can occur after ipsilateral CEA, possibly due to restored ciliary perfusion and increased aqueous production in the setting of unchanged outflow obstruction [21, 22].

In cases with 100% occlusion of the carotid arteries, a CEA is typically not performed, because it cares significant risks and has not been shown to decrease the risk of ischemic strokes [23]. While there have been cases where improving the blood flow to the ischemic eye has been shown to improve vision in OIS eyes [24, 25], visual prognosis at 1 year is poor [10]. Temporal artery to middle cerebral artery (STA-MCA) bypasses have been performed to improve vascularization. Kawaguchi reported promising results of STA-MCA on 44 patients with OIS: vision improved in 18 patients and remained stable in the other 26 patients; however, it is unclear how this procedure affected anterior segment neovascularization and IOP [26].

3.2　Ophthalmic Medical and Surgical Therapy

Treatment of NVG secondary to OIS consists of medical, surgical, and laser therapies. The goals of treatment are (1) control of IOP using IOP-lowering eye drops or oral medications, or IOP-lowering surgery, and (2) treatment of underlying retinal neovascularization with anti-vascular endothelial growth factor (anti-VEGF) therapy or panretinal photocoagulation. In cases of NVG secondary to OIS, decreasing IOP is not only paramount in protecting the optic nerve, but also essential for restoring blood flow in an eye which already has compromised perfusion pressure. Topical and oral IOP-lowering medications are used, and topical steroids and cycloplegics can be added if inflammation is present. Surgical IOP-lowering strategies for NVG secondary to OIS are similar to those that would be employed for NVG secondary to other etiologies. However, there may theoretically be a greater risk for postoperative hypotony given the poor ciliary body perfusion in OIS, but there is currently no evidence regarding outcomes of IOP-lowering surgery in eyes with NVG specifically secondary to OIS. Using an aqueous shunt with a smaller plate size and/or using reduced settings when performing cyclophotocoagulation may theoretically reduce the risk of hypotony.

Panretinal photocoagulation (PRP) is a treatment option for eyes with OIS with anterior and/or posterior segment neovascularization. The destruction of ischemic retina is thought to decrease the production of angiogenic growth factors which stimulate pathological neovascularization. While PRP has been shown to be effective in preventing and regressing NVI in a majority of eyes with PDR, only 36% of eyes with OIS have showed NVI regression after full PRP [10]. This may be due to persistent anterior segment ischemia [27] or uveal ischemia [28]. Mizener et al. noted that there was no capillary dropout on FA in 15 out of 15 patients with OIS and asserted that the effectiveness of PRP in PDR may not translate to OIS in the absence of capillary ischemia [13]. However, in cases where peripheral retinal ischemia is seen on FA, it is recommended that PRP should be performed [29].

Intravitreal anti-VEGF injections have been shown to regress NVI and decrease macular edema in the setting of OIS [30]. If the view to the posterior pole permits, PRP is sensible, however, intravitreal bevacizumab can be helpful in cases where corneal haze, poor dilation, hyphema, or vitreous hemorrhage preclude an adequate view for PRP.

4　Conclusion

NVG secondary to OIS is a relatively rare but devastating diagnosis, and evidence-based treatment is not clearly established. The symptoms of OIS are nonspecific and a diagnosis typically requires ruling out other causes of NVG, including diabetes and vascular occlusions. Most of the research on OIS stems from the retina and vascular surgery perspective, and evidence from the glaucoma perspective is lacking. For example, there is a paucity of data on how the angle anatomy and IOP respond to medical and surgical treatments in NVG secondary to OIS and whether the surgical IOP-lowering strategy for NVG from OIS differs from surgical planning for other causes of NVG. Further research from glaucoma and retinal specialists is needed to fully elucidate the pathophysiology and most effective treatment strategy for NVG secondary to OIS. Regardless of the relatively poor visual prognosis in eyes with OIS, early diagnosis of OIS and prompt referral for vascular workup can be potentially lifesaving.

References

1. Brown GC, Sharma S. Ocular ischemic syndrome. Retina. 2013;1091–103.
2. Mendrinos E, Machinis TG, Pournaras CJ. Ocular ischemic syndrome. Surv Ophthalmol. 2010;55:2–34.
3. Anguita R, Nazar C, Kobus R, Salinas A, Astete M. Bilateral ocular ischemic syndrome as a manifestation of Takayasu arteritis in children. Can J Ophthalmol. 2019;54:e105–8.
4. Papavasileiou E, Sobrin L, Papaliodis GN. Ocular ischemic syndrome presenting as retinal vasculitis in a patient with moyamoya syndrome. Retin Cases Brief Rep. 2015;9:170–2.
5. Brown GC, Magargal LE. The ocular ischemic syndrome: clinical, fluorescein angiographic and carotid angiographic features. Int Ophthalmol. 1988;11:239–51.
6. Kearns TP. Ophthalmology and the carotid artery. Am J Ophthalmol. 1979;88:714–22.
7. Kobayashi S, Hollenhorst RW, Sundt TM Jr. Retinal arterial pressure before and after surgery for carotid artery stenosis. Stroke. 1971;2:569–75.
8. Sturrock GD, Mueller HR. Chronic ocular ischaemia. Br J Ophthalmol. 1984;68:716–23.
9. Brown GC, Magargal LE, Schachat A, Shah H. Neovascular glaucoma. Etiologic considerations. Ophthalmology. 1984;91:315–20.
10. Sivalingam A, Brown GC, Magargal LE. The ocular ischemic syndrome. III. Visual prognosis and the effect of treatment. Int Ophthalmol. 1991;15:15–20.
11. Winterkorn JM, Teman AJ. Recurrent attacks of amaurosis fugax treated with calcium channel blocker. Ann Neurol. 1991;30:423–5.
12. Aasen J, Kerty E, Russell D, Bakke SJ, Nyberg-Hansen R. Amaurosis fugax: clinical, Doppler and angiographic findings. Acta Neurol Scand. 1988;77:450–5.
13. Mizener JB, Podhajsky P, Hayreh SS. Ocular ischemic syndrome. Ophthalmology. 1997;104:859–64.
14. Countee RW, Gnanadev A, Chavis P. Dilated episcleral arteries--a significant physical finding in assessment of patients with cerebrovascular insufficiency. Stroke. 1978;9:42–5.
15. Duker JS, Brown GC, Bosley TM, Colt CA, Reber R. Asymmetric proliferative diabetic retinopathy and carotid artery disease. Ophthalmology. 1990;97:869–74.
16. Sivalingam A, Brown GC, Magargal LE, Menduke H. The ocular ischemic syndrome. II. Mortality and systemic morbidity. Int Ophthalmol. 1989;13:187–91.
17. Cohn EJ Jr, Sandager GP, Benjamin ME, Lilly MP, Hanna DJ, Flinn WR. Assessment of ocular perfusion after carotid endarterectomy with color-flow duplex scanning. J Vasc Surg. 1999;29:665–71.
18. Geroulakos G, Botchway LT, Pai V, Wilkinson AR, Galloway JM. Effect of carotid endarterectomy on the ocular circulation and on ocular symptoms unrelated to emboli. Eur J Vasc Endovasc Surg. 1996;11:359–63.
19. Lauria AL, Koelling EE, Houghtaling PM, White PW (2020) Carotid endarterectomy for ocular ischemic syndrome: a case report and review of the literature. Ann Vasc Surg.
20. American Symptomatic Carotid N. Beneficial effect of carotid endarterectomy in symptomatic patients with high-grade carotid stenosis. N Engl J Med. 1991;325:445–53.
21. Kawano T, Saito K, Hidaka T, Kajihara N, Chuman H, Ohta H, Yokogami K, Takeshima H. Two patients with a rapid increase in the ocular pressure after carotid artery stenting for cervical internal carotid artery stenosis with ocular ischemic syndrome. J Neuroendovascular Therapy. 2018;12:553–9.
22. Ng E, Choong AM, Walker PJ. Neovascular glaucoma post carotid endarterectomy: a case report and review of the literature. Ann Vasc Dis. 2015;8:103–5.
23. EC/IC Bypass Study Group. Failure of extracranial-intracranial arterial bypass to reduce the risk of ischemic stroke. Results of an international randomized trial. N Engl J Med. 1985;313:1191–200.
24. Kiser WD, Gonder J, Magargal LE, Sanborn GE, Simeone F. Recovery of vision following treatment of the ocular ischemic syndrome. Ann Ophthalmol. 1983;15:305–10.
25. Higgins RA. Neovascular glaucoma associated with ocular hypoperfusion secondary to carotid artery disease. Aust J Ophthalmol. 1984;12:155–62.
26. Kawaguchi S, Iida J-I, Hashimoto H, Sakaki T. The role of STA-MCA bypass for the ocular ischemic syndrome due to the occlusive internal carotid artery diseases. Surg Cerebral Stroke. 2003;13:419–23.
27. Coppeto JR, Wand M, Bear L, Sciarra R. Neovascular glaucoma and carotid artery obstructive disease. Am J Ophthalmol. 1985;99:567–70.
28. Hayreh SS, Baines JA. Occlusion of the vortex veins. An experimental study. Br J Ophthalmol. 1973;57:217–38.
29. Malhotra R, Gregory-Evans K. Management of ocular ischaemic syndrome. Br J Ophthalmol. 2000;84:1428–31.
30. Amselem L, Montero J, Diaz-Llopis M, Pulido JS, Bakri SJ, Palomares P, Garcia-Delpech S. Intravitreal bevacizumab (Avastin) injection in ocular ischemic syndrome. Am J Ophthalmol. 2007;144:122–4.

Neovascular Glaucoma in Ocular Inflammatory Disease

Rachel A. Downes and Careen Y. Lowder

1 Background

Rubeosis iridis, the proliferation of new blood vessels on the iris, is a nonspecific reaction of the iris vasculature to a variety of noxious stimuli, including vascular, inflammatory, and neoplastic phenomena [1]. Neovascular glaucoma (NVG) occurs when such proliferation of fibrovascular tissue on the iris and in the angle directly obstructs aqueous outflow through the trabecular meshwork [2]. As the disease progresses, peripheral anterior synechiae can form, resulting in progressive synechial angle closure and elevated intraocular pressure (IOP) [2].

Neovascularization in the eye occurs when the homeostatic balance of pro-angiogenic (e.g., VEGF) and anti-angiogenic factors (e.g., pigment-epithelium-derived factor) shifts to favoring angiogenesis [3]. A 1998 study by Tripathi et al. assessed VEGF concentrations in aqueous samples from eyes with NVG, primary open-angle glaucoma (POAG), and cataracts [4]. The study found a significantly higher VEGF concentration in eyes with NVG compared to the other groups; specifically, VEGF concentration in eyes with NVG was 40-times higher than in those with POAG and 113-times higher than in

those with cataract [4]. In the NVG group, 12/12 eyes had NVG as the result of either proliferative diabetic retinopathy (PDR) or central retinal vein occlusion (CRVO) [4]. This is unsurprising, as retinal ischemia, most commonly in the form of PDR or CRVO, represents the etiology of NVG in up to 95% of cases [2, 5, 6]. Although the specific cause of retinal ischemia that incites NVG may vary from case to case, the current consensus is that VEGF is a final common mediator of neovascularization [7].

2 Neovascularization Secondary to Retinal Ischemia

Retinal ischemia occurs in numerous ocular inflammatory diseases, the result of thrombotic or obliterative vasculitis [8]. Thrombotic events can occur as the result of local endothelial injury or due to increased prothrombin, as is the case in Behçet's disease [8, 9]. In uveitic eyes with obliterative vasculitis, histologic studies have identified perivascular lymphocytic infiltration as well as the presence of CD4+ T cells within and around affected retinal vessels [8, 10, 11]. Regardless of the specific mechanism by which retinal ischemia occurs, the result is generally the same: upregulation of VEGF and thus induction of neovascularization [7, 8].

R. A. Downes · C. Y. Lowder (✉)
Cole Eye Institute, Cleveland Clinic,
Cleveland, OH, USA
e-mail: LOWDERC@ccf.org

© The Author(s), under exclusive license to Springer Nature Switzerland AG 2022
M. Qiu (ed.), *Neovascular Glaucoma*, Essentials in Ophthalmology,
https://doi.org/10.1007/978-3-031-11720-6_9

3 Neovascularization in the Absence of Retinal Ischemia

Although retinal ischemia is the most common inciting factor that gives rise to NVG, in ocular inflammatory diseases, neovascularization and NVG may occur in the absence of identifiable retinal ischemia [2, 12–14]. The specific mechanism by which this neovascularization occurs is not entirely clear, but there is evidence to suggest that cytokines and other mediators in the inflammatory cascade play a significant role in VEGF regulation [14, 15]. Specifically, nuclear factor-$\kappa\beta$,interleukin-1β, tumor necrosis factor-α, transforming growth factor-β2, interleukin-6, and interleukin-8 have all been implicated in the regulation of VEGF [15–21]. The interplay between these inflammatory mediators and VEGF may explain the occurrence of NVG in instances of uveitis without evident ischemia. Providing further evidence for this theory, a 2001 study by Fine et al. quantified and compared the levels of VEGF in eyes with uveitis with and without CME [22]. The study found a significantly greater level of VEGF in the uveitic eyes with CME, suggesting that VEGF may be upregulated sufficiently to cause a measurable effect in some but not all eyes with inflammatory disease [22].

4 NVG in Specific Ocular Inflammatory Diseases

Given the link between ischemia and VEGF and the central role of VEGF in neovascularization, it is unsurprising that most documented cases of NVG in uveitis have occurred in the setting retinal ischemia. NVG has been documented to be a sequela of ischemic vasculitis in inflammatory ocular diseases including sarcoidosis, cytomegalovirus infection, herpes zoster ophthalmicus, and neurofibromatosis [23–26] Myriad other ocular inflammatory disorders are associated with retinal ischemia and thus may result in NVG, including tuberculosis, West Nile virus,

Behçet's disease, multiple sclerosis, systemic lupus erythematosus, antiphospholipid antibody syndrome, Takayasu's disease, granulomatosis with polyangiitis, dermatomyositis, Churg–Strauss syndrome, Crohn's disease, polyarteritis nodosa, and Susac syndrome [8].

More rarely, there have been reports of NVG in the setting of ocular inflammatory disease without evidence of retinal vasculitis. Gaskin et al. published a case of a patient with NVG secondary to chronic low-grade panuveitis due to sarcoidosis [13]. The patient's flares consisted of granulomatous inflammation of the anterior chamber, left eye greater than right, requiring sub-Tenon's dexamethasone injections [13]. At a follow-up visit, the patient was noted to have neovascularization of the angle and the iris of the left eye; fluorescein angiography did not reveal any signs of retinal ischemia [13]. The authors postulate that the patient's chronic, aggressive, granulomatous inflammation provided an angiogenic stimulus sufficient to promote neovascularization even in the absence of ischemia-driven modulators [13].

5 Managing NVG in Ocular Inflammatory Diseases

Therapeutic strategies for NVG in ocular inflammatory disease are often multimodal, including topical IOP-lowering medication, panretinal photocoagulation (when retinal ischemia is evident), intravitreal anti-VEGF therapy, IOP-lowering surgery, and anti-inflammatory therapy including steroids and/or steroid-sparing immunomodulatory treatments [27, 28]. In contrast to NVG secondary to purely vascular processes such as PDR and CRVO, in NVG associated with inflammatory diseases, tools that target underlying inflammation are likely to be the most important and most effective components of a treatment plan [14]. Particularly in cases without retinal ischemia, addressing the inflammatory cascade that upregulates VEGF and thus fosters neovascularization may obviate the need for anti-VEGF treatment [14].

6 Conclusions

NVG in ocular inflammatory disease is a rare but clinically important phenomenon. To optimally treat high intraocular pressure (IOP) in patients with uveitis, it is critical to thoroughly examine the iris and perform gonioscopy to examine the angle to rule out neovascularization before attributing IOP elevations to a steroid response or secondary open-angle glaucoma. Early detection of NVG in this group enables targeted, timely interventions and ultimately ensures optimal visual outcomes. Additional research will be necessary to fully understand the pathophysiology of NVG in ocular inflammatory disease and to elucidate an evidence-based treatment strategy for this group.

References

1. Laatikainen L. Vascular changes in the iris in chronic anterior uveitis. Br J Ophthalmol. 1979;63(3):145–9.
2. Hayreh SS. Neovascular glaucoma. Prog Retin Eye Res. 2007;26(5):470–85.
3. Wang JW, et al. Short-term effect of intravitreal ranibizumab on intraocular concentrations of vascular endothelial growth factor-A and pigment epithelium-derived factor in neovascular glaucoma. Clin Exp Ophthalmol. 2014.
4. Tripathi RC, Li J, Tripathi BJ, Chalam KV, Adamis AP. Increased level of vascular endothelial growth factor in aqueous humor of patients with neovascular glaucoma. Ophthalmology. 1998;105(2):232–7. https://doi.org/10.1016/s0161-6420(98)92782-8.
5. Fong DS, Raizman MB. Spontaneous hyphema associated with anterior uveitis. Br J Ophthalmol. 1993;77(10):635–8.
6. Brown GC, Magargal LE, Schachat A, Shah H. Neovascular glaucoma; etiological considerations. Ophthalmology. 1984;91:315–20.
7. Rosenbaum DM, Rosenbaum PS, Gupta A, Michaelson MD, Hall DH, Kessler JA. Retinal ischemia leads to apoptosis which is ameliorated by aurintricarboxylic acid. Vis Res. 1997;37(24):3445–51.
8. Talat L, Lightman S, Tomkins-Netzer O. Ischemic retinal vasculitis and its management. J Ophthalmol. 2014;2014:197675.
9. Hughes EH, Dick AD. The pathology and pathogenesis of retinal vasculitis. Neuropathol Appl Neurobiol. 2003;29(4):325–40.
10. Gass JD, Olson CL. Sarcoidosis with optic nerve and retinal involvement. Arch Ophthalmol. 1976;94(6):945–50.
11. Eichenbaum JW, Friedman AH, Mamelok AE. A clinical and histopathological review of intermediate uveitis ("pars planitis"). Bull N Y Acad Med. 1988;64(2):165–74.
12. Fardeau C, Champion E, Massamba N, LeHoang P. Uveitic macular edema. Eye (Lond). 2016;30(10):1277–92.
13. Gaskin BJ, Danesh-Meyer HV. Neovascular glaucoma and sarcoidosis. Eye (Lond). 2005;19(5):599–601.
14. Sora D, Takayama K, Taguchi M, Sato T, Sakurai Y, Kanda T, Takeuchi M. Topical corticosteroid-resolved Rubeosis Iridis with neovascular glaucoma caused by noninfectious granulomatous uveitis. Case Rep Ophthalmol. 2018;9:243–7.
15. Gulati S, N, Forooghian F, Lieberman R, Jabs DA. Vascular endothelial growth factor inhibition in uveitis: a systematic review. Br J Ophthalmol. 2011 Feb;95(2):162–5.
16. Huang S, Robinson JB, Deguzman A, et al. Blockade of nuclear factor-kappaB signaling inhibits angiogenesis and tumorigenicity of human ovarian cancer cells by suppressing expression of vascular endothelial growth factor and interleukin 8. Cancer Res. 2000;60:5334–9.
17. Bian ZM, Elner SG, Elner VM. Regulation of VEGF mRNA expression and protein secretion by TGF-beta2 in human retinal pigment epithelial cells. Exp Eye Res. 2007;84:812–22.
18. Sola-Villa D, Camacho M, Sola R, et al. IL-1beta induces VEGF, independently of PGE2 induction, mainly through the PI3-K/mTOR pathway in renal mesangial cells. Kidney Int. 2006;70:1935–41.
19. Cha HS, Bae EK, Koh JH, et al. Tumor necrosis factor-alpha induces vascular endothelial growth factor-C expression in rheumatoid synoviocytes. J Rheumatol. 2007;34:16–9.
20. Cohen T, Nahari D, Cerem LW, et al. Interleukin 6 induces the expression of vascular endothelial growth factor. J Biol Chem. 1996;271:736–41.
21. Li M, Zhang Y, Feurino LW, et al. Interleukin-8 increases vascular endothelial growth factor and neuropilin expression and stimulates ERK activation in human pancreatic cancer. Cancer Sci. 2008;99:733–7.
22. Fine HF, Baffi J, Reed GF, et al. Aqueous humor and plasma vascular endothelial growth factor in uveitis-associated cystoid macular edema. Am J Ophthalmol. 2001;132:794–6.

23. Lobo A, Barton K, Minassian D, Du Bois RM, Lightman S. Visual loss in sarcoid-related uveitis. Clin Exp Ophthalmol. 2003;31:310–6.

24. Babu K, Murthy KR, Sudarshan S, Biswas J. Bilateral arteritis with cytomegalovirus retinitis in a patient infected with human immunodeficiency virus. Retin Cases Brief Rep. 2010;4(1):31–3.

25. Ahmad SS, Suan ALL, Alexander SM. Herpes zoster ophthalmicus, central retinal artery occlusion, and neovascular glaucoma in an Immunocompetent individual. J Ophthalmic Vis Res. 2019;14(1):97–100.

26. Pichi F, Morara M, Lembo A, Ciardella AP, Meduri A, Nucci P. Neovascular glaucoma induced by peripheral retinal ischemia in neurofibromatosis type 1: management and imaging features. Case Rep Ophthalmol. 2013;4(1):69–73.

27. Qureshi K, Kashani S, Kelly SP. Intracameral bevacizumab for rubeotic glaucoma secondary to retinal vein occlusion. Int Ophthalmol. 2009;29(6):537–9.

28. Olmos LC, Lee RK. Medical and surgical treatment of neovascular glaucoma. Int Ophthalmol Clin. 2011;51(3):27–36.

Neovascular Glaucoma in Chronic Retinal Detachments

Aaron Priluck, Loka Thangamathesvaran, and Ravi Pandit

1 Introduction

Retinal detachments have long been known to cause ischemic complications of the anterior and posterior segment [1]. Although tractional retinal detachments arising from primary retinal vascular disorders can result from and lead to retinal ischemia, this chapter will focus primarily on rhegmatogenous retinal detachments (RRD). RRD are associated with a wide range of biochemical and vascular derangements that can lead to anterior segment neovascularization and ultimately neovascular glaucoma (NVG). Moreover, the surgical approaches to repair such RRD may themselves induce changes that may predispose to NVG. This chapter will review the pathogenesis, epidemiology, and treatment strategies for NVG associated with RRD.

2 Biochemical Changes

Amino acids and their metabolites play a critical role in maintaining retinal health and promoting tissue repair. Imbalances in this milieu following

Aaron Priluck and Loka Thangamathesvaran contributed equally with all other contributors.

A. Priluck · L. Thangamathesvaran · R. Pandit (✉)
Wilmer Eye Institute, Johns Hopkins University
School of Medicine, Baltimore, MD, USA

RRD lead to upregulation of growth factors contributing to aberrant vasculature patterns and vitreoretinal abnormalities [2]. After development of a retinal break, there is a breakdown of the uveo-vascular barrier, resulting in an influx of inflammatory cells, and altering the expression of cytokines and amino acids to promote an overall pro-inflammatory environment [3, 4]. There is a high variability in the expression of these biochemicals reflecting the anatomical variations in the retinal breaks [3]. This pro-inflammatory environment promotes leukocyte recruitment, wound healing, and angiogenesis [5–10]. Several studies have compared the concentration of amino acids in vitreous samples between patients with and without RRD with several identified differences between these groups [2].

Patients with RRD have elevated levels of glutamate [2, 11]. Glutamate is the primary excitatory amino acid neurotransmitter within the retina and excess levels can result in excitotoxicity leading to DNA damage, cell death, and ultimately global ischemia [12–14]. Animal studies have evaluated the role of intravitreal injections of excitatory amino acid receptor antagonists in the context of RRD. These studies have shown a decrease in neuronal loss and protection against excitotoxic death with administration of these injections [13].

Dopamine levels are also elevated in vitreous samples following RRD [15]. There are two postulated mechanisms for how this increase contributes to retinal damage. First, cytosolic dopamine can undergo spontaneous oxidation to produce reactive oxygen species, which have been shown to damage RPE cells [16, 17]. Second, RPE cells have dopamine receptors which when bound to dopamine can alter cAMP levels [18]. cAMP is a pro-apoptotic factor that can lead to RPE death [19].

Several studies have shown elevation in angiogenic factors such as interleukin 8 (IL-8) and vascular endothelial growth factor (VEGF) following RRD [2, 20]. VEGF and IL-8 promote proinflammatory conditions via several mechanisms. Both IL-8 and VEGF increase endothelial cell migration and proliferation contributing to angiogenesis [21, 22]. VEGF also promotes the release of glutamate, with changes as described above [23]. Overexpression of these factors is found in other ischemic retinal processes such as proliferative diabetic retinopathy [24, 25] and retinal artery occlusions [26].

3   Peripheral Vascular Changes

Anatomic variations in peripheral retinal vascular patterns have also been noted in patients with RRD [27]. These patterns include peripheral non-perfusion, abrupt discontinuity of peripheral retinal vasculature, circumferential vascular loops, and wedge-shaped avascular notches [27].

Vascular discontinuity has been shown to correlate with lattice degeneration beyond the area of premature termination. The pattern of abrupt ending has also been noted in other pathologic processes including myopia [28], central retinal vein occlusion [29], and familial exudative vitreoretinopathy [30]. Circumferential vascular loops have been proposed to originate as a response to retinal ischemia following RRD [27, 31].

Avascularity and lack of supportive cellular populations may potentiate the development of retinal breaks. Astrocytes and microglial cells help maintain the integrity of retinal vasculature and prevent leakage; absence of these cells is noted in avascular retina predisposing to the development of incompetent vasculature in the peripheral retina [32]. Avascularity is noted more frequently in patients with high myopia [32]. There have been several hypotheses to suggest why myopic individuals are more predisposed to peripheral non-perfusion. First, as the eye elongates, peripheral avascular retina can stretch, resulting in peripheral areas that are weak and prone to atrophy [27]. An alternative hypothesis speculates that some patients are born with abnormal peripheral retinal vasculature. Vascularity of the peripheral retina has been proposed to be associated with emmetropization; therefore, patients with avascular peripheral retinas are predisposed to development of myopia and associated complications [33, 34]. These "pre-morbid ischemia" theories may explain why RRD associated with atrophic holes are far more likely to have peripheral ischemia than those associated with horseshoe tears (84.6% vs. 21.4%) [35].

Once a RRD has developed, there is an increase in the release of endothelin-1, a powerful vasoconstrictor, which induces further vascular alterations [36].

4   Macular Vascular Changes

Changes in macula flow patterns vary based on macular involvement ("macula-on" or "macula-off"). In macula-on RRD, in the immediate period following RRD both prior to surgical intervention and in the short-term following surgery, there is a reduction in vascular perfusion compared to control patients [37]. However, following surgery, macular flow has been shown to be restored back to normal [37, 38]. In contrast, studies evaluating vascular changes in macula-off RRD have noted substantial, permanent changes even after successful surgical repair. Several studies have shown reduction in velocity density in both the superficial capillary plexus, deep capillary plexus, and choriocapillaris [39, 40]. Although following surgery, there is improvement in macular perfusion, it does not reach the value of the fellow, unaffected, eye. The difference is more pronounced in the deep capillary plexus, in comparison with superficial capillary plexus, with the suggestion that the deep capillary plexus supplies more of the retina affected by RRD [39]. This has a functional correlation, as decreased foveal velocity density has been shown to correlate with reduced final visual acuity [40]. However, given the posterior and occasionally transient (in macula-on circumstances) reduction in blood flow, these changes alone would not be anticipated to lead to NVG.

In summary, retinal vascular pathology may contribute to the major risk factors for RRD, which in turn may induce further retinal vascular pathology. This cascade of changes can lead to the development of NVG.

5 Epidemiology

RRD can cause peripheral retinal ischemia as described above, with pro-angiogenic factors that may subsequently diffuse to adjacent anterior segment structures, resulting in neovascularization of the iris (NVI), neovascularization of the angle (NVA), and ultimately NVG [41].

In a case series, nine patients with longstanding RRD (duration ranging from 1 to 18 years) were reported to have retinal neovascularization in the location of detached retina without involvement of attached retina [35]. Many other case reports also document retinal neovascularization associated with chronic RRD [42–44].

There is strong experimental evidence that RRD causes NVI. In an animal model, Stefansson et al. demonstrated that cats undergoing simultaneous vitrectomy, lensectomy, and induced RRD all developed NVI. No NVI was observed in eyes that underwent vitrectomy and lensectomy without RRD or in the untreated control group, implicating the RRD as the sentinel event in the ischemic cascade. The NVI observed in this experimental group typically became clinically visible 1–2 months after surgery [45]. Observational human studies have demonstrated that untreated RRD can also lead to NVI. In a case series of 22 patients who did not undergo

surgery for RRD repair for various reasons, five patients (23%) developed NVI with the average RRD duration being 9.6 years [46]. In a case series from Japan, 36 (1.3%) of 2853 eyes with RRD developed NVI during the course of treatment, and 34 of the 36 patients had persistent RRD at the time of onset of NVI [47]. Also notably, all 36 eyes with RRD that developed NVI had either no prior vitreoretinal surgery, an unsuccessful vitreoretinal surgery, or a vitreoretinal surgery that was complicated by mild anterior segment necrosis or vortex vein damage, implying that failure to successfully treat RRD without complication led to development of NVI [47]. Similarly, in a case series of seven eyes of seven nondiabetic patients, NVI developed after re-detachment following scleral buckle repair of RRD. The authors noted that NVI was generally identified 3–26 weeks after peripheral retinal re-detachment postoperatively [48].

Nevertheless, RRD is a rare cause of NVI; thus, a patient who presents with NVI is unlikely to have RRD as the underlying cause. In a retrospective study of all patients with NVI seen at a Korean hospital, chronic RRD accounted for only 3.2% of patients with NVI. Proliferative diabetic retinopathy and retinal vein occlusion accounted for the vast majority of NVI in their cohort, which is consistent with the NVG literature [49]. Retrospective reviews of 208 NVG patients from a tertiary eye hospital in the United States and 337 NVG patients from a tertiary eye hospital in Saudi Arabia reported that RRD was the presumed etiology of the NVG in only 1.5% and 3.6% of cases, respectively, while proliferative diabetic retinopathy and retinal vein occlusion again accounted for the majority of cases [50, 51].

Untreated RRD can also lead to NVA. While the incidence of NVA secondary to RRD is not specifically known, in general the development of NVA parallels the development of NVI [52]. In the aforementioned study by Stefansson et al., two of the eight eyes of the cats in the experimental group that developed NVI also developed histological NVA at 6–12 months [45]. The fibrovascular membranes of NVA can obstruct aqueous outflow and result in elevated intraocular pressure (IOP). As the disease progresses, the fibrovascular membrane can contract and form peripheral anterior synechiae, which eventually results in progressive synechial angle closure.

Although symptomatic RRD occurring in developed countries are typically treated expeditiously before development of NVG, rapid diagnosis and timely surgical access remain ongoing challenges in developing countries, with 44–70% of patients in such settings undergoing surgery more than 1 month after symptom onset [53]. In addition, up 5% of all RRD may be asymptomatic and therefore remain untreated until incidentally discovered. Characteristics of chronic, often undiagnosed, and therefore untreated RRD include atrophic retinal breaks, inferior retinal breaks, inferior retinal detachments, absence of posterior vitreous detachment, and young age [54, 55].

To avoid neovascular complications from RRD, timely diagnosis and repair should be pursued.

6   Surgical Management

The definitive treatment for the ischemic sequelae of RRD is retinal reattachment. In a 1998 case series of 7 eyes of patients without primary retinal vascular disease who developed NVI after primary retinal reattachment surgery, three (42%) went on to develop NVG. Of the four eyes that underwent a revision retinal reattachment procedure, anterior proliferative retinopathy was found in all cases, and rubeosis regressed in all cases of successful reattachment. In contrast, NVI and subsequent complications persisted in cases that did not undergo secondary repair, or cases in which secondary repair failed to reattach the retina. The final visual acuity, as expected, was better in the eyes with successful retinal reattachment, with those eyes maintaining Snellen acuity (20/70–20/400) compared to those who remained detached (hand motions to light perception). It is interesting to note that a high encircling scleral buckle was present in all seven cases [48].

Several studies have demonstrated anterior retinal ischemia after scleral buckling [56]. In a study by Ogasawara et al. of 7 young patients (mean age 32 years) without retinal vascular dis-

ease who underwent uncomplicated scleral buckling procedure 1–7 years (mean 4 years) prior, retinal arterial blood flow was 50% lower than the contralateral eye; in the two patients in whom the buckling elements were removed, blood flow increased by 44 and 73% [57]. It is important to note that patients may retain good vision despite decreased retinal perfusion, and thus, a high index of suspicion is required in RRD repaired in this manner [58]. In select cases of symptomatic retinal ischemia after scleral buckling with successful retinal reattachment, removal of the scleral buckle can be considered after careful consideration of risks and benefits.

In cases of RRD with scarred and non-salvageable peripheral retina, a pars plana lensectomy and vitrectomy with retinectomy may be performed to access and subsequently excise diseased anterior retinal tissue, respectively. While this can relieve peripheral RRDs that can lead to ischemia, there is also high potential to induce or worsen ischemia by transecting blood supply to the peripheral retina. In a study by Bourke et al. of 20 consecutive patients who underwent successful retinal reattachment with retinectomy, 10 (50%) demonstrated anterior retinal neovascularization and 9 (18%) were noted to have NVI. The authors suggested aggressive removal of all retina anterior to the retinectomy and prophylactic peripheral laser photocoagulation (PRP) in non-retinectomized areas to mitigate against this complication [59]. Interestingly, vitrectomy and/or lensectomy required for RRD repair may allow increased diffusion of pro-angiogenic factors to the anterior segment [60]. Conversely, silicone oil may be protective in this regard, though this tamponade brings a host of other complications, including acute and chronic elevated IOP due to non-neovascular reasons [61, 62].

While laser retinopexy of peripheral RRD may avoid the complications of incisional surgery, this procedure halts progression of RRD but does not reverse it, and ischemia in detached (albeit barricaded) retina may continue to progress [63, 64].

Adjunctive cryotherapy directly to peripheral retinal neovascularization (e.g., not to the retinal breaks as a means of retinopexy) has been shown in a small case series to hasten regression of neovascularization compared to retinal reattachment alone (2 weeks vs. 2–3 months) [35].

Thus, the full spectrum of retinal repair procedures can both address RRD-associated retinal ischemia and NVG but also potentiate this phenomenon by a multitude of mechanisms.

7 Medical Management

The use of anti-VEGF monotherapy can be considered in cases of chronic untreated RRD. Singh et al. reported on a case of a patient with good visual acuity, macular attachment, but 8 clock hours of peripheral RRD with iris neovascularization in whom bevacizumab was used in an attempt to avoid further surgery. Although the neovascularization regressed after injection, it recurred 10 weeks after the injection, and the patient ultimately required RRD repair. The neovascularization resolved permanently after repair with vitrectomy and retinectomy [65]. An anti-VEGF approach could be considered in patients with high surgical risk, although the optimal anti-VEGF treatment algorithms are not well studied in this context. Likely, chronic follow-up and treatment would be required.

In non-RRD-associated ischemic ocular conditions, PRP has offered durable benefits in prevention and treatment of NVG [66]. Although PRP may be considered in cases of NVG induced by surgical methods of RRD repair, PRP is typically not possible in setting of ongoing RRD due lack of apposition between the outer retina and RPE; attempts to achieve photocoagulation in this setting (e.g., increasing laser power or duration) may induce retinal necrosis and further ischemia [67]. In contrast, trans-scleral cryotherapy can achieve an ablative effect through subretinal fluid [68]. Thus, isolated cryotherapy may be an appropriate, non-invasive, and durable option in cases of NVG secondary to peripheral retinal detachments where operative repair is not possible. Moreover, cryotherapy has also been demonstrated to augment the effect of intravitreal bevacizumab and PRP for the treatment of NVG in other ischemic conditions and thus a multimodal approach may be employed, tailored to the underlying cause of NVG after RRD [65].

8 Conclusion

RRD is a rare but potent cause of retinal ischemia and subsequent NVG. Moreover, RRD risk factors such as myopia, atrophic holes, and lattice degeneration may be associated with pre-existing peripheral retinal ischemia; such eyes may already be predisposed to NVG even prior to development of RRD. Acute retinal breaks and subsequent RRD induce numerous retinal vascular changes, inflammation, and ischemia in both macula-on and macula-off settings. Chronic untreated RRD confers a high risk of NVG, but timely repair can largely reverse the ischemic process. However, accurate diagnosis and timely treatment of RRD remain a challenge in resource-limited settings. Many of the surgical treatments for RRD may induce new retinal ischemia despite successful repair and facilitate the diffusion of pro-angiogenic factors to the anterior segment, resulting in NVG by a different mechanism than the initial RRD. Alternatively, post-operative NVG may be a sign of a new, recurrent RRD. In office cryotherapy and intravitreal anti-VEGF medications can be considered in NVG cases where operative repair of underlying RRD is not possible.

References

1. Schulze RR. Rubeosis iridis. Am J Ophthalmol. 1967;63(3):487–95.
2. Yalcinbayir O, Buyukuysal RL, Gelisken O, Buyukuysal C, Can B. Amino acid and vascular endothelial growth factor levels in subretinal fluid in rhegmatogenous retinal detachment. Mol Vis. 2014;20:1357–65.
3. Garweg JG, Zandi S, Pfister I, Rieben R, Skowronska M, Tappeiner C. Cytokine profiles of phakic and pseudophakic eyes with primary retinal detachment. Acta Ophthalmol. 2019;97(4):e580–e8.
4. Hollborn M, Francke M, Iandiev I, Bühner E, Foja C, Kohen L, et al. Early activation of inflammation- and immune response-related genes after experimental detachment of the porcine retina. Invest Ophthalmol Vis Sci. 2008;49(3):1262–73.
5. Shinkai A, Yoshisue H, Koike M, Shoji E, Nakagawa S, Saito A, et al. A novel human CC chemokine, eotaxin-3, which is expressed in IL-4-stimulated vascular endothelial cells, exhibits potent activity toward eosinophils. J Immunol. 1999;163(3):1602–10.
6. Chen J, Vistica BP, Takase H, Ham DI, Fariss RN, Wawrousek EF, et al. A unique pattern of up- and down-regulation of chemokine receptor CXCR3 on

inflammation-inducing Th1 cells. Eur J Immunol. 2004;34(10):2885–94.

7. Chen W, Zhao B, Jiang R, Zhang R, Wang Y, Wu H, et al. Cytokine expression profile in aqueous humor and sera of patients with acute anterior uveitis. Curr Mol Med. 2015;15(6):543–9.

8. Hooks JJ, Nagineni CN, Hooper LC, Hayashi K, Detrick B. IFN-beta provides immuno-protection in the retina by inhibiting ICAM-1 and CXCL9 in retinal pigment epithelial cells. J Immunol. 2008;180(6):3789–96.

9. Radeke MJ, Peterson KE, Johnson LV, Anderson DH. Disease susceptibility of the human macula: differential gene transcription in the retinal pigmented epithelium/choroid. Exp Eye Res. 2007;85(3):366–80.

10. Turner MD, Nedjai B, Hurst T, Pennington DJ. Cytokines and chemokines: at the crossroads of cell signalling and inflammatory disease. Biochim Biophys Acta. 2014;1843(11):2563–82.

11. Diederen RM, La Heij EC, Deutz NE, Kijlstra A, Kessels AG, van Eijk HM, et al. Increased glutamate levels in the vitreous of patients with retinal detachment. Exp Eye Res. 2006;83(1):45–50.

12. Thoreson WB, Witkovsky P. Glutamate receptors and circuits in the vertebrate retina. Prog Retin Eye Res. 1999;18(6):765–810.

13. Mehta A, Prabhakar M, Kumar P, Deshmukh R, Sharma PL. Excitotoxicity: bridge to various triggers in neurodegenerative disorders. Eur J Pharmacol. 2013;698(1–3):6–18.

14. Bertram KM, Bula DV, Pulido JS, Shippy SA, Gautam S, Lu MJ, et al. Amino-acid levels in subretinal and vitreous fluid of patients with retinal detachment. Eye (Lond). 2008;22(4):582–9.

15. Martucci A, Cesareo M, Pinazo-Durán MD, Di Pierro M, Di Marino M, Nucci C, et al. Is there a relationship between dopamine and rhegmatogenous retinal detachment? Neural Regen Res. 2020;15(2):311–4.

16. Miyazaki I, Asanuma M. Dopaminergic neuron-specific oxidative stress caused by dopamine itself. Acta Med Okayama. 2008;62(3):141–50.

17. Akeo K, Ebenstein DB, Dorey CK. Dopa and oxygen inhibit proliferation of retinal pigment epithelial cells, fibroblasts and endothelial cells in vitro. Exp Eye Res. 1989;49(3):335–46.

18. Gallemore RP, Steinberg RH. Effects of dopamine on the chick retinal pigment epithelium. Membrane potentials and light-evoked responses. Invest Ophthalmol Vis Sci. 1990;31(1):67–80.

19. Kolb H, Linberg KA, Fisher SK. Neurons of the human retina: a Golgi study. J Comp Neurol. 1992;318(2):147–87.

20. Rasier R, Gormus U, Artunay O, Yuzbasioglu E, Oncel M, Bahcecioglu H. Vitreous levels of VEGF, IL-8, and TNF-alpha in retinal detachment. Curr Eye Res. 2010;35(6):505–9.

21. Senger DR, Galli SJ, Dvorak AM, Perruzzi CA, Harvey VS, Dvorak HF. Tumor cells secrete a vascular permeability factor that promotes accumulation of ascites fluid. Science. 1983;219(4587):983–5.

22. Leung DW, Cachianes G, Kuang WJ, Goeddel DV, Ferrara N. Vascular endothelial growth factor is a secreted angiogenic mitogen. Science. 1989;246(4935):1306–9.

23. Diederen RM. Biochemical and clinical factors in rhegmatogenous retinal detachment: Citeseer; 2007.

24. Yuuki T, Kanda T, Kimura Y, Kotajima N, Tamura J, Kobayashi I, et al. Inflammatory cytokines in vitreous fluid and serum of patients with diabetic vitreoretinopathy. J Diabetes Complicat. 2001;15(5):257–9.

25. Hernández C, Segura RM, Fonollosa A, Carrasco E, Francisco G, Simó R. Interleukin-8, monocyte chemoattractant protein-1 and IL-10 in the vitreous fluid of patients with proliferative diabetic retinopathy. Diabet Med. 2005;22(6):719–22.

26. Kramer M, Goldenberg-Cohen N, Axer-Siegel R, Weinberger D, Cohen Y, Monselise Y. Inflammatory reaction in acute retinal artery occlusion: cytokine levels in aqueous humor and serum. Ocul Immunol Inflamm. 2005;13(4):305–10.

27. Chen SN, Hwang JF, Wu WC. Peripheral retinal vascular patterns in patients with Rhegmatogenous retinal detachment in Taiwan. PLoS One. 2016;11(2):e0149176.

28. Kaneko Y, Moriyama M, Hirahara S, Ogura Y, Ohno-Matsui K. Areas of nonperfusion in peripheral retina of eyes with pathologic myopia detected by ultrawidefield fluorescein angiography. Invest Ophthalmol Vis Sci. 2014;55(3):1432–9.

29. Spaide RF. Peripheral areas of nonperfusion in treated central retinal vein occlusion as imaged by wide-field fluorescein angiography. Retina. 2011;31(5):829–37.

30. Kashani AH, Brown KT, Chang E, Drenser KA, Capone A, Trese MT. Diversity of retinal vascular anomalies in patients with familial exudative vitreoretinopathy. Ophthalmology. 2014;121(11):2220–7.

31. Spitznas M, Bornfeld N. The architecture of the most peripheral retinal vessels. Albrecht Von Graefes Arch Klin Exp Ophthalmol. 1977;203(3–4):217–29.

32. Provis JM. Development of the primate retinal vasculature. Prog Retin Eye Res. 2001;20(6):799–821.

33. Smith EL. Prentice award lecture 2010: a case for peripheral optical treatment strategies for myopia. Optom Vis Sci. 2011;88(9):1029–44.

34. Chen TC, Tsai TH, Shih YF, Yeh PT, Yang CH, Hu FC, et al. Long-term evaluation of refractive status and optical components in eyes of children born prematurely. Invest Ophthalmol Vis Sci. 2010;51(12):6140–8.

35. Bonnet M. Peripheral neovascularization complicating rhegmatogenous retinal detachments of long duration. Graefes Arch Clin Exp Ophthalmol. 1987;225(1):59–62.

36. Arroyo JG, Yang L, Bula D, Chen DF. Photoreceptor apoptosis in human retinal detachment. Am J Ophthalmol. 2005;139(4):605–10.

37. Eshita T, Shinoda K, Kimura I, Kitamura S, Ishida S, Inoue M, et al. Retinal blood flow in the macular area before and after scleral buckling procedures for rhegmatogenous retinal detachment without macular involvement. Jpn J Ophthalmol. 2004;48(4):358–63.

38. Yoshikawa Y, Shoji T, Kanno J, Ibuki H, Ozaki K, Ishii H, et al. Evaluation of microvascular changes in the macular area of eyes with rhegmatogenous retinal detachment without macular involvement using swept-source optical coherence tomography angiography. Clin Ophthalmol. 2018;12:2059–67.
39. McKay KM, Vingopoulos F, Wang JC, Papakostas TD, Silverman RF, Marmalidou A, et al. Retinal microvasculature changes after repair of macula-off retinal detachment assessed with optical coherence tomography angiography. Clin Ophthalmol. 2020;14:1759–67.
40. Wang H, Xu X, Sun X, Ma Y, Sun T. Macular perfusion changes assessed with optical coherence tomography angiography after vitrectomy for rhegmatogenous retinal detachment. Graefes Arch Clin Exp Ophthalmol. 2019;257(4):733–40.
41. Lee P, Wang CC, Adamis AP. Ocular neovascularization: an epidemiologic review. Surv Ophthalmol. 1998;43(3):245–69.
42. Labriola LT, Brant AM, Eller AW. Chronic retinal detachment with secondary retinal macrocyst and peripheral neovascularization. Semin Ophthalmol. 2009;24(1):2–4.
43. Felder KS, Brockhurst RJ. Retinal neovascularization complicating rhegmatogenous retinal detachment of long duration. Am J Ophthalmol. 1982;93(6):773–6.
44. Georgalas I, Paraskevopoulos T, Symmeonidis C, Petrou P, Koutsandrea C. Peripheral sea-fan retinal neovascularization as a manifestation of chronic rhegmatogenous retinal detachment and surgical management. BMC Ophthalmol. 2014;14:112.
45. Stefansson E, Landers MB, Wolbarsht ML, Klintworth GK. Neovascularization of the iris: an experimental model in cats. Invest Ophthalmol Vis Sci. 1984;25(3):361–4.
46. Ivanisević M. The natural history of untreated rhegmatogenous retinal detachment. Ophthalmologica. 1997;211(2):90–2.
47. Tanaka S, Ideta H, Yonemoto J, Sasaki K, Hirose A, Oka C. Neovascularization of the iris in rhegmatogenous retinal detachment. Am J Ophthalmol. 1991;112(6):632–4.
48. Barile GR, Chang S, Horowitz JD, Reppucci VS, Schiff WM, Wong DT. Neovascular complications associated with rubeosis iridis and peripheral retinal detachment after retinal detachment surgery. Am J Ophthalmol. 1998;126(3):379–89.
49. Jeong YC, Hwang YH. Etiology and features of eyes with Rubeosis Iridis among Korean patients: a population-based single center study. PLoS One. 2016;11(8):e0160662.
50. Brown GC, Magargal LE, Schachat A, Shah H. Neovascular glaucoma. Etiologic considerations. Ophthalmology. 1984;91(4):315–20.
51. Al-Shamsi HN, Dueker DK, Nowilaty SR, Al-Shahwan SA. Neovascular glaucoma at king khaled eye specialist hospital - etiologic considerations. Middle East Afr J Ophthalmol. 2009;16(1):15–9.
52. Hayreh SS, Rojas P, Podhajsky P, Montague P, Woolson RF. Ocular neovascularization with retinal vascular occlusion-III. Incidence of ocular neovascularization with retinal vein occlusion. Ophthalmology. 1983;90(5):488–506.
53. Yorston D, Jalali S. Retinal detachment in developing countries. Eye (Lond). 2002;16(4):353–8.
54. Brod RD, Flynn HW. Asymptomatic rhegmatogenous retinal detachment. Curr Opin Ophthalmol. 1996;7(3):1–6.
55. Li YM, Fang W, Jin XH, Li JK, Zhai J, Feng LG. Risk factors related to chronic rhegmatogenous retinal detachment. Int J Ophthalmol. 2012;5(1):92–6.
56. Enghelberg M, Chalam KV. Ultra wide field angiography documented peripheral retinal eovascularization as cause of vitreous hemorrhage after scleral buckle surgery. J Surg Case Rep. 2020;2020(6):rjaa142.
57. Ogasawara H, Feke GT, Yoshida A, Milbocker MT, Weiter JJ, McMeel JW. Retinal blood flow alterations associated with scleral buckling and encircling procedures. Br J Ophthalmol. 1992;76(5):275–9.
58. Regillo CD, Sergott RC, Brown GC. Successful scleral buckling procedures decrease central retinal artery blood flow velocity. Ophthalmology. 1993;100(7):1044–9.
59. Bourke RD, Cooling RJ. Vascular consequences of retinectomy. Arch Ophthalmol. 1996;114(2):155–60.
60. Itakura H, Kishi S, Kotajima N, Murakami M. Persistent secretion of vascular endothelial growth factor into the vitreous cavity in proliferative diabetic retinopathy after vitrectomy. Ophthalmology. 2004;111(10):1880–4.
61. Batman C, Ozdamar Y. The effect of bevacizumab for anterior segment neovascularization after silicone oil removal in eyes with previous vitreoretinal surgery. Eye (Lond). 2010;24(7):1243–6.
62. Nicolai M, Lassandro N, Franceschi A, Rosati A, De Turris S, Pelliccioni P, et al. Intraocular pressure rise linked to silicone oil in retinal surgery: a review. Vision (Basel). 2020;4(3).
63. Shukla D, Maheshwari R, Kim R. Barrage laser photocoagulation for macula-sparing asymptomatic clinical rhegmatogenous retinal detachments. Eye (Lond). 2007;21(6):742–5.
64. Greenberg PB, Baumal CR. Laser therapy for rhegmatogenous retinal detachment. Curr Opin Ophthalmol. 2001;12(3):171–4.
65. Singh A, Stewart JM. Intraocular bevacizumab for iris neovascularization in a silicone oil-filled eye. Retin Cases Brief Rep. 2008;2(3):253–5.
66. Rodrigues GB, Abe RY, Zangalli C, Sodre SL, Donini FA, Costa DC, et al. Neovascular glaucoma: a review. Int J Retina Vitreous. 2016;2:26.
67. Canaan SA. Photocoagulation in retinal diseases. J Natl Med Assoc. 1962;54:71–2.
68. Ryan's retina. In: Schachat AP, Wilkinson CP, Hinton DR, Sadda SR, Wiedemann P, editors. 6th ed. p. 1895.

Neovascular Glaucoma in Ocular Tumors and Radiation

Matthew P. Nicholas, Annapurna Singh, and Arun D. Singh

1 Introduction

Neovascular glaucoma (NVG) is an extraordinarily aggressive form of secondary glaucoma characterized by elevated intraocular pressure (IOP) and anterior segment neovascularization. In the early stages of anterior segment neovascularization, there is neovascularization of the iris (NVI, also called rubeosis iridis). As the disease progresses, the neovascularization extends into the iridocorneal angle (NVA) and obstructs aqueous outflow, resulting in elevated IOP. The NVA causes a fibrovascular membrane to occlude the trabecular meshwork (TM), and eventually, peripheral anterior synechiae (PAS) can develop and cause synechial angle closure and profoundly elevated IOP [1, 2]. Fragile, immature neovessels are also prone to hemorrhaging, causing hyphema that can also obstruct aqueous outflow at the TM.

NVG is principally associated with severe retinal ischemia, typically due to vascular disease such as proliferative diabetic retinopathy (PDR), central retinal vein occlusion (CRVO), ocular ischemic syndrome (OIS), and more rarely, due to ocular inflammatory disease or chronic retinal detachment (RD) (which causes ischemia due to separation of the retina from the choriocapillaris) [1, 2]. The anterior segment neovascularization that causes NVG is driven by posterior-to-anterior diffusion of vascular endothelial growth factor (VEGF) produced by the ischemic retina. However, NVG may arise due to other etiologies, including intraocular tumors. Malignant tumors require angiogenesis in order to grow, and the same angiogenesis employed by the tumor may promote anterior segment neovascularization. Tumors most frequently associated with NVG include retinoblastoma (RB), malignant uveal melanoma, ciliary body (CB) medulloepithelioma, and uveal metastases. In some cases, NVG may be the presenting finding, and neoplasia should be suspected in any case of NVG for which a more likely etiology cannot be established. Finally, NVG is a potential complication of radiation retinopathy, which may arise following radiotherapy to the eye, head, or neck. Radiation-associated NVG closely resembles NVG seen in the setting of PDR.

2 Neovascular Glaucoma Due to Intraocular Tumors

2.1 General Clinical Features and Diagnosis

NVG may present with eye pain due to elevated IOP, and vision may be decreased due to microcystic corneal edema, dispersed hyphema, vitreous hemorrhage, diminished retinal perfusion,

M. P. Nicholas · A. Singh · A. D. Singh (✉)
Cole Eye Institute, Cleveland Clinic,
Cleveland, OH, USA
e-mail: singha@ccf.org

© The Author(s), under exclusive license to Springer Nature Switzerland AG 2022
M. Qiu (ed.), *Neovascular Glaucoma*, Essentials in Ophthalmology,
https://doi.org/10.1007/978-3-031-11720-6_11

and, in the later stages, glaucomatous optic neuropathy. NVI, which is usually most prominent along the pupillary border, is almost always visible on slit-lamp examination, but may be confirmed by iris fluorescein angiography (FA). However, NVI is not synonymous with NVG, and examination of the angle via gonioscopy is critical to assess for the presence of NVA and for separate or concomitant causes of IOP elevation, such as angle closure due to mass effect, direct tumor invasion of angle structures, and pigment deposition (suggesting melanomalytic glaucoma). CB masses may sometimes be directly visualized on gonioscopy after pupillary dilation. Signs of anterior chamber inflammation may also be present.

If a tumor is suspected, additional testing such as scleral transillumination, B-scan ultrasound, and/or ultrasound biomicroscopy (UBM) may be helpful in identifying a mass not readily visible on examination. A dilated fundus examination should always be performed to evaluate for the presence of tumors, RD, retinal ischemia, and/or posterior segment neovascularization. FA and optical coherence tomography (OCT) angiography can be useful to assess retinal perfusion and identify retinal and iris neovascularization [3]. Finally, as with all glaucomas, assessment of the optic nerve head and optic nerve function should be performed. Unfortunately, intraocular malignancies presenting with NVG often necessitate enucleation, so detailed evaluation with OCT and automated visual fields may be unnecessary.

2.2   Retinoblastoma

RB is a relatively rare tumor (in the United States, approximately 200–300 new cases per year), but is the most common ocular malignancy in children [4]. Diagnosis occurs at an average age of 2 years old and is rare in children older than 6 years of age [4]. Although the mortality is low in developed countries (3–5%), mortality in lower-income regions (where prevalence is unfortunately higher due to higher birth rates) can be as high as 70% [5]. RB should be suspected in any child with leukocoria, elevated IOP, or unexplained poor vision and must be ruled out in any pediatric patient with NVI or NVG. On fundus examination, RB appears as a dome-shaped, elevated, whitish retinal mass and is characterized by internal calcifications. These can be readily identified with B-scan ultrasound.

NVI is common in advanced RB. In one histopathologic series of 149 enucleated eyes with RB, approximately 30% were found to have NVI; among the subset of 34 eyes (23%) with known elevated IOP, 77% had NVI on histopathology [6]. Almost all of the eyes with NVI exhibited posterior pole and vitreous involvement of the tumor. A separate clinical analysis of 303 eyes by Shields et al. yielded similar results: 17% of the enucleated eyes with RB had a history of elevated IOP, and among the subset of eyes with known elevated IOP, 74% of those eyes had NVI on histopathology [7]. Fast-growing RB tumors have a tendency to outgrow their blood supplies, leading to tumor necrosis. VEGF expression is increased in necrotic regions of the tumor, and the extent of the necrosis is predictive of NVI formation [8]. Optic nerve invasion and choroidal invasion, both of which are also associated with metastatic risk [5], are also correlated with NVI [8].

Any child suspected of having retinoblastoma should be referred promptly to an experienced ocular oncologist. Ocular hypotensive therapy (except brimonidine, which is contraindicated in young children) may be appropriate for comfort in some cases, but the NVG is of secondary importance compared to containment of the tumor. IOP-lowering surgeries are contraindicated given the potential for tumor dissemination [9]. NVG in the setting of RB confers a "group E" categorization according to the International Classification of Retinoblastoma [10, 11]. These eyes are invariably enucleated and may require adjuvant chemotherapy if high-risk features (e.g., retrolaminar optic nerve involvement or massive choroidal invasion) are found on histopathologic examination [12] (Fig. 1) [13].

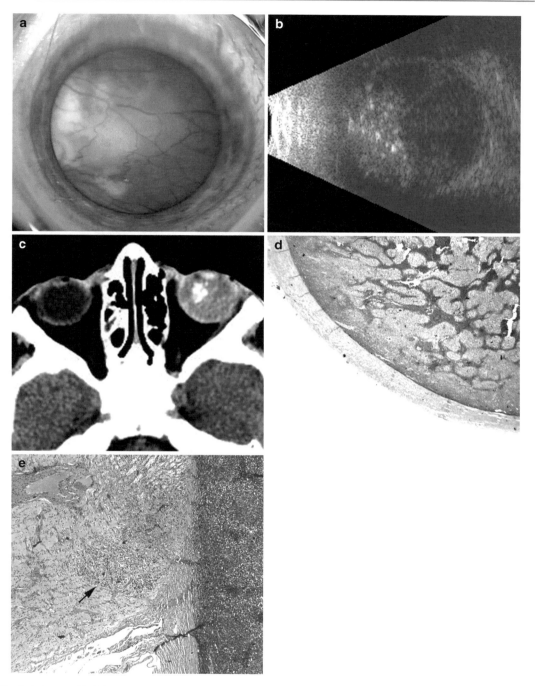

Fig. 1 A 3 year old child presented with pain and redness of the left of 1 week duration. About a month prior to the presentation, the parents had noticed a whitish discoloration of the pupil. On examination, the left eye showed diffuse conjunctival congestion and leukocoria. The cornea was hazy and there was iris neovascularizarion (**a**) with secondary glaucoma (IOP 34 mmHg). Ultrasonographic examination revealed a calcific intraocular mass, suggestive of a retinoblastoma (**b**). This was confirmed by a computerized tomogram (**c**). Following detailed counselling about various therapeutic options, enucleation of the left eye was performed. Histopathologic examination confirmed the presence of a necrotic retinoblastoma, filling almost the whole globe, and iris neovascularization. There was massive choroidal involvement, (**d**) and the tumor extended into the retrolaminar part of the optic nerve, though the cut end of the nerve was uninvolved (**e**). Four weeks later, adjuvant chemotherapy was initiated

2.3   Medulloepithelioma

Intraocular medulloepithelioma, which may be benign or malignant, is a rare, non-hereditary embryonal tumor arising from the primitive medullary epithelium. It almost always develops in the nonpigmented epithelium of the pars plicata of the CB, but rarely may occur in the iris, retina, or optic nerve head. Here, we will discuss CB medulloepithelioma. Like retinoblastoma, medulloepithelioma occurs almost exclusively in young children (median 2–5 years old) [14] and should be considered in all cases of NVI/NVG in this age group. It is rarely (5%) associated with pleuropulmonary blastoma [14].

On examination, the tumor is a light gray or pink, vascularized mass extending from the CB, sometimes with iris involvement and usually with characteristic intratumoral cysts. UBM and anterior segment OCT demonstrating these cysts can be helpful in diagnosis. Occasionally, the cysts can dislodge and become free-floating in the anterior chamber [14–16]. Medulloepithelioma is initially misdiagnosed in up to 88% of cases (and therefore frequently mismanaged [14, 16, 17]), likely due to the difficulty in visualizing the tumor until the CB mass is relatively large [14]. Ectropion uveae and corectopia may be present. Because of the proximity of the CB to the crystalline lens, cataract is common [14, 16], and ectopia lentis is variably present as well (in rare cases, as the only presenting sign [18]). NVI can be seen in approximately 20–50% of cases of medulloepithelioma, with most of these eyes exhibiting NVG as well [14, 16]. Medulloepithelioma also has a predilection for the formation of vascularized membranes along the hyaloid face (retrolental neoplastic cyclitic membranes, seen in about half of cases [14]) and may be associated with vitreous hemorrhage [19] (Fig. 2).

Careful evaluation for medulloepithelioma should be undertaken in any child with NVI/ NVG or retrolental neoplastic cyclitic membranes, and any incisional procedure (e.g., IOP-lowering or cataract surgery) should be deferred until the diagnosis is certain and any underlying tumor is treated. As with retinoblastoma, NVG is

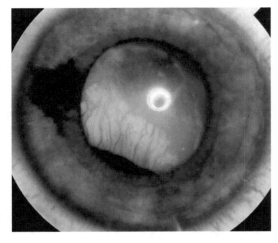

Fig. 2 A 38-month-old girl presented with leukocoria of 2 months duration. On examination, lens coloboma and a vascularized retrolental sheet (cyclitic membrane) were noted. A pigmented mass was seen in the ciliary body region from 6 to 8 o'clock position. Tumor recurred after excision necessitating enucleation. Histopathologically, the lesion was confirmed to be malignant teratoid medulloepithelioma. (Reprinted from Singh A, Singh AD, Shields CL, Shields JA. Iris neovascularization in children as a manifestation of underlying medulloepithelioma. J Pediatr Ophthalmol Strabismus. 2001;38(4):224–8. With permission from Slack Incorporated.)

more often seen in advanced cases of medulloepithelioma. Enucleation is usually required, though plaque brachytherapy may allow preservation of the globe in select cases [14, 19].

2.4   Uveal Malignant Melanoma

Uveal malignant melanoma comprises melanomas of the choroid (90%), CB (6%), and iris (4%) [20]. It is the most common intraocular malignancy in adults, with an incidence of 5.2 per million, a peak age of presentation around 60 years, and a strong predilection for Caucasians (98%) [21]. We will focus on choroidal malignant melanoma (CMM), which typically presents as a dark, elevated mass. Prompt diagnosis is critical, as CMM is associated not only with vision-threatening complications, but also life-threatening metastatic potential (usually by hematogenous spread to the liver).

IOP elevation is uncommon in uveal malignant melanomas and was present in only 3% of eyes with uveal malignant melanoma in a large series of 2111 eyes. Among the subset of eyes with elevated IOP, only approximately 35% were due principally to NVG (with remainder due in roughly equal parts to angle closure, pigment dispersion, and tumor invasion of the angle) [7]. Among the cases of NVG secondary to uveal melanoma, 95% were in eyes with CMM [7]. NVG is very rare in CB or iris melanomas, which tend to cause elevated IOP by direct angle invasion or pigment deposition in the TM [7], though cases of NVG secondary to iris melanoma have been reported [22].

As with other tumors, NVI/NVG may be the presenting signs of uveal melanoma [23], sometimes leading to initial mismanagement that can increase the risk of metastasis and secondary complications. NVG secondary to CMM is seen predominantly in cases of large, advanced tumors, due to either lack of ophthalmic care or misdiagnosis. Enucleation is often required.

In addition to arising as a secondary complication of untreated CMM, NVG may also be seen following globe-sparing radiotherapy for CMM, which has mostly replaced enucleation for medium-sized tumors (10–15 mm in diameter, 3–5 mm in height), and even some larger ones [21, 24, 25]. Interestingly, post-radiation NVG in these cases seems to be due to effects of the residual CMM (so-called "toxic tumor syndrome") rather than solely from radiation retinopathy (discussed below), as tumor resection (which is only rarely performed due to the potential complications) in some cases appears to resolve anterior segment neovascularization and IOP elevation (and associated exudative RD) [26] and reduce the risk of future NVG [27].

Treatment for NVG following radiotherapy for CMM typically includes intravitreal anti-VEGF agents [28, 29], and conventional treatment with ocular antihypertensives and glaucoma filtering surgery. Any incisional IOP-lowering surgery should be considered only after careful assessment (serial monitoring with examination, photos, and A-scan ultrasound measurement of tumor thickness) and confirmation of regression of the treated tumor, since tumor seeding has been observed after filtering procedures in eyes with undiagnosed uveal melanoma [9, 30, 31]. Theoretically, incisional IOP-lowering surgery should be safe following effective tumor treatment and its successful use has been reported [32, 33]. However, there have been reports of tumor recurrence with involvement of filtering surgery sites, even after apparently effective tumor treatment [34, 35]. For example, Sweeny et al. [34] reported tumor extension into a Baerveldt glaucoma implant capsule more than 8 years after apparently effective radioiodine plaque brachytherapy (followed by failed trabeculectomy and then aqueous shunt several months after radiotherapy). The eye was enucleated in this case, but the patient subsequently developed metastases to the orbit (suspected to be due to the aqueous shunt surgery, given the apparently local spread and the relatively quick failure of the trabeculectomy), brain, and liver.

Cases of metastasis following incisional surgery despite prior radiotherapy suggest the need for caution in performing filtering surgery in eyes with a history of uveal melanoma, especially that involving the iris or CB. However, we are not aware of any known cases of metastasis via a filtering surgery site following treatment of CMM, which, as mentioned earlier, accounts for nearly all melanoma-associated NVG. Nevertheless, cyclophotocoagulation (CPC) may be a more prudent choice than incisional surgery following treatment of uveal melanoma, especially in eyes with limited visual potential. CPC has been used successfully for the treatment of NVG (discussed in detail in a separate chapter) and with some success (in terms of vision and globe preservation, as well as pain reduction) in glaucoma secondary to uveal melanoma [36–38] and can be titrated via consecutive treatments. There are little published data on the use of CPC specifically for NVG secondary to uveal melanoma [39].

2.5   Uveal Metastasis

The most common primary tumors to metastasize to the uveal tract are breast (47%) and lung (21%)

carcinomas [40]. The choroid is the most frequent site of metastasis (88%), likely due to its high vascularity, though most patients with uveal metastasis likely remain asymptomatic and do not seek ophthalmic care [41]. IOP elevation is rare in eyes with uveal metastasis (5%) and is typically due to angle closure secondary to mass effect or direct tumor invasion of the TM, rather than due to NVG [7, 42]. When it does occur, NVG typically results from iris metastasis, which is frequently associated with NVI [42] and may occur concomitantly with the other aforementioned mechanisms (Fig. 3).

Systemic chemotherapy for the primary malignancy can be helpful in decreasing the ocular tumor burden. Regression of anterior segment neovascularization and reduction in tumor size have been reported with intracameral administration of anti-VEGF therapy (bevacizumab) [43, 44]. Given the relatively poor long-term survival in patients with metastatic disease, conservative measures are usually preferable.

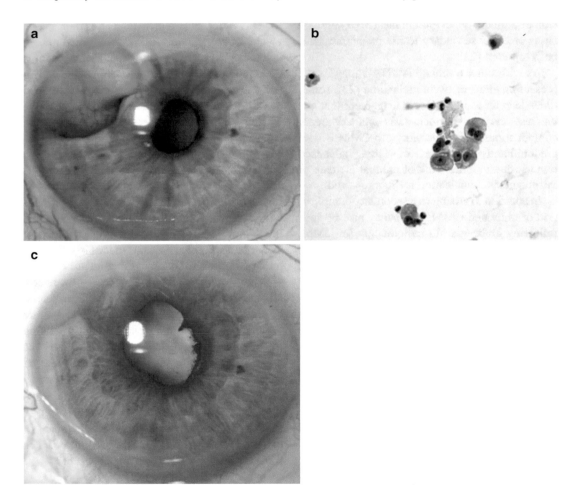

Fig. 3 A 68 year old man initially presented with left hip pain which led to a diagnosis of left renal mass with widespread bone metastasis. Left radical nephrectomy showed evidence of clear cell type renal cell carcinoma (grade 4). He continued to progress slowly over the next 4 years despite being treated with several investigational drugs developing ocular pain. On examination visual acuity was 20/200 with normal intraocular pressure. A kidney shaped vascular mass was visible in the iridociliary region (**a**). Anterior segment fluorescein angiography confirmed vascularity of the lesion and fine NVI. Four weeks following treatment with Iodine-125 plaque radiotherapy and single intracameral bevacizumab injection, marked regression of the lesion is evident (**b**). FNAB of metastatic renal cell carcinoma illustrates the characteristic features of clear cell renal cell carcinoma (**c**). Note the abundant finely vacuolated cytoplasm surrounding nuclei with prominent nucleoli. (Reprinted from Biscotti CV, Singh AD. Uveal metastases. Monogr Clin Cytol. 2012;21:17–30. With permission from Karger Publishers. Copyright © 2011, Karger Publishers.)

2.6 Benign Intraocular Tumors

NVG is rarely seen in association with benign intraocular tumors. When present, NVG is usually secondary to chronic RD, such as the exudative RD sometimes seen with retinal capillary hemangioblastomas in von Hippel-Lindau disease (familial cerebello-retinal angiomatosis) [45]. Management consists of treating the underlying neoplasm (e.g., via radiation, cryotherapy, laser photocoagulation, or photodynamic therapy) in order to resolve the RD and thereby reduce the ischemic drive for VEGF production. In the absence of RD, NVG has also been reported in association with benign retinal vasoproliferative tumor, and excisional biopsy via pars plana vitrectomy in this case led to regression of NVI and normalization of IOP [46] (Fig. 4). Following treatment of benign tumors, persistently elevated IOP can be managed with the usual medical and/or surgical strategies. Rarely, NVG associated with benign tumors may lead to intractable IOP elevation, and eventually, a blind, painful eye requiring evisceration or enucleation.

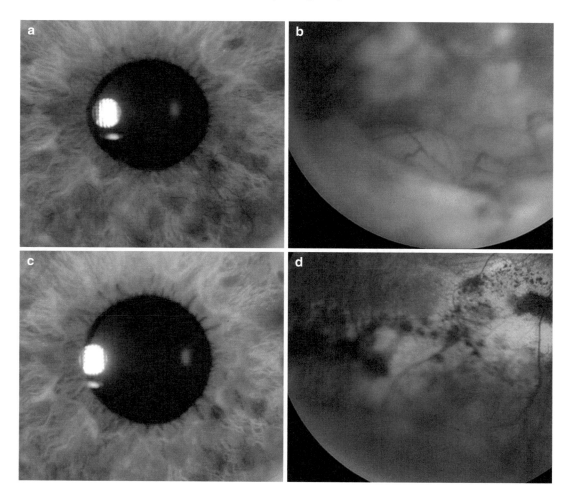

Fig. 4 Slit lamp photograph of the right eye at presentation demonstrating multiple Lisch nodules and florid neovascularization of the iris (**a**). On gonioscopic examination there was 360 degree neovascularization of the angle. In the inferior fundus there was a pink, elevated vascular mass with surrounding lipid exudate, consistent with vasoproliferative tumor (**b**). After treatment with cryotherapy and two intravitreal injections of bevacizumab, the neovascularization of the iris resolved almost completely (**c**). The vasoproliferative tumor appeared less vascular with chorioretinal atrophy and hyperpigmentation of the posterior margin (**d**). Note resolution of lipid exudates. (Reprinted from Hood CT, Janku L, Lowder CY, Singh AD. Retinal vasoproliferative tumor in association with neurofibromatosis type 1. J Pediatr Ophthalmol Strabismus. https://doi.org/10.3928/01913913-20090616-05. Epub 2009 Jun 25. PMID: 19645388. With permission from Slack Incorporated)

3 Neovascular Glaucoma Due to Radiation Retinopathy

Radiation retinopathy (RR) is a predictable, dose-related complication of radiation treatment of ocular malignancies (most commonly CMM), but may result from a sufficient dose of radiation to the head or neck for any reason. RR may manifest within months or many years after radiation exposure. Larger tumors confer a higher RR risk due to the higher radiation doses required to treat them [47, 48].

Clinically, RR closely resembles diabetic retinopathy, with microaneurysms, intraretinal hemorrhages, hard exudates, cotton wool spots, and macular edema. Like diabetic retinopathy, RR is thought to arise due to ischemia resulting from microvascular damage to endothelial cells [49] and may progress to a proliferative phase (PRR) that can be complicated by NVG (Fig. 5). Pre-existing diabetes mellitus, young age, and tumor/treatment proximity to the optic nerve are all risk factors for developing PRR [50].

Treatment of PRR and associated NVG is analogous to NVG treatment in PDR, namely intravitreal anti-VEGF injections and panretinal photocoagulation (discussed in more detail in other chapters in this book focusing on PDR, anti-VEGF, and PRP), though PRR may be more relentless than PDR. IOP-lowering surgery may be necessary to adequately control IOP in the setting of NVG secondary to PRR. In one small series of 12 patients with radiation-related NVG who received periodic intravitreal bevacizumab, 6 eventually required enucleation (4 due to pain), but 6 reported good pain control and 4 were reported to have normalized IOP despite decline in visual acuity [51].

4 Conclusion

NVG is an uncommon, but well-established sequela of intraocular malignancies. It may be the presenting sign of a not-yet diagnosed intraocular tumor. As such, appropriate clinical suspicion and thorough evaluation (especially prior to any surgical intervention) are warranted in all cases. Because NVG is frequently a sign of chronicity and advanced disease, the eye is often unsalvageable at the time of diagnosis. Management, therefore, often centers on timely enucleation to prevent metastasis, and the NVG itself is of secondary importance. In contrast, for NVG associated with benign tumors (usually secondary to chronic exudative RD) or radiation

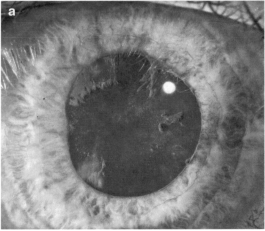
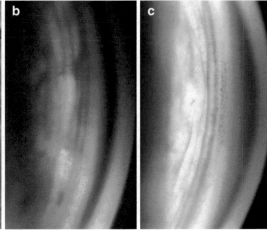

Fig. 5 Radiation retinopathy. Neovascular glaucoma following radiation therapy (**a**). Goniophotograph of another case showing neovascularization and bleeding in the anterior chamber angle (**b**). Eight weeks after treatment with pan retinal photocoagulation and intravireal injection of bevacizumab (1.25 mg/0.05 ml. Note that the angle neovascularization and hyphema has resolved completely (**c**). (Kamrava M, Lamb J, Soberón V, McCannel TA. Ocular complications of radiotherapy. In Clinical Ophthalmic Oncology. Volume 1. Basic Principles. Eds Singh AD, Damato, BE. Springer- Nature, Heidleberg 2019. Chapter 12. With permission from Springer-Nature)

retinopathy, enucleation or evisceration are only rarely necessary. When indicated, enucleation or evisceration in the setting of a benign intraocular tumor is usually a result of end-stage NVG rather than the underlying inciting pathology. Consequently, the goal in these cases is maximal preservation of vision by (1) suppressing the underlying neovascular drive with anti-VEGF or panretinal photocoagulation and (2) medical and/ or surgical IOP control. Early recognition remains key in order to minimize irreversible glaucomatous optic neuropathy.

References

1. Hayreh SS. Neovacular glaucoma. Prog Retin Eye Res. 2007;26(5):470–85.
2. Rodrigues GB, Abe RY, Zangalli C, Sodre SL, Donini FA, Costa DC, et al. Neovascular glaucoma: a review. Int J Retina Vitreous [Internet]. 2016 Nov 14 [cited 2020 Oct 19];2. Available from: https://www.ncbi.nlm.nih.gov/pmc/articles/PMC5116372/
3. Roberts PK, Goldstein DA, Fawzi AA. Anterior segment optical coherence tomography angiography for identification of iris vasculature and staging of iris neovascularization: a pilot study. Curr Eye Res. 2017;42(8):1136–42.
4. Key Statistics for Retinoblastoma [Internet]. The American Cancer Society. 2021 [cited 2021 Jun 13]. Available from: https://www.cancer.org/cancer/retinoblastoma/about/key-statistics.html
5. Dimaras H, Kimani K, Dimba EA, Gronsdahl P, White A, Chan HS, et al. Retinoblastoma. Lancet. 2012;379(9824):1436–46.
6. Yoshizumi MO, Thomas JV, Smith TR. Glaucoma-inducing mechanisms in eyes with retinoblastoma. Arch Ophthalmol. 1978;96(1):105–10.
7. Shields CL, Shields JA, Shields MB, Augsburger JJ. Prevalence and mechanisms of secondary intraocular pressure elevation in eyes with intraocular tumors. Ophthalmology. 1987;94(7):839–46.
8. Pe'er J, Neufeld M, Baras M, Gnessin H, Itin A, Keshet E. Rubeosis iridis in retinoblastoma. Histologic findings and the possible role of vascular endothelial growth factor in its induction. Ophthalmology. 1997;104(8):1251–8.
9. Grossniklaus HE, Brown RH, Stulting RD, Blasberg RD. Iris melanoma seeding through a trabeculectomy site. Arch Ophthalmol. 1990;108(9):1287–90.
10. Shields CL, Mashayekhi A, Demirci H, Meadows AT, Shields JA. Practical approach to management of retinoblastoma. Arch Ophthalmol. 2004;122(5):729–35.
11. Linn MA. Intraocular retinoblastoma: the case for a new group classification. Ophthalmol Clin N Am. 2005;18(1):41–53, viii.
12. Kim JW. Retinoblastoma: evidence for postenucleation adjuvant chemotherapy. Int Ophthalmol Clin. 2015;55(1):77–96.
13. Chévez-Barrios P, Eagle RC, Krailo M, Piao J, Albert DM, Gao Y, et al. Study of unilateral retinoblastoma with and without histopathologic high-risk features and the role of adjuvant chemotherapy: a children's oncology group study. J Clin Oncol. 2019;37(31):2883–91.
14. Kaliki S, Shields CL, Eagle RC, Vemuganti GK, Almeida A, Manjandavida FP, et al. Ciliary body medulloepithelioma: analysis of 41 cases. Ophthalmology. 2013;120(12):2552–9.
15. Spicer WTH, Greeves RA. Multiple cysts in the anterior chamber derived from a congenital cystic growth of the ciliary epithelium. Proc R Soc Med. 1915;8(Sect Ophthalmol):9–26.
16. Broughton WL, Zimmerman LE. A clinicopathologic study of 56 cases of intraocular medulloepitheliomas. Am J Ophthalmol. 1978;85(3):407–18.
17. Shields JA, Eagle RC, Shields CL, Potter PD. Congenital neoplasms of the nonpigmented ciliary epithelium (medulloepithelioma). Ophthalmology. 1996;103(12):1998–2006.
18. Gupta NK, Simon JW, Walton DS, Augsburger JJ. Bilateral ectopia lentis as a presenting feature of medulloepithelioma. J Am Assoc Pediatric Ophthalmol Strabismus. 2001;5(4):255–7.
19. Attiku Y, Rishi P, Biswas J, Krishnakumar S. Plaque radiation for ciliary body medulloepithelioma presenting with neovascular glaucoma and vitreous hemorrhage in 13-year-old Asian girl. Am J Ophthalmol Case Rep [Internet]. 2020 Apr 23 [cited 2020 Oct 19];18. Available from: https://www.ncbi.nlm.nih.gov/pmc/articles/PMC7191537/
20. Kaliki S, Shields CL. Uveal melanoma: relatively rare but deadly cancer. Eye (Lond). 2017;31(2):241–57.
21. Singh AD, Turell ME, Topham AK. Uveal melanoma: trends in incidence, treatment, and survival. Ophthalmology. 2011;118(9):1881–5.
22. Bianciotto C, Shields CL, Kang B, Shields JA. Treatment of iris melanoma and secondary neovascular glaucoma using bevacizumab and plaque radiotherapy. Arch Ophthalmol. 2008;126(4):578–9.
23. Sahu S, Bhutia TW, Shrestha V, Singh SK, Puri LR. Large choroidal melanoma presenting as neovascular glaucoma. GMS Ophthalmol Cases [Internet]. 2019 May 31 [cited 2020 Oct 19];9. Available from: https://www.ncbi.nlm.nih.gov/pmc/articles/PMC6607447/
24. Bell DJ, Wilson MW. Choroidal melanoma: natural history and management options. Cancer Control. 2004;11(5):296–303.
25. Chattopadhyay C, Kim DW, Gombos DS, Oba J, Qin Y, Williams MD, et al. Uveal melanoma: from diagnosis to treatment and the science in between. Cancer. 2016;122(15):2299–312.
26. Konstantinidis L, Groenewald C, Coupland SE, Damato B. Trans-scleral local resection of toxic cho-

roidal melanoma after proton beam radiotherapy. Br J Ophthalmol. 2014;98(6):775–9.

27. Cassoux N, Cayette S, Plancher C, Lumbroso-Le Rouic L, Levy-Gabriel C, Asselain B, et al. Choroidal melanoma: does endoresection prevent neovascular glaucoma in patient treated with proton beam irradiation? Retina. 2013;33(7):1441–7.

28. Vásquez LM, Somani S, Altomare F, Simpson ER. Intracameral bevacizumab in the treatment of neovascular glaucoma and exudative retinal detachment after brachytherapy in choroidal melanoma. Can J Ophthalmol. 2009;44(1):106–7.

29. Dunavoelgyi R, Zehetmayer M, Simader C, Schmidt-Erfurth U. Rapid improvement of radiation-induced neovascular glaucoma and exudative retinal detachment after a single intravitreal ranibizumab injection. Clin Exp Ophthalmol. 2007;35(9):878–80.

30. Pasternak S, Erwenne CM, Nicolela MT. Subconjunctival spread of ciliary body melanoma after glaucoma filtering surgery: a clinicopathological case report. Can J Ophthalmol. 2005;40(1):69–71.

31. Singer PR, Krupin T, Smith ME, Becker B. Recurrent orbital and metastatic melanoma in a patient undergoing previous glaucoma surgery. Am J Ophthalmol. 1979;87(6):766–8.

32. Sharkawi E, Oleszczuk JD, Bergin C, Zografos L. Baerveldt shunts in the treatment of glaucoma secondary to anterior uveal melanoma and proton beam radiotherapy. Br J Ophthalmol. 2012;96(8):1104–7.

33. Fatehi N, McCannel TA, Giaconi J, Caprioli J, Law SK, Nouri-Mahdavi K. Outcomes of glaucoma drainage device surgery in eyes with treated uveal melanoma. OOP. 2019;5(1):20–7.

34. Sweeney AR, Keene CD, Klesert TR, Jian-Amadi A, Chen PP. Orbital extension of anterior uveal melanoma after Baerveldt tube shunt implantation. Can J Ophthalmol. 2014;49(6):e133–5.

35. Tay E, Cree IA, Hungerford J, Franks W. Recurrence of treated ciliary body melanoma following trabeculectomy. Clin Exp Ophthalmol. 2009;37(5):503–5.

36. Piirtola A, Puska P, Kivelä T. Red laser Cyclophotocoagulation in the treatment of secondary glaucoma in eyes with uveal melanoma. J Glaucoma. 2014;23(1):50–5.

37. Girkin CA, Goldberg I, Mansberger SL, Shields JA, Shields CL. Management of iris melanoma with secondary glaucoma. J Glaucoma. 2002;11(1):71–4.

38. Shukla AG, Vaidya S, Yaghy A, Razeghinejad R, Mantravadi AV, Myers JS, et al. Transscleral cyclophotocoagulation for glaucoma in the setting of uveal melanoma. Ophthalmol Glaucoma. 2020.

39. Shukla AG, Vaidya S, Yaghy A, Razeghinejad R, Mantravadi AV, Myers JS, Kaliki S, Shields CL. Transscleral Cyclophotocoagulation for Glaucoma in the Setting of Uveal Melanoma. Ophthalmol Glaucoma. 2020;S2589–4196(20)30256–8.

40. Shields CL, Shields JA, Gross NE, Schwartz GP, Lally SE. Survey of 520 eyes with uveal metastases. Ophthalmology. 1997;104(8):1265–76.

41. Cohen VML. Ocular metastases. Eye (Lond). 2013;27(2):137–41.

42. Ferry AP, Font RL. Carcinoma metastatic to the eye and orbit II. A clinicopathological study of 26 patients with carcinoma metastatic to the anterior segment of the eye. Arch Ophthalmol. 1975;93(7):472–82.

43. Hidaka T, Chuman H, Nao-i N. A case report of intravitreal bevacizumab for iris metastasis of small cell lung carcinoma with Neovascular glaucoma. Case Rep Ophthalmol. 2018;9(2):401–4.

44. Vale S, Montalvo L, Baez E, Oliver AL. Intravitreal bevacizumab as therapy for refractory neovascular glaucoma secondary to iris metastasis of breast carcinoma. Am J Ophthalmol Case Rep. 2018;9:45–7.

45. Ruppert MD, Gavin M, Mitchell KT, Peiris AN. Ocular manifestations of von Hippel-Lindau Disease. Cureus [Internet]. [cited 2021 Jun 14];11(8). Available from https://www.ncbi.nlm.nih.gov/pmc/articles/PMC6776162/

46. Nakamura Y, Takeda N, Mochizuki M. A case of vasoproliferative retinal tumor complicated by neovascular glaucoma. Retin Cases Brief Rep. 2013;7(4):338–42.

47. Summanen P, Immonen I, Kivelä T, Tommila P, Heikkonen J, Tarkkanen A. Radiation related complications after ruthenium plaque radiotherapy of uveal melanoma. Br J Ophthalmol. 1996;80(8):732–9.

48. Miguel D, de Frutos-Baraja JM, López-Lara F, Saornil MA, García-Álvarez C, Alonso P, et al. Radiobiological doses, tumor, and treatment features influence on outcomes after episcleral brachytherapy. A 20-year retrospective analysis from a single-institution: part II. J Contemp Brachytherapy. 2018;10(4):347–59.

49. Archer DB, Amoaku WM, Gardiner TA. Radiation retinopathy--clinical, histopathological, ultrastructural and experimental correlations. Eye (Lond). 1991;5(Pt 2):239–51.

50. Bianciotto C, Shields CL, Pirondini C, Mashayekhi A, Furuta M, Shields JA. Proliferative radiation retinopathy after plaque radiotherapy for uveal melanoma. Ophthalmology. 2010;117(5):1005–12.

51. Nagendran ST, Finger PT. Anti-VEGF intravitreal bevacizumab for radiation-associated neovascular glaucoma. Ophthalmic Surg Lasers Imaging Retina. 2015;46(2):201–7.

Treatment Goals in Neovascular Glaucoma

Humberto Salazar and Swarup S. Swaminathan

1 Introduction

Neovascular glaucoma (NVG) is a severe complication of a variety of ocular diseases, typically those associated with retinal ischemia. Regardless of the underlying etiology, NVG often conveys a poor prognosis; most eyes with NVG either present with or eventually develop severe visual disability [1, 2]. Optic nerve damage due to the rapid and extreme rise in intraocular pressure (IOP) that occurs in NVG leads to a significant reduction in visual acuity (VA), which is often already affected by the underlying retinal pathology. Elevated IOP typically causes considerable eye pain in addition to vision loss, which leads these patients to seek care.

Management of NVG consists of two overarching goals: treatment of the underlying retinal pathology and IOP reduction. Anti-neovascular therapies and aggressive management of the retinal disease are of utmost importance in any stage of NVG to target the primary etiology of this condition [3]. Multiple factors, such as clinical presentation, severity of other ocular conditions, and the patient's activities of daily living must be assessed when considering surgical options and treatment goals. Assessing visual potential is of particular importance in guiding the intensity of management. This chapter discusses the different treatment goals that guide the management of NVG and the factors that must be considered when establishing these goals.

2 Disease Staging

The clinical presentation of NVG is extremely variable, with differing degrees of vision loss, pain, and IOP elevation. Several classification systems of NVG have been used in research and clinical practice to standardize disease staging and management [4–6]. These systems are based on clinical presentation, with a strong emphasis on gonioscopy. Appropriate staging of NVG helps guide treatment options, treatment goals, and overall prognosis, all of which are strongly dependent on the severity of disease.

Several classification systems include neovascularization of the iris (NVI) and neovascularization of the angle (NVA) without elevated IOP within their classification schemes. In this chapter, we consider anterior segment neovascularization without elevated IOP to not be overt NVG, but rather an important precursor to NVG that warrants aggressive treatment of the underlying retinal disease to prevent progression to NVG. The earliest stages of NVG can be characterized by elevated IOP in the presence of NVI and possibly NVA but an otherwise open irido-

H. Salazar · S. S. Swaminathan (✉)
Bascom Palmer Eye Institute, University of Miami Miller School of Medicine, Miami, FL, USA
e-mail: sswaminathan@med.miami.edu

© The Author(s), under exclusive license to Springer Nature Switzerland AG 2022
M. Qiu (ed.), *Neovascular Glaucoma*, Essentials in Ophthalmology,
https://doi.org/10.1007/978-3-031-11720-6_12

corneal angle on gonioscopy. Small focal peripheral anterior synechiae (PAS) may be starting to develop. At this stage, a mostly invisible fibrovascular membrane has formed over the trabecular meshwork, thereby preventing sufficient egress of aqueous humor and elevating the IOP [3]. VA can be variably affected depending on the acuity of onset and the corneal edema caused by IOP elevation. However, eyes with the earliest stages of NVG typically have a good prognosis given that iridocorneal angle and optic nerve damage is minimal, and thus, VA typically returns to baseline once the IOP is controlled. Antivascular endothelial growth factor (VEGF) therapy is essential for controlling the neovascular drive, while IOP-lowering medications are key to preventing optic nerve damage. NVG in the earliest stages constitutes the minority of diagnosed cases, because most patients do not present for evaluation until more advanced disease stages. Mild elevation in IOP typically does not cause ocular pain or a decrease in VA; these patients do not acutely seek ophthalmic care. Additionally, NVI and NVA in patients with elevated IOP are not always detected in retina clinics, as most patients are dilated and gonioscopy is not typically performed. These factors often delay the referral to glaucoma specialists at this early stage.

As NVG progresses, the clinical picture can be characterized by elevated IOP, the presence of NVI and NVA, and early contraction of the fibrovascular membrane, which leads to PAS formation and progressive synechial angle closure [4]. Because the iridocorneal angle is still partially open, eyes at this stage typically respond to topical IOP-lowering medications, especially after potential regression of the fibrovascular membrane with anti-VEGF therapy. Although surgery is frequently necessary for long-term IOP control, medical IOP management can help temporarily delay surgery until NVA has regressed. By extension, as NVG progresses and reaches the most severe stage, clinical features include an iridocorneal angle that has become completely or almost completely closed due to PAS. Because of the extensive iridocorneal angle closure, eyes at this stage do not respond sufficiently to topical IOP-lowering medications and frequently require urgent surgical intervention to prevent further optic neuropathy.

Most patients seek acute care at later disease stages due to the associated decrease in vision and ocular pain. Clinical manifestations, specifically the severity of pain and degree of vision loss, can be highly variable at any stage but are typically more severe at later stages of the disease. Microcystic corneal edema caused by acute IOP elevation is a significant contributor to decreased vision. While some patients present with an IOP in the 30–40 mmHg range with mild discomfort and mildly decreased vision, others may present with an IOP in the 50–60 mmHg range, severe pain, and VA of hand motion or worse. Associated exam findings may include hyphema, anterior chamber cells and flare, vitreous hemorrhage, and tractional retinal detachment due to neovascular retinal disease. Vision loss can rapidly progress at these later stages of disease if left untreated.

3   Goals of Acute Management of NVG

Initial treatment of NVG aims to suppress the neovascular drive with pan-retinal photocoagulation (PRP) and/or anti-VEGF injection, in addition to topical and possibly oral IOP-lowering medications. Eyes that present in the earlier stages of disease may have regression of the fibrovascular membrane after initial PRP and/or anti-VEGF injection and may retain relatively normal angle anatomy, thereby preventing the development of extensive peripheral anterior synechiae and subsequent chronic angle-closure glaucoma (CACG) [7]. However, the window of time between the onset of NVA and subsequent synechial angle closure is relatively short. Therefore, immediate anti-VEGF treatment can potentially save the portions of the angle that are still open from closing due to synechiae.

The initial goal of IOP management in the acute NVG setting is a reduction to a more physiologic level, approximately around 20–30 mmHg, which can halt further vision loss and resolve pain.

IOP can be initially lowered with the use of topical and/or oral IOP-lowering medications. Given that these patients often have multiple systemic diseases that can affect other organ systems, care must be taken to avoid contraindicated medications (e.g., the use of acetazolamide would be inappropriate in a patient with severe kidney disease). In NVG eyes with angles that are still mostly open, topical and/or oral IOP-lowering medications may be sufficient to maintain a physiologic IOP. However, in NVG eyes with angles that have already become nearly completely closed, medical therapy is often insufficient, and these eyes often require IOP-lowering surgery to achieve an adequate and sustained IOP reduction [8]. If surgery cannot be performed immediately, topical and/or oral IOP-lowering medications should be continued until surgical intervention is possible. Modest IOP reduction in this interim period can not only reduce the risk and extent of glaucomatous optic neuropathy but may also help avoid postoperative suprachoroidal hemorrhage, for which rapid IOP reduction is a known risk factor [9–11]. These patients are often already at greater risk for this devastating complication, as they are more likely to have coexisting cardiovascular conditions for which they are prescribed blood thinners.

4   Assessing Visual Potential

One of the most important factors that guide the overall management of NVG is the assessment of the eye's visual potential. The aggressiveness of both anti-neovascular therapy and IOP reduction depends on the amount of vision that remains and how much can be potentially recovered. In eyes with good visual potential, initial treatment should encompass all previously discussed therapies. In contrast, in eyes with confirmed no light perception (NLP) and no potential of recovering vision, the goal of care should be significantly modified to that of maintaining comfort. However, there is a wide spectrum of possibilities in between these extreme examples, and in those cases, appropriately assessing the visual potential is key to guiding management.

Knowledge of a prior baseline VA can be helpful in these assessments. Eyes with good baseline VA prior to the development of NVG can potentially recover some vision with treatment of NVG and other causes of vision loss [12]. In contrast, eyes with poor baseline VA and poor overall visual potential prior to the development of NVG have a poorer prognosis and may at best return to the previous limited VA with appropriate treatment if detected early. Unfortunately, many patients presenting with NVG have not previously seen an eye provider and are unaware of their underlying systemic and ocular diseases. Therefore, an accurate prior baseline VA is often unknown.

When evaluating visual potential, it is essential to thoroughly account for reversible etiologies of decreased vision. Providers should treat any vision-limiting conditions while initiating anti-VEGF treatment to subsequently assess the eye's true visual potential. Common reversible causes of decreased vision in the setting of NVG include corneal edema, acute optic nerve hypoperfusion, hyphema, cataract, and vitreous hemorrhage [13]. Extremely elevated IOP (i.e., greater than 50 mmHg) can cause significantly decreased vision due to hypoperfusion of the optic nerve resulting from the difference between the IOP and diastolic blood pressure [14]. Microcystic corneal edema may also contribute to decreased vision. Lowering the IOP to a physiologic level using a combination of topical and/or oral IOP-lowering medications and anterior chamber paracentesis can potentially improve vision in the acute setting and allow for a more accurate assessment of VA and visual potential. It is not uncommon for an eye to improve from light perception vision to counting fingers after the acutely elevated IOP is rapidly normalized. Glycerin may also be applied to the cornea to temporarily resolve microcystic edema. Anterior chamber paracentesis must be performed conservatively and with care, as sudden and rapid IOP reduction can lead fragile neovascular vessels to shear, resulting in a hyphema. Decompression retinopathy has also been reported after anterior chamber paracentesis in which rapid IOP reduction results in new retinal hemorrhages [15]. In eyes with a significant cataract, visual potential can be tested with potential acuity meter testing. A combination of these techniques is often required to obtain the best estimate of visual potential.

Unfortunately, some reversible causes of vision loss cannot be rapidly corrected, such as vitreous hemorrhage or dense cataracts. Assessment of visual potential in these cases should be ongoing, and the visual potential should not be assumed to be poor until all concurrent conditions are treated and optimized. If vitreous hemorrhage is present, ocular ultrasonography can be useful to evaluate the status of the retina and to rule out any contraindications to intravitreal injection [16]. Intravitreal anti-VEGF injection can help treat the underlying cause of the vitreous hemorrhage, but reassessing VA to gauge the impact of the anti-VEGF injection can take several weeks. While cataract extraction, vitrectomy, and other surgical procedures would help gauge visual potential, performing these procedures quickly is often impractical in the setting of an acute NVG presentation.

The extent of functional vision can be assessed using various exam techniques. Directional light perception, which can be very useful for ambulation, can be tested by shining a muscle light toward the eye from different directions and assessing if the patient can detect the location of the light source. Relative light brightness also can be used as a proxy for optic nerve function [17]. The patient is asked to describe the brightness of the muscle light in comparison with the fellow eye. Naturally, this test requires a relatively healthy fellow eye. Additionally, simply testing whether the patient can distinguish a door frame with the NVG eye can also provide insight into the amount of visual function. Ultimately, it is best to err on the side of assuming better visual potential than may be present to ensure that the patient is provided with the best chance to recover vision. Objectively "poor" VA can still provide functional ambulatory vision to patients, so management options should be extensively discussed with the patient in these cases.

5 Surgical Therapies: Using Visual Potential as a Guide

5.1 Eyes with Good Visual Potential

Eyes with functional visual potential should be treated with prompt and aggressive anti-neovascular and IOP-lowering treatment, including surgery if necessary. Trabeculectomy was historically used in the treatment of NVG eyes. However, with mounting evidence that failure rates are higher in NVG, trabeculectomy is no longer a common surgery in this setting [18]. Aqueous shunts are a common surgical strategy in NVG eyes with good visual potential, and both valved and non-valved aqueous shunts can be used [19–25]. With the recent advent of micro-incisional glaucoma surgery (MIGS), there may also be a growing role for angle surgery in NVG. This strategy may be considered in NVG eyes with angles that remain visibly open after initial anti-VEGF therapy but have persistently elevated IOP due to membrane formation over the trabecular meshwork. However, the concept of angle surgery in NVG has not been formally studied yet and must be carefully weighed against the theoretically increased risk of hyphema if occult NVA remains.

Disease stage and response to topical IOP-lowering medications can further help determine an appropriate surgical strategy. As previously mentioned, NVG eyes with elevated IOP and partially open angles typically respond well to medical IOP-lowering therapy. It may be favorable to treat these eyes with anti-VEGF therapy alone at first and control the IOP medically to delay surgery until the NVA is regressed and there is no more active neovascularization. This can prevent aqueous shunt failure due to obstruction by persistent fibrovascular membrane in the iridocorneal angle. In contrast, NVG eyes with total or nearly total synechial angle closure typically do not respond to medical IOP-lowering therapy. These eyes often require immediate surgical intervention to lower the IOP and prevent optic nerve damage; however, it may also be preferable to delay aqueous shunt surgery until after regression of NVA to prevent failure. Although many glaucoma specialists opt to perform immediate tube shunt surgery along with anti-VEGF therapy, others prefer to begin with trans-scleral cyclophotocoagulation (CPC). CPC was historically reserved for eyes with poor visual potential because of the increased risk of prolonged inflammation and macular edema, but recent literature supports improved CPC outcomes with modified laser settings [26]. "Gentle" CPC (i.e., treatment of only 180 degrees or reduced laser settings) can be performed in these eyes to control IOP while anti-VEGF therapy takes effect, followed by incisional surgery if target IOP is not reached once the neovascularization has regressed and the eye is not as inflamed [27]. CPC is also an alternative for patients with reasonable visual potential but who are poor surgical candidates due to other comorbidities or personal factors that preclude them from having incisional surgery. CPC can be repeated more than once if the desired IOP is not achieved on the first attempt.

In the postoperative period, it is important to remain vigilant to detect and treat common complications if they arise. Aside from suprachoroidal hemorrhage, choroidal effusions can also occur after IOP-lowering surgery due to the rapid decrease in IOP [28]. Prior to surgery, treatment with topical and/or oral IOP-lowering medications can help reduce the magnitude of this sudden decrease in IOP. If there is active anterior segment neovascularization at the time of aqueous shunt insertion, bleeding can occur and a blood clot can occlude the tube tip, resulting in a IOP spike. This transient IOP elevation can usually be controlled with topical IOP-lowering medications while awaiting dissolution of the clot. Intracameral tPA injection can also be used to help dissolve the clot in these situations. Additionally, as previously described, aqueous shunt failure can occur in setting of active neovascularization due to obstruction by fibrovascular membrane. Ideally, an anti-VEGF injection should be administered as early as possible preoperatively to regress most of the anterior seg-

ment neovascularization by the time of surgery and decrease the risk of aqueousc shunt failure, hyphema, and other complications [29].

5.2 Eyes with Poor Visual Potential

Eyes with poor visual potential may not require such aggressive anti-neovascular and IOP-lowering treatment, as the goal in these eyes is to relieve pain and keep the eye comfortable. Although optimizing the visual outcome is still desirable, the risks of incisional glaucoma surgery may not outweigh the benefits of aggressive IOP reduction. CPC is often preferred over an aqueous shunt in NVG eyes with very poor visual potential, since it is a much less invasive procedure and can help achieve acceptable IOP reduction with resolution of pain [30]. It is imperative to perform a thorough assessment, as previously described, prior to determining that an eye has poor visual potential and pursuing a corresponding treatment strategy.

In eyes confirmed to have NLP vision, the goal of treatment is pain control. Topical and/or oral IOP-lowering medications are occasionally sufficient to relieve pain. Topical steroid and cycloplegic eyedrops can also be used as adjunctive therapy for pain management. CPC may be used in these eyes if the pain is thought to be a result of the elevated IOP, as well as to reduce long-term dependence on oral carbonic anhydrase inhibitors. If medical or laser IOP-lowering therapy does not adequately address the pain, other options for pain control include injection of retrobulbar alcohol or chlorpromazine [31]. Enucleation is typically reserved for refractory cases.

6 Goals of Chronic Management of NVG

Patients with NVG should be followed long-term by both retina and glaucoma providers to continue anti-VEGF therapy and monitor IOP control. Treatment of the underlying neovascular disease is essential to preventing recurrent NVA and subsequent loss of remaining trabecular meshwork function. Many eyes with NVG develop some extent of PAS and a secondary CACG, which requires long-term management by glaucoma providers. The relative severity of angle closure and optic neuropathy can vary depending on the stage of NVG at the time of the initial presentation and treatment.

Patients with NVG should be immediately referred to a primary care provider, if they do not already have one, for aggressive management of coexisting systemic diseases. Many patients with NVG have uncontrolled systemic conditions such as diabetes mellitus and essential hypertension and unfortunately often have other systemic complications of these diseases, such as kidney disease, heart disease, and neuropathy. Patients with NVG have a significantly elevated mortality rate and thus require intensive treatment of their systemic diseases [8, 32].

6.1 Baseline and Longitudinal Evaluation

After stabilizing the acute issues, a new "baseline" evaluation is important for assessing the extent of vision loss, staging the severity of glaucomatous optic neuropathy, setting a target IOP, and determining future progression. The assessment should begin with a complete ocular examination including measurement of best-corrected VA, IOP, slit lamp biomicroscopy, undilated gonioscopy, and dilated fundoscopy of both eyes. Any uncontrolled concurrent ocular diseases that can contribute to decreased vision and that could confound this new baseline assessment should be noted and treated. A thorough gonioscopic examination should be performed, specifically documenting the location and extent of synechial angle closure for future comparison. Baseline gonioscopic photographs can be particularly useful for this purpose. Notably, it is essential to perform gonioscopy in the fellow unaffected eye to ensure a healthy iridocorneal angle and the absence of early neovasculariza-

tion, which is especially pertinent to bilateral retinal conditions such as proliferative diabetic retinopathy [33, 34].

The optic nerve examination is of particular importance to determine the severity of glaucomatous optic neuropathy. However, optic nerve anatomy is often distorted by tractional membranes, neovascularization of the disc, or overlying vitreous hemorrhage, which can make it difficult to assess the severity of cupping (Fig. 1). Comparing the optic nerve to the contralateral eye can occasionally be helpful, although this assessment is only valuable if the fellow eye is relatively healthy. Cupping of the unaffected fellow eye may suggest underlying primary openangle glaucoma, which is a known risk factor for central retinal vein occlusion and consequent NVG [35]. Pallor of the affected neuroretinal rim indicates significant optic nerve damage, which may or may not be glaucomatous in nature. Vascular insult to the optic nerve head given potential underlying systemic conditions and hypoperfusion due to prior IOP elevations should be considered. Regardless of the anatomy, base-

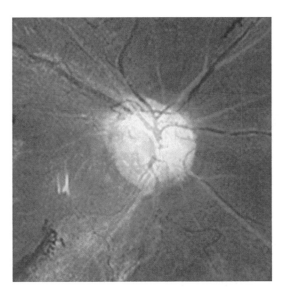

Fig. 1 Optic nerve photograph of a patient with neovascular glaucoma, demonstrating disc pallor, neovascularization of the disc, sclerotic vessels, and mild tractional membranes. It is often challenging to determine an accurate cup-to-disk ratio in these eyes given the impact of these findings on the optic nerve head

line optic nerve photographs are useful for future comparison when assessing for progressive cupping on subsequent examinations.

Standard automated perimetry (SAP) is traditionally used to determine the severity of decreased vision from glaucomatous optic neuropathy and to monitor for progression and stability in response to treatment. Clinicians use different classification systems to stage glaucomatous disease severity, such as the Hodapp-Anderson-Parrish (HAP) criteria and the Advanced Glaucoma Intervention Study (AGIS) scoring system [36]. Additionally, these criteria are often used to set a target IOP. The most common SAP test settings are a 24–2 test pattern with a size III stimulus using the Swedish Interactive Thresholding Algorithm (SITA) standard algorithm. However, the use of perimetric testing for staging disease severity in NVG is difficult due to multiple confounders. Macular edema, macular ischemia, retinal atrophy, scarring from PRP, tractional retinal detachments, and vitreous hemorrhage can all create extensive nonspecific visual field defects that can be difficult to differentiate from glaucomatous scotomas (Fig. 2). In addition, visual fields in NVG eyes with poor VA are typically unreliable or demonstrate general depression [37]. Reliability can sometimes be improved by modifying test parameters, such as performing a 10–2 protocol, switching to the larger size V testing stimulus, and using the SITA-Fast or SITA-Faster algorithms. Although perimetric testing in NVG eyes is often of unclear value for staging purposes, they can still be helpful for monitoring disease progression if they are reproducible. However, changes in the status of the patient's underlying retinal disease (e.g., fluctuating amounts of macular edema) can also impact perimetric testing.

Optic nerve head imaging is another key component in the assessment of glaucoma. Optical coherence tomography (OCT) images evaluating the thickness of the retinal nerve fiber layer (RNFL) and ganglion cell layer (GCL) are typically used at the time of baseline glaucoma evaluation and to monitor for subsequent glaucomatous progression [38]. Unlike perimetry, OCT imaging does not depend upon the subjective partici-

pation of the patient and thus can be obtained with greater consistency in eyes with poorer VA. However, there are multiple challenges to obtaining reliable OCTs. Scan quality can be affected by disturbances in the ocular media, such as corneal punctate epithelial erosions, cataracts, or vitreous hemorrhage. In addition, the OCT image can be significantly confounded by underlying retinal pathology and other concurrent ocular diseases frequently seen in NVG (Figs. 3 and 4). In the setting of retinal vascular disease, thinning of the RNFL and GCL can be caused by inner retinal ischemia and atrophy; distinguishing between a retinal and a glaucomatous etiology of inner retinal thinning in these eyes can prove to be challenging. Optic nerve head edema, which can occur in uncontrolled diabetes or hypertension, can cause artifactual thickening of the RNFL and GCL. In addition, macular edema, retinal exudates, and scarring can distort the retinal anatomy and lead to poor segmentation by the OCT software [39]. Patients with diabetic macular edema have also been shown to have thickened temporal RNFL measurements due to mild inner retinal edema, which is an example of how retinal disease can influence parameters used to assess glaucomatous progression [40]. Similar to perimetry, structural imaging can be potentially helpful in monitoring longitudinal changes in these retinal layers although fluctuations in the degree of retinal disease can affect these evaluations.

Given the dynamic changes that can occur in the initial period after the acute onset of NVG, we recommend obtaining baseline perimetry, OCT, and optic nerve photographs approximately 2–3 months after initial presentation and treatment. This time frame will allow for stabilization of IOP and retinal disease, thereby increasing the probability of obtaining more reliable testing. Baseline perimetry may need to be repeated to account for the learning effect and improve reliability, and OCT testing may need to be repeated after significant improvements in the clarity of optical media (e.g., cleared vitreous hemorrhage, cataract removal).

Initially, NVG patients should be examined monthly to monitor the VA, IOP, regression or

Central 24-2 Threshold Test

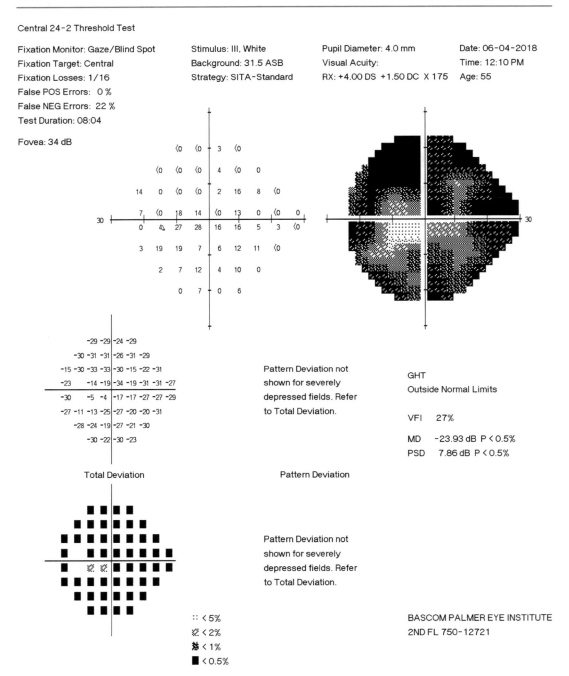

Fixation Monitor: Gaze/Blind Spot   Stimulus: III, White   Pupil Diameter: 4.0 mm   Date: 06-04-2018
Fixation Target: Central   Background: 31.5 ASB   Visual Acuity: Time: 12:10 PM
Fixation Losses: 1/16   Strategy: SITA-Standard   RX: +4.00 DS +1.50 DC X 175   Age: 55
False POS Errors: 0 %
False NEG Errors: 22 %
Test Duration: 08:04

Fovea: 34 dB

Pattern Deviation not
shown for severely
depressed fields. Refer
to Total Deviation.

GHT
Outside Normal Limits

VFI   27%

MD   -23.93 dB P < 0.5%
PSD   7.86 dB P < 0.5%

Total Deviation   Pattern Deviation

Pattern Deviation not
shown for severely
depressed fields. Refer
to Total Deviation.

BASCOM PALMER EYE INSTITUTE
2ND FL 750-12721

:: < 5%
⚇ < 2%
❃ < 1%
■ < 0.5%

Fig. 2 Standard automated perimetry of a patient with neovascular glaucoma in the left eye. While a mostly reliable test, one can note the subtle "clover leaf" pattern present and the dense superior and inferior arcuate scotomas. This patient had a highly ischemic central retinal vein occlusion, which required extensive pan-retinal photocoagulation. She was also noted to have severe macular ischemia on fluorescein angiography. The underlying retinal pathology makes it difficult to attribute the perimetric findings to a glaucomatous process

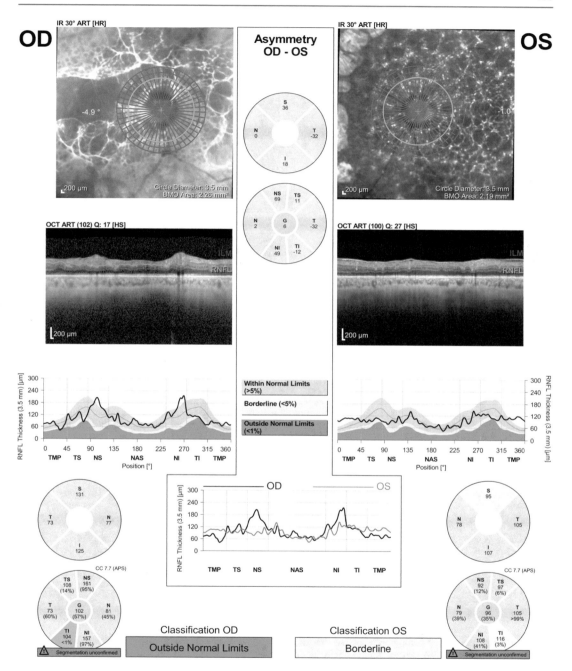

Fig. 3 Optical coherence tomography of the retinal nerve fiber layer (RNFL) in a patient with bilateral proliferative diabetic retinopathy and neovascular glaucoma in the left eye. RNFL thickness in both eyes is distorted due to peripapillary epiretinal membranes and mild retinal edema. Caution must be exercised when trending RNFL thickness values in such eyes. Of note, the signal quality is affected by an unstable ocular tear film, as noted in the top infrared images

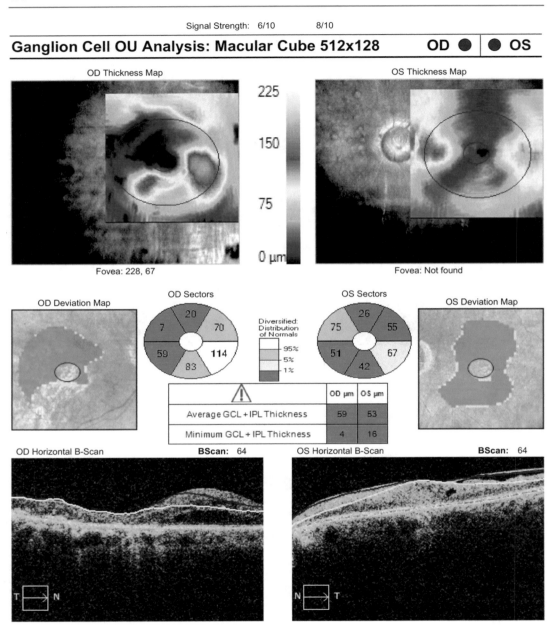

Fig. 4 Optical coherence tomography of the macular ganglion cell-inner plexiform layers (GCIPL) in a patient with bilateral proliferative diabetic retinopathy and neovascular glaucoma in the right eye. While the deviation map of the right eye suggests temporal thinning, as commonly seen in glaucoma, and deviation map of the left eye suggests diffuse thinning, evaluation of the B-scans below demonstrates aberrant layer segmentation in both eyes with severe retinal atrophy in the right eye. Such confounders must be carefully considered when assessing neovascular glaucoma patients

recurrence of NVA, extent of PAS, and response to treatment of the underlying retinal disease. If monthly anti-VEGF injections are given by a retina specialist, gonioscopic examination can be performed in longer intervals given the low risk of recurrent NV. Structural and functional testing with OCT and perimetry should initially be repeated at least every 3 months to create a robust baseline. The same parameters that were used in the baseline visual field should be used in subsequent tests to allow for adequate comparison. However, parameters may need to be altered if there is any significant change in the status of the patient's other ocular conditions. A new baseline should be established every time the target IOP is modified and/or after any surgical procedure is performed. The optic nerve should be evaluated at each visit and compared to baseline photos to monitor for progressive cupping.

After the patient is deemed to be stable, the frequency of follow-up visits can be gradually extended to every 6 months. Some patients may require many frequent visits before their disease becomes stabilized. On the other hand, some patients may achieve stability indefinitely with minimal glaucomatous optic neuropathy after the initial NVG treatment. If treated aggressively and promptly, these eyes may not necessarily go on to develop synechial angle closure and thus can be monitored less frequently from a glaucoma provider's standpoint.

6.2 Determination of a Target IOP

Setting a target IOP for an eye with NVG is important to guide management and establish treatment goals. Lower targets may require more aggressive medical or surgical therapy to reach, and therefore, the benefits of achieving a low target IOP must be weighed against the risks of treatment. The target IOP is not a static number, but rather a dynamic goal that should be reassessed and modified in response to treatment and to changes in visual potential. If the retinal disease is controlled and does not significantly confound visual field testing and structural optic

nerve imaging, disease stage can be established based on the baseline glaucoma evaluation using any of the published glaucoma classification systems [36]. Most classification systems for primary open-angle glaucoma recommend a specific amount or percentage of IOP reduction depending on the disease stage and that calculated number can be used to set the initial target IOP. This concept may not be applicable in many cases since it is often not possible to use perimetry to stage disease severity and guide target IOPs in NVG, as discussed above. Therefore, we recommend using the optic nerve status and the visual potential of the eye as a guide. For the vast majority of NVG eyes, we believe that a reasonable initial target IOP would be in the high teens. A lower target IOP, such as in the low teens, may be needed in NVG eyes that have more severe optic nerve cupping, or in eyes that have underlying primary open-angle glaucoma. On the other hand, a higher target IOP, such as in the low to mid-20s, might be beneficial for some NVG eyes. For example, patients with extremely high IOP on initial presentation who are on antiplatelet or anticoagulant medications may fare better with a higher target IOP, given the risk of suprachoroidal hemorrhage with a sudden and large decrease in IOP. In addition, if the underlying retinal disease is particularly severe and is thought to be the main cause of profound vision loss, it may also be reasonable to establish a higher target IOP (for example low 20s), since progressive IOP-related vision loss at such pressures is unlikely. Finally, eyes with very poor visual potential may also benefit from a higher target IOP, or by using pain to guide treatment rather than a target IOP.

Other patient factors that should be taken into consideration when setting a target IOP include surgical candidacy, overall health, life expectancy, and patient preferences regarding medical and surgical treatment. Patients who are poor surgical candidates or who have a short life expectancy may not require a low target IOP. The risks and benefits of a given target IOP and the treatments that would be necessary to achieve this target should be thoroughly discussed with patients before making treatment decisions.

7 Conclusion

The two main goals of both acute and chronic treatment of NVG are to treat the underlying retinal ischemic disease and to control the IOP to prevent vision loss from progressive glaucomatous optic neuropathy. The initial therapy may vary depending on the stage of NVG, but most eyes require a combination of PRP, intravitreal anti-VEGF injection, and medical and surgical IOP-lowering treatment. Assessing the visual potential of NVG eyes is extremely important in guiding the choice of a surgical procedure and longitudinal IOP management. It is essential to account for all potentially reversible causes of vision loss when assessing visual potential. When the visual potential is unclear, it is recommended to err toward more aggressive treatment to provide the best chance for visual recovery. After initial treatment, NVG eyes require long-term treatment of the underlying retinal disease and management of IOP. Baseline glaucoma structural and functional testing should be performed but may be significantly confounded by multiple factors. A target IOP should be set according to this initial evaluation, particularly the optic nerve appearance and overall visual potential. Eyes with NVG frequently require a combination of long-term medical and surgical IOP-lowering treatments to achieve the target IOP, which should be continuously reassessed. Judicious management of NVG is essential to maintaining functional vision throughout the patient's lifetime—the overarching goal of glaucoma management.

References

1. Cronemberger S, Lourenco LF, Silva LC, Calixto N, Pires MC. Prognosis of glaucoma in relation to blindness at a university hospital. Arq Bras Oftalmol. 2009;72(2):199–204.
2. Lazcano-Gomez G, J RS, Lynch A, L NB, Martinez K, Turati M, et al. Neovascular glaucoma: a retrospective review from a tertiary eye care center in Mexico. J Curr Glaucoma Pract. 2017;11(2):48–51.
3. Hayreh SS. Neovascular glaucoma. Prog Retin Eye Res. 2007;26(5):470–85.
4. Shazly TA, Latina MA. Neovascular glaucoma: etiology, diagnosis and prognosis. Semin Ophthalmol. 2009;24(2):113–21.
5. SooHoo JR, Seibold LK, Pantcheva MB, Kahook MY. Aflibercept for the treatment of neovascular glaucoma. Clin Exp Ophthalmol. 2015;43(9):803–7.
6. Teich SA, Walsh JB. A grading system for iris neovascularization. Prognostic implications for treatment. Ophthalmology. 1981;88(11):1102–6.
7. Simha A, Aziz K, Braganza A, Abraham L, Samuel P, Lindsley KB. Anti-vascular endothelial growth factor for neovascular glaucoma. Cochrane Database Syst Rev. 2020;2(2):Cd007920.
8. Sánchez-Tabernero S, Juberías JR, Artells N, Crespo-Millas S, Meneses C, Muñoz-Moreno MF, et al. Management and systemic implications of diabetic neovascular glaucoma. Ophthalmic Res. 2019;62(2):111–5.
9. Risk factors for suprachoroidal hemorrhage after filtering surgery. The fluorouracil filtering surgery study group. Am J Ophthalmol. 1992;113(5):501–7.
10. Jeganathan VS, Ghosh S, Ruddle JB, Gupta V, Coote MA, Crowston JG. Risk factors for delayed suprachoroidal haemorrhage following glaucoma surgery. Br J Ophthalmol. 2008;92(10):1393–6.
11. Learned D, Eliott D. Management of delayed suprachoroidal hemorrhage after glaucoma surgery. Semin Ophthalmol. 2018;33(1):59–63.
12. Liao N, Li C, Jiang H, Fang A, Zhou S, Wang Q. Neovascular glaucoma: a retrospective review from a tertiary center in China. BMC Ophthalmol. 2016;16:14.
13. Havens SJ, Gulati V. Neovascular glaucoma. Dev Ophthalmol. 2016;55:196–204.
14. Wen JC, Chen CL, Rezaei KA, Chao JR, Vemulakonda A, Luttrell I, et al. Optic nerve head perfusion before and after intravitreal antivascular growth factor injections using optical coherence tomography-based microangiography. J Glaucoma. 2019;28(3):188–93.
15. Kim ES, Yu SY, Han SB, Kim M. Decompression retinopathy after intravitreal bevacizumab and anterior chamber paracentesis in a patient with neovascular glaucoma. Indian J Ophthalmol. 2016;64(11):861–3.
16. Sandinha MT, Kotagiri AK, Owen RI, Geenen C, Steel DH. Accuracy of B-scan ultrasonography in acute fundus obscuring vitreous hemorrhage using a standardized scanning protocol and a dedicated ophthalmic ultrasonographer. Clin Ophthalmol. 2017;11:1365–70.
17. Browning DJ, Buckley EG. Reliability of brightness comparison testing in predicting afferent pupillary defects. Arch Ophthalmol. 1988;106(3):341–3.
18. Takihara Y, Inatani M, Fukushima M, Iwao K, Iwao M, Tanihara H. Trabeculectomy with mitomycin C for neovascular glaucoma: prognostic factors for surgical failure. Am J Ophthalmol. 2009;147(5):912–8, 8.e1.
19. Budenz DL, Barton K, Gedde SJ, Feuer WJ, Schiffman J, Costa VP, et al. Five-year treatment outcomes in the Ahmed Baerveldt comparison study. Ophthalmology. 2015;122(2):308–16.

20. Cheng Y, Liu XH, Shen X, Zhong YS. Ahmed valve implantation for neovascular glaucoma after 23-gauge vitrectomy in eyes with proliferative diabetic retinopathy. Int J Ophthalmol. 2013;6(3):316–20.
21. Gedde SJ. Personal communication regarding the results of the Ahmed Baerveldt comparison study. Miami: Bascom Palmer Eye Institute; 2021.
22. Shalaby WS, Myers JS, Razeghinejad R, Katz LJ, Pro M, Dale E, et al. Outcomes of valved and nonvalved tube shunts in neovascular glaucoma. Ophthalmol Glaucoma. 2020.
23. Shchomak Z, Cordeiro Sousa D, Leal I, Abegão PL. Surgical treatment of neovascular glaucoma: a systematic review and meta-analysis. Graefes Arch Clin Exp Ophthalmol. 2019;257(6):1079–89.
24. Simsek T, Bilgeç MD. Ahmed glaucoma valve implantation versus suprachoroidal silicone tube implantation following the injection of bevacizumab into the anterior chamber in patients with neovascular glaucoma. Graefes Arch Clin Exp Ophthalmol. 2019;257(4):799–804.
25. Suda M, Nakanishi H, Akagi T, Murakami T, Suzuma K, Suda K, et al. Baerveldt or Ahmed glaucoma valve implantation with pars plana tube insertion in Japanese eyes with neovascular glaucoma: 1-year outcomes. Clin Ophthalmol. 2018;12:2439–49.
26. Ndulue JK, Rahmatnejad K, Sanvicente C, Wizov SS, Moster MR. Evolution of cyclophotocoagulation. J Ophthalmic Vis Res. 2018;13(1):55–61.
27. Sarrafpour S, Saleh D, Ayoub S, Radcliffe NM. Micropulse transscleral cyclophotocoagulation: a look at long-term effectiveness and outcomes. Ophthalmol Glaucoma. 2019;2(3):167–71.
28. Schrieber C, Liu Y. Choroidal effusions after glaucoma surgery. Curr Opin Ophthalmol. 2015;26(2):134–42.
29. Hwang HB, Han JW, Yim HB, Lee NY. Beneficial effects of adjuvant intravitreal bevacizumab injection on outcomes of Ahmed glaucoma valve implantation in patients with neovascular glaucoma: systematic literature review. J Ocul Pharmacol Ther. 2015;31(4):198–203.
30. Schwartz K, Budenz D. Current management of glaucoma. Curr Opin Ophthalmol. 2004;15(2):119–26.
31. Idowu OO, Ashraf DC, Kalin-Hajdu E, Ryan MC, Kersten RC, Vagefi MR. Efficacy of care for blind painful eyes. Ophthalmic Plast Reconstr Surg. 2019;35(2):182–6.
32. Blanc JP, Molteno AC, Fuller JR, Bevin TH, Herbison P. Life expectancy of patients with neovascular glaucoma drained by Molteno implants. Clin Exp Ophthalmol. 2004;32(4):360–3.
33. Nielsen NV. The prevalence of glaucoma and ocular hypertension in type 1 and 2 diabetes mellitus. An epidemiological study of diabetes mellitus on the island of Falster, Denmark. Acta Ophthalmol. 1983;61(4):662–72.
34. Ohrt V. The frequency of rubeosis iridis in diabetic patients. Acta Ophthalmol. 1971;49(2):301–7.
35. Yin X, Li J, Zhang B, Lu P. Association of glaucoma with risk of retinal vein occlusion: a meta-analysis. Acta Ophthalmol. 2019;97(7):652–9.
36. Brusini P, Johnson CA. Staging functional damage in glaucoma: review of different classification methods. Surv Ophthalmol. 2007;52(2):156–79.
37. Tan NYQ, Tham YC, Koh V, Nguyen DQ, Cheung CY, Aung T, et al. The effect of testing reliability on visual field sensitivity in normal eyes: the Singapore Chinese eye study. Ophthalmology. 2018;125(1):15–21.
38. Kotowski J, Wollstein G, Folio LS, Ishikawa H, Schuman JS. Clinical use of OCT in assessing glaucoma progression. Ophthalmic Surg Lasers Imaging. 2011;42(Suppl 0):S6–14.
39. Patel PJ, Chen FK, da Cruz L, Tufail A. Segmentation error in stratus optical coherence tomography for neovascular age-related macular degeneration. Invest Ophthalmol Vis Sci. 2009;50(1):399–404.
40. Hwang DJ, Lee EJ, Lee SY, Park KH, Woo SJ. Effect of diabetic macular edema on peripapillary retinal nerve fiber layer thickness profiles. Invest Ophthalmol Vis Sci. 2014;55(7):4213–9.

Panretinal Photocoagulation for Neovascular Glaucoma

Anna G. Mackin, Nathalie Massamba, and Dimitra Skondra

1   Introduction

For decades, panretinal photocoagulation (PRP) has been a standard of care procedure for managing anterior segment neovascularization associated with retinal vascular diseases, including proliferative diabetic retinopathy (PDR), retinal vein occlusion, central retinal artery occlusion (CRAO), and ocular ischemic syndrome (OIS) most commonly stemming from carotid artery occlusive disease. In 1974, Callahan first described regression of anterior segment neovascularization in response to PRP in a patient with PDR [1]. PRP has proven to be effective in the earlier stages of neovascular glaucoma (NVG), characterized by iris neovascularization (NVI) without elevated intraocular pressure (IOP), as well as more advanced stages of NVG characterized by angle neovascularization (NVA), elevated IOP, and peripheral anterior synechiae

A. G. Mackin
Department of Ophthalmology and Visual Science,
The University of Chicago, Chicago, IL, USA

N. Massamba
Department of Ophthalmology, Handicap, and Vision,
Pitie Salpetriere Hospital, Sorbonne University,
Paris, France

D. Skondra (✉)
Department of Ophthalmology and Visual Science,
The University of Chicago, Chicago, IL, USA

J. Terry Ernest Ocular Imaging Center, The
University of Chicago, Chicago, IL, USA
e-mail: dskondra@bsd.uchicago.edu

(PAS) [2]. In the current era of anti-vascular endothelial growth factor (VEGF) agents that are widely used to treat retinal vascular disorders, PRP has not lost its relevance. PRP remains essential in the management paradigm of NVG due to its safety and long-lasting efficacy.

2   Mechanism of Action

Retinal ischemia is a key feature in the pathogenesis of retinal vascular diseases [3]. Retinal vessel damage in these conditions leads to tissue hypoxia, and increased hypoxia-inducible factor-1 (HIF-1) levels [4]. As a key transcription factor, upregulated HIF-1 leads to increased expression of hypoxia-regulated genes, including VEGF, placental growth factor (PlGF), platelet-derived growth factor-B (PDGF-B), and stromal-derived growth factor-1 (SDF-1) that together stimulate the growth of new vessels [5]. PRP functions to halt this cascade by reducing the global retinal oxygen demand. By causing thermal burns and tissue coagulation, PRP destroys some of the peripheral ischemic retina and eliminates the angiogenic factors it produces, thereby decreasing the vasoproliferative drive [6]. PRP is also thought to improve retinal oxygenation by facilitating oxygen diffusion from the choroid [6, 7]. It has also been proposed that PRP interferes with neovascularization by altering the balance between the matrix metalloproteinases and their

M. Qiu (ed.), *Neovascular Glaucoma*, Essentials in Ophthalmology,
https://doi.org/10.1007/978-3-031-11720-6_13

inhibitors produced by the retinal pigment epithelium [7]. These changes take several weeks to take effect; anterior segment neovascularization typically regresses within 4 weeks after PRP in the majority of patients, but in some cases may take between 2 and 30 months to disappear [8].

3   Clinical Indications and Procedure

3.1   Proliferative Diabetic Retinopathy

In 1976, the first Diabetic Retinopathy Study (DRS) reported that PRP reduced the risk of severe vision loss in patients with high-risk PDR by more than 50% [9]. The same year, Little et al. reported that argon laser PRP in eyes with PDR and anterior segment neovascularization resulted in regression of the NVI and NVA [10]. Since that time, PRP has been the treatment of choice for patients with high-risk PDR. Eyes with high-risk PDR without anterior segment neovascularization have a lower risk of developing NVG after PRP [11, 12]. Furthermore, eyes with PDR that already have anterior segment neovascularization at the time of PRP were reported to have a significant regression of the NVI and NVA after PRP [10, 13].

In the DRS protocol, PRP was initially administered with a xenon arc or argon blue-green (488 nm) laser sequentially delivering at least 1500 discrete gray-white spots at 100–200 millisecond duration and 100–500 micron diameter, scattered outside the vascular arcades. Because of less discomfort compared to higher-wavelength lasers, argon was the dominant modality for PRP until Blumenkranz and colleagues developed a novel frequency-doubled 532-nm-wavelength Nd:YAG laser. The PASCAL (PAttern SCAn Laser; Topcon Medical Laser Systems, Santa Clara, California, USA), a commercially available version of this laser, rapidly delivers a grid of up to 56 shorter duration laser pulses following a single foot pedal depression thus allowing for a faster PRP procedure [14]. The shorter pulse duration also results in a different mechanism of cellular injury transitioning from thermal dena-

turation at higher pulse durations to microbubble formation around melanosomes at shorter pulse durations [15]. Shorter laser pulse duration limits laser spot expansion and collateral laser damage [16, 17], and is significantly more comfortable for the patient [18]. There is also a lower risk of overlapping laser burns, because the PASCAL 20 millisecond duration laser burns show a healing response over time [19, 20].

A retrospective study by Chappelow et al. compared DRS-style PRP administered with an argon laser to a PASCAL PRP treatment delivering the same number and size of spots in an array of short 20 millisecond pulses; this study demonstrated that patients treated using the PASCAL had poorer regression of neovascularization and more recurrences compared to patients treated with argon laser [7]. There was also a higher rate of NVI and NVG in the PASCAL group; however, this relationship did not show statistical significance [7]. On the other hand, the Manchester Pascal Study reported a favorable regression of neovascularization following the 20 millisecond PASCAL PRP; however, significantly higher laser dosimetry and ablation areas were described, requiring on average 6924 PRP spots and a 836 mm^2 ablation area to achieve complete disease regression in severe PDR [19]. The Diabetic Retinopathy Clinical Research Network Protocol S data demonstrated that patients treated with pattern laser had a significantly higher rate of anterior segment neovascularization and NVG at 2-year follow-up compared to patients treated with single spot conventional laser [21]. However, it was highlighted that many patients in the pattern laser group had a substantially lower total treatment area than the conventional laser group and thus were undertreated [22]. Multiple authors have concluded that pattern laser PRP can be as effective as conventional argon PRP with a more favorable side effect profile; however, the settings require adjustment based on the severity of disease in order to achieve an adequate treatment area [17, 22, 23]. Figure 1 shows an Optos fundus photograph of the right eye of a patient with PDR and anterior segment neovascularization treated effectively with a combination of pattern and conventional PRP (Fig. 1).

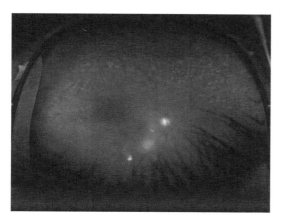

Fig. 1 Optos fundus photograph of the right eye of a patient with proliferative diabetic retinopathy and associated anterior chamber neovascularization treated effectively with a combination of pattern and conventional PRP

Anti-VEGF injections are now widely used for the management of PDR. Several randomized clinical trials have demonstrated that monthly ranibizumab is non-inferior in prevention of NVI and NVG compared to PRP [24, 25], while resulting in less peripheral visual field loss [25, 26]. However, pragmatic real-world data suggest that the long-lasting effect of PRP is superior to anti-VEGF alone in the long-term prevention of anterior segment neovascularization [27], since many patients become lost to follow-up and are not able to adhere to a strict anti-VEGF injection schedule outside of a clinical trial. Serial anti-VEGF injections may be useful as an adjunct to PRP, especially since the therapeutic effects of PRP do not take place immediately, and multiple sessions may be required to complete adequate PRP.

3.2 Central Retinal Vein Occlusion

In 1977, Laatikainen et al. published the results of the first prospective randomized controlled trial of PRP in patients with central retinal vein occlusion (CRVO) without NVG, demonstrating that PRP decreased the rate of NVI and NVG in patients with ischemic CRVO [28, 29]. The results also

suggested that PRP was not indicated in patients with non-ischemic CRVO, since none of these patients developed NVI or NVG at 1-year follow-up [28]. Shortly thereafter, the benefit of PRP in significantly decreasing the risk of NVG in patients with ischemic CRVO was supported by other studies [30, 31]. At the same time, several studies suggested that the degree of retinal non-perfusion was directly related to anterior segment neovascularization [30, 32]. The pivotal Central Vein Occlusion Study (CVOS) subsequently provided evidence regarding whether or not early prophylactic PRP could definitively prevent anterior segment neovascularization in eyes with ischemic CRVO [8]. This study enrolled patients within 1 year of CRVO diagnosis who had at least 10 disk areas of retinal non-perfusion on fluorescein angiogram. The results published in 1995 demonstrated that early prophylactic PRP did not definitively prevent anterior segment neovascularization, whereas prompt PRP treatment was effective in treating de novo anterior segment neovascularization. Furthermore, the study demonstrated more robust regression of anterior segment neovascularization in PRP-naive eyes compared to eyes previously treated with prophylactic PRP. As a result, CVOS advocated against early prophylactic PRP as long as patients could be monitored closely and treated promptly in case of NVI or NVA development [33]. The importance of close follow-up was further highlighted by the fact that up to 16% of patients with non-ischemic disease converted to ischemia within 4 months after diagnosis [34]. Since the publication of CVOS, other studies including systematic literature reviews have supported the finding that PRP cannot definitively prevent anterior segment neovascularization in patients with ischemic CRVO; however, PRP is effective in regressing NVI and NVA and reducing the rate of neovascular glaucoma [35, 36]. Recent studies have suggested the use of anti-VEGF injections as an adjunct to PRP in patients who develop NVG due to ischemic CRVO in order to achieve a more rapid regression of anterior segment neovascularization [37, 38].

3.3   Retinal Artery Occlusion

Anterior segment neovascularization is reported to develop in 3.0–28.2% of patients with CRAO and PRP has been reported to be the gold standard treatment [39, 40]. Studies have shown that anterior segment neovascularization secondary to CRAO tends to occur relatively early, ranging from 1 to 16 weeks after CRAO diagnosis [40–42]. The first retrospective review of the efficacy of PRP for anterior segment neovascularization following CRAO was published in 1989 by Duker and Brown [42]. Among all eyes with NVI (regardless of NVG), PRP led to NVI regression in 65%. Among the subgroup of eyes with NVI without NVG or PAS, early PRP led to NVI regression in 89%. On the other hand, among the subgroup of eyes with NVI with NVG, late PRP led to NVI regression in only 38% [42]. Although there is no evidence to date that prophylactic PRP following CRAO definitively prevents the onset of neovascularization, early PRP upon first diagnosis of anterior or posterior segment neovascularization is critical in the prevention of progression to NVG. In the anti-VEGF era, there are subsequent reports of treating open-angle NVG associated with CRAO using intravitreal bevacizumab followed by PRP within 2–4 weeks, resulting in regression of anterior segment neovascularization and adequate IOP control with medical management alone [43, 44]. This treatment, however, may not be sufficient in patients with more advanced stages of NVG after the development of synechial angle closure, which commonly requires surgical intervention to achieve IOP control. The surgical options for IOP lowering in NVG will be discussed at length in other chapters. Early close follow-up for patients with new CRAO is critical to promptly identify and treat any neovascularization and prevent progression to more advanced disease.

3.4   Ocular Ischemic Syndrome

In 1984, Carter published the first report of PRP to manage anterior segment neovascularization due to common carotid artery occlusion not ame-nable to endarterectomy [45]. Since then, PRP has become a standard of care treatment for patients with OIS and anterior segment neovascularization associated with evidence of retinal ischemia [46]. Since uveal ischemia without retinal ischemia can occur in the setting of OIS, PRP is only indicated in the presence of retinal capillary non-perfusion as shown on fluorescein angiography [46], and only 36% of NVG eyes with OIS have NVI regression following full PRP treatment [47]. There is currently a paucity of data regarding how the angle anatomy and IOP respond to PRP in NVG secondary to OIS versus NVG secondary to other etiologies, and whether the surgical IOP-lowering strategy differs in the setting of OIS. As such, it would be prudent to perform pre-operative PRP in eyes with NVG secondary to OIS undergoing IOP-lowering surgery. There are currently no available reports of combination intravitreal anti-VEGF and PRP therapy for the treatment of anterior segment neovascularization in OIS.

3.5   Combination Treatment with Anti-VEGF Agents and PRP

Much of the data about the efficacy of PRP for treating ischemic retinal pathology is from before the advent of anti-VEGF. In the modern anti-VEGF era, there is strong evidence that intraocular injection of anti-VEGF agents induces a more rapid regression of anterior segment neovascularization compared to PRP, and this will be discussed in more detail in the chapter focusing on anti-VEGF for NVG. A retrospective case control study comparing same-day anti-VEGF combined with PRP versus PRP alone for the management of neovascular glaucoma reported that a group of 11 patients receiving anti-VEGF combined with PRP (9 with open angles, 2 with closed angles) had a significantly greater and faster regression of anterior segment neovascularization, and better IOP control, compared to a group of 12 patients receiving PRP alone (6 with open angles, 1 with a closed angle, and 5 with no gonioscopy available) [38]. All the patients in the combination therapy group achieved complete NVI regression with the mean time to regression of 12 days, compared to 17% of patients in the PRP group who achieved complete NVI regression with the mean time to regression of 127 days. A prospective randomized controlled trial of prompt PRP for NVG compared to intravitreal bevacizumab injection followed by PRP within 1 week also demonstrated that anti-VEGF combined with PRP in 10 subjects (3 with closed angles) induced faster regression of anterior segment NV compared to PRP alone in 9 subjects (2 with closed angles). Patients receiving anti-VEGF combined with PRP had regression of anterior segment neovascularization within 1 week after the injection, whereas patients receiving PRP alone did not have regression of anterior segment neovascularization until after 4 weeks [37]. This difference may be less relevant for patients in the earliest stages of NVG without any development of fibrovascular membrane in the angle or PAS since IOP may normalize after the NVA eventually regresses. However, the difference of several weeks may be critical for patients in the more advanced stages of NVG who are at risk of progressing from open-angle NVG to closed-angle NVG with profoundly elevated IOP that is more difficult to manage medically and is more likely to require IOP-lowering surgery. In these patients, prompt anti-VEGF in combination with PRP may regress their NVA more rapidly than PRP alone and therefore possibly prevent the progression to angle-closure NVG. The surgical options for IOP lowering in NVG will be discussed at length in other chapters.

3.6   Limitations and Complications

PRP requires adequate visualization of the retina, so NVG patients with media opacity such as corneal edema, hyphema, mature cataract, or vitreous hemorrhage may not be able to undergo PRP adequately, or at all. Complications of extensive PRP can include ciliochoroidal effusion, which has been reported in as many as 90% of patients following PRP with a high laser burn intensity,

and is thought to occur as a result of choriocapillaris disruption and fluid transudation [48]. Although transient, ciliochoroidal effusions can be minimized by dividing the full PRP treatment across two or more sessions spaced approximately 2 weeks apart, or using a multispot laser delivery system [49]. If the PRP sessions are spaced apart by more than 1 month, interval monthly anti-VEGF may be required to provide some anti-neovascular effect, until full PRP can be completed [50]. Intensive PRP treatment can lead to the breakdown of RPE barrier and resultant fluid exudation causing exudative retinal detachment [51, 52]. The incidence of exudative retinal detachment is low with multispot laser delivery systems [49, 53]. In the majority of cases, exudation is transient and self-limiting; however, there are reports of intravitreal anti-VEGF and corticosteroid injections needed to treat exudative retinal detachments associated with intensive PRP [52, 54]. Loss of peripheral visual field following PRP has been reported across all indicated conditions [25, 55]. The reported risk of visual field loss sufficient to preclude driving ranges from 11% to 50% [56]. The highest risk is reported in patients treated with the xenon arc laser, which is no longer in common practice. Multispot laser delivery systems result in less peripheral visual field loss, with the majority of patients able to preserve peripheral visual field compatible with driving [56]. Visual field loss from PRP may confound visual field testing in the monitoring of glaucoma progression. Furthermore, there are reports of decreased retinal function measured by ERG following PRP, specifically a reduction in a- and b-wave amplitudes of combined cone-rod responses [37, 57]. However, underlying retinal ischemia and optic nerve ischemia are the major determinants of worsening full-field ERG parameters in patients with NVG [37, 58]. A decrease in night vision has also been described following PRP [59]; however, this finding is confounded by the natural history of progressive diabetic retinopathy and other retinal vascular conditions, with some data suggesting preservation of rod function following PRP compared to untreated progressive PDR [60]. Another complication of PRP is exacerbation of existing macular edema, which is often associated with visual acuity loss and decreased contrast sensitivity [61, 62]. The risk of worsening macular edema is lower with 20 millisecond PASCAL PRP [23] and may be further ameliorated by concurrent anti-VEGF treatment [61, 63].

4 Conclusion

NVG is a severe complication of ischemic retinal pathology, and these vulnerable patients are often at high risk of becoming lost to follow-up, which can lead to devastating visual outcomes. While it is necessary for the glaucoma specialist to control the IOP to prevent vision loss from glaucomatous optic neuropathy, the retina specialist's priority is to control the underlying neovascular drive. Glaucoma and retina specialists should work collaboratively to rapidly regress neovascularization with anti-VEGF, prevent its recurrence with full PRP, and achieve IOP control while minimizing surgical complications. Combination treatment with PRP and anti-VEGF leverages their synergistic therapeutic benefits to regress NVI and NVA faster, reduce side effects, achieve a more robust IOP response, and ensure long-term disease control.

References

1. Callahan MA. Letter: photocoagulation and rubeosis iridis. Am J Ophthalmol. 1974;78(5):873–4. https://doi.org/10.1016/0002-9394(74)90338-9.
2. Rodrigues GB, Abe RY, Zangalli C, Sodre SL, Donini FA, Costa DC, et al. Neovascular glaucoma: a review. Int J Retina Vitreous. 2016;2:26. https://doi.org/10.1186/s40942-016-0051-x.
3. Campochiaro PA. Ocular neovascularization. J Mol Med (Berl). 2013;91(3):311–21. https://doi.org/10.1007/s00109-013-0993-5.
4. Shahulhameed S, Swain S, Jana S, Chhablani J, Ali MJ, Pappuru RR, et al. A robust model system for retinal hypoxia: live imaging of calcium dynamics and gene expression studies in primary human mixed retinal culture. Front Neurosci. 2019;13:1445. https://doi.org/10.3389/fnins.2019.01445.
5. Vadlapatla RK, Vadlapudi AD, Mitra AK. Hypoxia-inducible factor-1 (HIF-1): a potential target for intervention in ocular neovascular diseases. Curr Drug Targets. 2013;14(8):919–35. https://doi.org/10.2174/13894501113149990015.
6. Wilson AS, Hobbs BG, Shen WY, Speed TP, Schmidt U, Begley CG, et al. Argon laser photocoagulation-induced modification of gene expression in the retina. Invest Ophthalmol Vis Sci. 2003;44(4):1426–34. https://doi.org/10.1167/iovs.02-0622.
7. Chappelow AV, Tan K, Waheed NK, Kaiser PK. Panretinal photocoagulation for proliferative diabetic retinopathy: pattern scan laser versus argon laser. Am J Ophthalmol. 2012;153(1):137–42 e2. https://doi.org/10.1016/j.ajo.2011.05.035.
8. Central vein occlusion study of photocoagulation. Manual of operations. Central Vein Occlusion Study Group. Online J Curr Clin Trials. 1993;Doc No 92:[32,228 words; 678 paragraphs].
9. Preliminary report on effects of photocoagulation therapy. Am J Ophthalmol. 1976;81(4):383–96. https://doi.org/10.1016/0002-9394(76)90292-0.
10. Little HL, Rosenthal AR, Dellaporta A, Jacobson DR. The effect of pan-retinal photo-coagulation on rubeosis iridis. Am J Ophthalmol. 1976;81(6):804–9. https://doi.org/10.1016/0002-9394(76)90364-0.
11. Photocoagulation treatment of proliferative diabetic retinopathy. Clinical application of Diabetic Retinopathy Study (DRS) findings, DRS Report Number 8. The Diabetic Retinopathy Study Research Group. Ophthalmology. 1981;88(7):583–600.
12. Four risk factors for severe visual loss in diabetic retinopathy. The third report from the Diabetic Retinopathy Study. The Diabetic Retinopathy Study Research Group. Arch Ophthalmol. 1979;97(4):654–5. https://doi.org/10.1001/archopht.1979.01020010310003.
13. Havens SJ, Gulati V. Neovascular glaucoma. Dev Ophthalmol. 2016;55:196–204. https://doi.org/10.1159/000431196.
14. Blumenkranz MS, Yellachich D, Andersen DE, Wiltberger MW, Mordaunt D, Marcellino GR, et al. Semiautomated patterned scanning laser for retinal photocoagulation. Retina. 2006;26(3):370–6. https://doi.org/10.1097/00006982-200603000-00024.
15. Schuele G, Rumohr M, Huettmann G, Brinkmann R. RPE damage thresholds and mechanisms for laser exposure in the microsecond-to-millisecond time regimen. Invest Ophthalmol Vis Sci. 2005;46(2):714–9. https://doi.org/10.1167/iovs.04-0136.
16. Sanghvi C, McLauchlan R, Delgado C, Young L, Charles SJ, Marcellino G, et al. Initial experience with the Pascal photocoagulator: a pilot study of 75 procedures. Br J Ophthalmol. 2008;92(8):1061. https://doi.org/10.1136/bjo.2008.139568.
17. Nagpal M, Marlecha S, Nagpal K. Comparison of laser photocoagulation for diabetic retinopathy using 532-nm standard laser versus multispot pattern scan laser. Retina. 2010;30(3):452–8. https://doi.org/10.1097/IAE.0b013e3181c70127.
18. Muqit MM, Marcellino GR, Gray JC, McLauchlan R, Henson DB, Young LB, et al. Pain responses of Pascal 20 ms multi-spot and 100 ms single-spot panretinal

photocoagulation: Manchester Pascal Study, MAPASS report 2. Br J Ophthalmol. 2010;94(11):1493–8. https://doi.org/10.1136/bjo.2009.176677.

19. Muqit MM, Marcellino GR, Henson DB, Young LB, Turner GS, Stanga PE. Pascal panretinal laser ablation and regression analysis in proliferative diabetic retinopathy: Manchester Pascal Study Report 4. Eye. 2011;25(11):1447–56. https://doi.org/10.1038/eye.2011.188.

20. Muqit MM, Denniss J, Nourrit V, Marcellino GR, Henson DB, Schiessl I, et al. Spatial and spectral imaging of retinal laser photocoagulation burns. Invest Ophthalmol Vis Sci. 2011;52(2):994–1002. https://doi.org/10.1167/iovs.10-6309.

21. Bressler SB, Beaulieu WT, Glassman AR, Gross JG, Jampol LM, Melia M, et al. Factors associated with worsening proliferative diabetic retinopathy in eyes treated with panretinal photocoagulation or ranibizumab. Ophthalmology. 2017;124(4):431–9. https://doi.org/10.1016/j.ophtha.2016.12.005.

22. Thomas M, Rao RC, Johnson MW, Paulus YM. Re: Bressler et al.: Factors associated with worsening proliferative diabetic retinopathy in eyes treated with panretinal photocoagulation or ranibizumab (Ophthalmology. 2017;124:431–439). Ophthalmology. 2017;124(12):e87–e8. https://doi.org/10.1016/j.ophtha.2017.06.025.

23. Alasil T, Waheed NK. Pan retinal photocoagulation for proliferative diabetic retinopathy: pattern scan laser versus argon laser. Curr Opin Ophthalmol. 2014;25:3.

24. Sivaprasad S, Prevost AT, Vasconcelos JC, Riddell A, Murphy C, Kelly J, et al. Clinical efficacy of intravitreal aflibercept versus panretinal photocoagulation for best corrected visual acuity in patients with proliferative diabetic retinopathy at 52 weeks (CLARITY): a multicentre, single-blinded, randomised, controlled, phase 2b, non-inferiority trial. Lancet. 2017;389(10085):2193–203. https://doi.org/10.1016/S0140-6736(17)31193-5.

25. Writing Committee for the Diabetic Retinopathy Clinical Research N, Gross JG, Glassman AR, Jampol LM, Inusah S, Aiello LP, et al. Panretinal photocoagulation vs Intravitreous ranibizumab for proliferative diabetic retinopathy: a randomized clinical trial. JAMA. 2015;314(20):2137–46. https://doi.org/10.1001/jama.2015.15217.

26. Gross JG, Glassman AR, Liu D, Sun JK, Antoszyk AN, Baker CW, et al. Five-year outcomes of panretinal photocoagulation vs intravitreous ranibizumab for proliferative diabetic retinopathy: a randomized clinical trial. JAMA Ophthalmol. 2018;136(10):1138–48. https://doi.org/10.1001/jamaophthalmol.2018.3255.

27. Obeid A, Su D, Patel SN, Uhr JH, Borkar D, Gao X, et al. Outcomes of eyes lost to follow-up with proliferative diabetic retinopathy that received panretinal photocoagulation versus intravitreal anti–

vascular endothelial growth factor. Ophthalmology. 2019;126(3):407–13. https://doi.org/10.1016/j.ophtha.2018.07.027.

28. Laatikainen L, Kohner EM, Khoury D, Blach RK. Panretinal photocoagulation in central retinal vein occlusion: a randomised controlled clinical study. Br J Ophthalmol. 1977;61(12):741–53. https://doi.org/10.1136/bjo.61.12.741.

29. Laatikainen L. A prospective follow-up study of panretinal photocoagulation in preventing neovascular glaucoma following ischaemic central retinal vein occlusion. Graefe's Arch Clin Exp Ophthalmol. 1983;220(5):236–9. https://doi.org/10.1007/bf02308081.

30. May DR, Klein ML, Peyman GA, Raichand M. Xenon arc panretinal photocoagulation for central retinal vein occlusion: a randomised prospective study. Br J Ophthalmol. 1979;63(11):725–34. https://doi.org/10.1136/bjo.63.11.725.

31. Magargal LE, Brown GC, Augsburger JJ, Donoso LA. Efficacy of panretinal photocoagulation in preventing neovascular glaucoma following ischemic central retinal vein obstruction. Ophthalmology. 1982;89(7):780–4. https://doi.org/10.1016/s0161-6420(82)34724-7.

32. Laatikainen L, Blach RK. Behaviour of the iris vasculature in central retinal vein occlusion: a fluorescein angiographic study of the vascular response of the retina and the iris. Br J Ophthalmol. 1977;61(4):272–7. https://doi.org/10.1136/bjo.61.4.272.

33. A randomized clinical trial of early panretinal photocoagulation for ischemic central vein occlusion. The Central Vein Occlusion Study Group N report. Ophthalmology. 1995;102(10):1434–44.

34. Natural history and clinical management of central retinal vein occlusion. The Central Vein Occlusion Study Group. Arch Ophthalmol. 1997;115(4):486–91. https://doi.org/10.1001/archopht.1997.01100150488006.

35. Mohamed Q, McIntosh RL, Saw SM, Wong TY. Interventions for central retinal vein occlusion: an evidence-based systematic review. Ophthalmology. 2007;114(3):507-19., 24. https://doi.org/10.1016/j.ophtha.2006.11.011.

36. Bradshaw SE, Gala S, Nanavaty M, Shah A, Mwamburi M, Kefalas P. Systematic literature review of treatments for management of complications of ischemic central retinal vein occlusion. BMC Ophthalmol. 2016;16:104. https://doi.org/10.1186/s12886-016-0282-5.

37. Wittstrom E, Holmberg H, Hvarfner C, Andreasson S. Clinical and electrophysiologic outcome in patients with neovascular glaucoma treated with and without bevacizumab. Italy: Wichtig Editore; 2012. p. 563.

38. Ehlers JP, Spirn MJ, Lam A, Sivalingam A, Samuel MA, Tasman W. Combination intravitreal bevacizumab/panretinal photocoagulation versus panretinal

photocoagulation alone in the treatment of neovascular glaucoma. Retina (Philadelphia, Pa). 2008;28(5):696–702. https://doi.org/10.1097/IAE.0b013e3181679c0b.

39. Jung YH, Ahn SJ, Hong JH, Park KH, Han MK, Jung C, et al. Incidence and clinical features of neovascularization of the iris following acute central retinal artery occlusion. Korean J Ophthalmol: KJO. 2016;30(5):352–9. https://doi.org/10.3341/kjo.2016.30.5.352.

40. Rudkin AK, Lee AW, Chen CS. Ocular neovascularization following central retinal artery occlusion: prevalence and timing of onset. Eur J Ophthalmol. 2010;20(6):1042–6. https://doi.org/10.1177/112067211002000603.

41. Duker JS, Sivalingam A, Brown GC, Reber R. A prospective study of acute central retinal artery obstruction: the incidence of secondary ocular neovascularization. Arch Ophthalmol. 1991;109(3):339–42. https://doi.org/10.1001/archopht.1991.01080030041034.

42. Duker JS, Brown GC. The efficacy of panretinal photocoagulation for neovascularization of the iris after central retinal artery obstruction. Ophthalmology. 1989;96(1):92–5. https://doi.org/10.1016/s0161-6420(89)32946-0.

43. Sagong M, Kim J, Chang W. Intravitreal bevacizumab for the treatment of neovascular glaucoma associated with central retinal artery occlusion. Korean J Ophthalmol: KJO. 2009;23(3):215–8. https://doi.org/10.3341/kjo.2009.23.3.215.

44. Vatavuk Z, Bencic G, Mandic Z. Intravitreal bevacizumab for neovascular glaucoma following central retinal artery occlusion. Eur J Ophthalmol. 2007;17(2):269–71. https://doi.org/10.1177/112067210701700220.

45. Carter JE. Panretinal photocoagulation for progressive ocular neovascularization secondary to occlusion of the common carotid artery. Ann Ophthalmol. 1984;16(6):572–6.

46. Mizener JB, Podhajsky P, Hayreh SS. Ocular ischemic syndrome. Ophthalmology. 1997;104(5):859–64. https://doi.org/10.1016/S0161-6420(97)30221-8.

47. Brown GC, Sharma S, Brown MM. Ocular ischemic syndrome. In: Schachat AP, editor. Ryan's retina. 6th ed. Elsevier; 2018. p. 1227–39.

48. Yuki T, Kimura Y, Nanbu S, Kishi S, Shimizu K. Ciliary body and choroidal detachment after laser photocoagulation for diabetic retinopathy. A high-frequency ultrasound study. Ophthalmology. 1997;104(8):1259–64. https://doi.org/10.1016/s0161-6420(97)30149-3.

49. Reddy SV, Husain D. Panretinal photocoagulation: a review of complications. Semin Ophthalmol. 2018;33(1):83–8. https://doi.org/10.1080/08820538.2017.1353820.

50. Sun Y, Liang Y, Zhou P, Wu H, Hou X, Ren Z, et al. Anti-VEGF treatment is the key strategy for neovascular glaucoma management in the short term. BMC Ophthalmol. 2016;16(1):150. https://doi.org/10.1186/s12886-016-0327-9.

51. Doft BH, Blankenship GW. Single versus multiple treatment sessions of argon laser panretinal photocoagulation for proliferative diabetic retinopathy. Ophthalmology. 1982;89(7):772–9. https://doi.org/10.1016/s0161-6420(82)34734-x.

52. Schatz P, Aldayel A, Taskintuna I, Abdelkader E, Mura M. Serous retinal detachment after panretinal photocoagulation for proliferative diabetic retinopathy: a case report. J Med Case Rep. 2017;11(1):265. https://doi.org/10.1186/s13256-017-1424-y.

53. Sahto AA, Nangrejo KM, Siddique SJ, Abbassi AM. Incidence of complications in single vs multiple treatment sessions of green laser panretinal photocoagulation for proliferative diabetic retinopathy. Medical Channel. 2011;17(4):91–3.

54. Gharbiya M, Grandinetti F, Balacco GC. Intravitreal triamcinolone for macular detachment following panretinal photocoagulation. Eye. 2005;19(7):818–20. https://doi.org/10.1038/sj.eye.6701658.

55. Hayreh SS, Klugman MR, Podhajsky P, Servais GE, Perkins ES. Argon laser panretinal photocoagulation in ischemic central retinal vein occlusion. A 10-year prospective study. Graefe's Arch Clin Exp Ophthalmol. 1990;228(4):281–96. https://doi.org/10.1007/bf00920049.

56. Subash M, Comyn O, Samy A, Qatarneh D, Antonakis S, Mehat M, et al. The effect of multispot laser panretinal photocoagulation on retinal sensitivity and driving eligibility in patients with diabetic retinopathy. JAMA Ophthal. 2016;134(6):666–72. https://doi.org/10.1001/jamaophthalmol.2016.0629.

57. Frank RN. Visual fields and electroretinography following extensive photocoagulation. Arch Ophthalmol. 1975;93(8):591–8. https://doi.org/10.1001/archopht.1975.01010020575004.

58. Wittström E, Ponjavic V, Lövestam-Adrian M, Larsson J, Andréasson S. Electrophysiological evaluation and visual outcome in patients with central retinal vein occlusion, primary open-angle glaucoma and neovascular glaucoma. Acta Ophthalmol. 2010;88(1):86–90. https://doi.org/10.1111/j.1755-3768.2008.01424.x.

59. Seiberth V, Alexandridis E, Feng W. Function of the diabetic retina after panretinal argon laser coagulation. Graefe's Arch Clin Exp Ophthalmol. 1987;225(6):385–90. https://doi.org/10.1007/bf02334163.

60. Bavinger JC, Dunbar GE, Stem MS, Blachley TS, Kwark L, Farsiu S, et al. The effects of diabetic retinopathy and pan-retinal photocoagulation on photoreceptor cell function as assessed by dark adaptometry. Invest Ophthalmol Vis Sci. 2016;57(1):208–17. https://doi.org/10.1167/iovs.15-17281.

61. Googe J, Brucker AJ, Bressler NM, Qin H, Aiello LP, Antoszyk A, et al. Randomized trial evaluating short-term effects of intravitreal ranibizumab or triamcino-

lone acetonide on macular edema after focal/grid laser for diabetic macular edema in eyes also receiving panretinal photocoagulation. Retina. 2011;31(6):1009–27. https://doi.org/10.1097/IAE.0b013e318217d739.

62. Brucker AJ, Qin H, Antoszyk AN, Beck RW, Bressler NM, Browning DJ, et al. Observational study of the development of diabetic macular edema following panretinal (scatter) photocoagulation given in 1 or 4 sittings. Arch Ophthalmol. 2009;127(2):132–40. https://doi.org/10.1001/archophthalmol.2008.565.

63. Preti RC, Ramirez LM, Monteiro ML, Carra MK, Pelayes DE, Takahashi WY. Contrast sensitivity evaluation in high risk proliferative diabetic retinopathy treated with panretinal photocoagulation associated or not with intravitreal bevacizumab injections: a randomised clinical trial. Br J Ophthalmol. 2013;97(7):885–9. https://doi.org/10.1136/bjophthalmol-2012-302675.

Anti-Vascular Endothelial Growth Factor for Neovascular Glaucoma

Narine Viruni and Cindy X. Cai

1 Introduction and Anti-VEGF Mechanism of Action

Neovascular glaucoma (NVG) is an aggressive form of secondary glaucoma that develops in response to posterior segment ischemia. It is associated with the production of pro-angiogenic factors that promote neovascularization of the iris (NVI) and iridocorneal angle (NVA), which obstructs aqueous outflow through the trabecular meshwork, resulting in elevated intraocular pressure (IOP). Neovascularization is a complex process that involves various pro-angiogenic and anti-angiogenic factors. Vascular endothelial growth factor (VEGF) is a hypoxia-induced angiogenic factor that plays a major role in mediating neovascularization [1–4]. Intravitreal injections of recombinant human VEGF have been shown to produce NVI, and prolonged exposure to VEGF leads to NVG in a non-human primate model [3]. Increased levels of VEGF have been identified in the aqueous humor of human eyes with NVG [5]. Historically, panretinal photocoagulation (PRP) has been the treatment of choice in controlling the VEGF signal in eyes with retinal ischemia [6, 7], and the role of PRP in managing NVG will be discussed in detail in another

chapter. However, PRP alone may not completely halt anterior segment neovascularization in every patient [8] or may not be possible due to media opacity. Anti-VEGF antibodies directly block the pro-angiogenic factors leading to neovascularization and are important in the treatment of NVG [9, 10].

VEGF is a member of a family of proteins including VEGF-A, VEGF-B, VEGF-C, VEGF-D, and placental growth factor, of which VEGF-A plays the dominant role in regulating angiogenesis [11]. Several agents have been developed to target VEGF-A. Bevacizumab is a neutralizing recombinant humanized monoclonal antibody designed to inhibit all major isoforms of human VEGF-A and is approved by the U.S. Food and Drug Administration for the treatment of metastatic colorectal, non-small cell lung cancer, and other malignancies [12]. Intravitreal bevacizumab is used off-label to treat VEGF-mediated ocular diseases, including NVG [13]. Ranibizumab is an antigen-binding fragment (Fab) of a humanized monoclonal antibody that binds to the VEGF-A receptors VEGFR1 and VEGFR2 thereby blocking the interaction of VEGF-A with these receptors [14]. Aflibercept is a recombinant fusion protein of portions of VEGF receptors 1 and 2 that binds to and inhibits VEGF-A and placental growth factor (PGF) [15]. Brolucizumab is a humanized monoclonal single-chain antibody fragment that binds to the three major isoforms of VEGF-A thereby pre-

N. Viruni · C. X. Cai (✉)
Wilmer Eye Institute, Johns Hopkins University,
Baltimore, MD, USA
e-mail: ccai6@jhmi.edu

© The Author(s), under exclusive license to Springer Nature Switzerland AG 2022
M. Qiu (ed.), *Neovascular Glaucoma*, Essentials in Ophthalmology,
https://doi.org/10.1007/978-3-031-11720-6_14

venting interaction with receptors VEGFR-1 and VEGFR-2 [16]. The majority of studies involving anti-VEGF in treatment of NVG utilize bevacizumab, but ranibizumab and aflibercept have also been reported.

2 Role of Anti-VEGF in Various Stages of NVG

The clinical manifestation of NVG exists on a spectrum that has historically been divided into four stages: (1) the prerubeosis stage, in which there is no visible anterior segment neovascularization, and the IOP is normal, (2) the pre-glaucoma stage, in which there is visible anterior segment neovascularization, and the IOP is normal, (3) the open-angle NVG stage, in which there is anterior segment neovascularization, the IOP is elevated, and the angle is still open without peripheral anterior synechiae, and (4) the closed-angle NVG stage, in which there is anterior segment neovascularization, the IOP is elevated, and the angle has become synechially closed due to peripheral anterior synechiae [17, 18]. Of note, the open-angle and closed-angle NVG stages refer to elevated IOP with or without true glaucomatous optic neuropathy; however, the historical convention is to refer to these stages as "NVG," and for the purpose of this chapter, this terminology will be used. Future consensus panels are needed to determine whether neovascular "ocular hypertension" may be a more descriptive term in the setting of elevated IOP without true glaucomatous optic neuropathy.

2.1 Anti-VEGF Therapy in Prerubeosis Stage of NVG

Prerubeosis stage refers to a precursor stage to NVG, in which there is no visible anterior segment neovascularization or IOP elevation. Patients with any ischemic retinal diseases are inherently at risk for developing neovascular complications, including NVG. Chronic VEGF suppression in eyes undergoing anti-VEGF ther-

apy for other indications (e.g., macular edema, vitreous hemorrhage) could result in decreased risk for anterior segment neovascularization. Eyes with moderate and severe non-proliferative diabetic retinopathy undergoing aflibercept injections have been reported to be at lower risk for developing proliferative complications including NVI/NVA and NVG [19].

2.2 Anti-VEGF Therapy in Pre-Glaucoma Stage of NVG

Administration of intravitreal or intracameral anti-VEGF can lead to rapid regression of NVI within days of treatment [18, 20–26]. In the most detailed study of the effects of anti-VEGF in the pre-glaucoma stage of NVG using iris fluorescein angiography, Luke et al. reported that intravitreal anti-VEGF injections combined with PRP resulted in 70% complete and 30% partial regression of NVI at 2 weeks of follow-up [21]. Although 90% of NVI recurred, repeat anti-VEGF injections were administered, and complete or partial regression of NVI was sustained through 12 months of follow-up. No patients developed NVA, elevated IOP, or required IOP-lowering surgery during 12 months of follow-up.

2.3 Anti-VEGF Therapy in Open-Angle Stage of NVG

Intravitreal anti-VEGF can be effective in reducing anterior segment neovascularization and normalizing IOP in eyes with open-angle NVG, especially when the anti-VEGF injections are administered on a scheduled basis. Soohoo et al. evaluated the effects of serial intravitreal anti-VEGF injections on four eyes with either (1) newly diagnosed NVI and NVA with normal IOP or (2) NVI and NVA with elevated IOP but no synechial angle closure [27]. Patients received an anti-VEGF injection at the initial diagnosis and received additional scheduled anti-VEGF injections at 4 weeks, 8 weeks, and every 8 weeks thereafter for a total of 52 weeks. All eyes demonstrated rapid regression of NVI and NVA with normalization of the IOP as early as 1 day following treatment. An average of 6.8 injections were given. IOP control was maintained on topical IOP-lowering medications without any eyes requiring IOP-lowering surgery, and this effect was sustained through 52 weeks of follow-up. In this small series of 4 patients, 1 patient already had prior PRP, and no patients received additional PRP during the follow-up period, demonstrating the therapeutic effect from anti-VEGF alone. These results suggest that anti-VEGF, if initiated early and administered regularly, may have the potential to delay or avoid the need for IOP-lowering surgery in NVG eyes with open angles.

On the other hand, when anti-VEGF injections were administered for open-angle NVG on an as-needed basis for recurrent NVI with elevated IOP, as compared to a scheduled basis regardless of NVI or IOP status, lower success rates have been reported. In a retrospective case series by Wakabayashi et al., eyes with NVI, elevated IOP, and open angles were treated with an intravitreal anti-VEGF injection [18]. Rapid regression of NVI and normalization of IOP occurred in 71% of eyes within 1 week after a single injection. Subsequently, 58% developed recurrent NVI with elevated IOP, requiring another anti-VEGF injection; the interval between the initial anti-VEGF and NVI recurrence ranged from 29 to 120 days. In this series, 71% of patients underwent additional PRP, 29% required IOP-lowering surgery within 6 months despite anti-VEGF injections, and 41% eventually required IOP-lowering surgery during a mean follow-up of 13 months.

The key difference between the Soohoo study and the Wakabayashi study is that the Soohoo study employed the strategy of administering serial anti-VEGF on a scheduled basis, for an average of 6.8 injections over the course of 12 months. In contrast, the Wakabayashi study employed the strategy of administering repeated anti-VEGF injections only on an as-needed basis when there was recurrent NVI and elevated IOP, for an average of two injections over the course of 6 months. In this setting, many eyes developed recurrent NVI, NVA, and elevated IOP, and

41% progressed to require IOP-lowering surgery. The results from these two studies suggest that regularly scheduled serial anti-VEGF injections in open-angle NVG has the potential to prevent NVI/NVA recurrence, IOP elevation, disease progression, and need for IOP-lowering surgery.

2.4 Anti-VEGF Therapy in Closed-Angle Stage of NVG

Although still effective for regressing anterior and posterior segment neovascularization, anti-VEGF injections may be less effective for normalizing IOP or reducing the need for IOP-lowering surgery in NVG eyes that have already developed extensive synechial angle closure [18, 21, 28–32]. In a prospective interventional case series, Luke et al. investigated intravitreal anti-VEGF injections as an adjunct to PRP in eyes with NVI, NVA, and elevated IOP [21]. All patients received intravitreal anti-VEGF in combination with PRP at baseline, and injections were repeated if there was recurrent, persistent, or worsening NVA. At 14 days after initial injection, 70% had complete NVI regression and 30% had unchanged rubeosis status. The baseline IOP was 41.4 ± 13.4 mmHg which decreased to 13.9 ± 3.4 mmHg by 12 months of follow-up. In eyes that did not already have complete synechial angle closure at baseline, adjuvant anti-VEGF injections prevented progressive synechial angle closure. However, eyes that already had extensive synechial angle closure at baseline, anti-VEGF injections did not normalize the IOP, and these eyes required IOP-lowering surgery for adequate IOP control.

Similar findings were reported in the aforementioned study by Wakabayashi et al. [18] In NVG eyes with $\geq 270°$ synechial angle closure, anti-VEGF injections led to NVI regression but did not normalize the IOP. Despite repeated intravitreal anti-VEGF injections and additional PRP, 93% of eyes with closed-angle NVG required IOP-lowering surgery within 2 months. In contrast, among NVG eyes with <90° synechial angle closure, only 41% of eyes required IOP-lowering surgery to achieve IOP control. The mean interval between intravitreal anti-VEGF and IOP-lowering surgery was significantly shorter in the closed-angle NVG group compared to the open-angle NVG group (11 days compared to 195 days, respectively). The results from these studies suggest that while anti-VEGF is ubiquitously effective at regressing neovascularization in all stages of NVG, anti-VEGF is not as effective in lowering IOP in NVG eyes with extensive synechial closure compared to NVG eyes with angles that are still mostly open. These results call attention to the window of opportunity that exists in NVG eyes with open angles to administer anti-VEGF promptly to prevent synechial angle closure and need for IOP-lowering surgery.

3 Anti-VEGF Route of Administration

Anti-VEGF can be administered intravitreally, intracamerally, subconjunctivally, and topically in the setting of NVG. Pharmacokinetic studies of anti-VEGF in rabbit models suggest that intravitreal injection of anti-VEGF achieves the highest concentrations of the medication in the iris, ciliary body, retina, and choroid [33]. Intracameral administration can have a similar clinical effect in reducing anterior segment neovascularization compared to intravitreal injection [34]. Subconjunctival administration of anti-VEGF achieves acceptable levels, while topical administration appears to have poor distribution in target tissues [33].

3.1 Intravitreal Anti-VEGF Monotherapy

The most common route of administration of anti-VEGF is intravitreal. Intravitreal bevacizumab 1.25 mg/0.05 mL, ranibizumab 0.5 mg/0.05 mL, and aflibercept 2.0 mg/0.05 have all been reported in the context of NVG. Regression of NVI appears as early as 1 day after the treatment [27, 34] with recurrences of NVI appearing anywhere between 4 days and 15 months [13, 18, 20, 21, 27–30, 35,

36] after the initial treatment, though the presence of NVI at 4 days may represent incomplete regression rather than NVI recurrence. Overall, 44% of eyes in the pre-glaucoma stage of NVG recur by 6 months whereas 71% of eyes in the open-angle stage of NVG recur by 6 months [18].

3.2 Intracameral Anti-VEGF Monotherapy

Intracameral anti-VEGF appears to be as effective as intravitreal anti-VEGF in regressing NVI. Grover et al. reported that intracameral anti-VEGF reduces aqueous VEGF concentrations by 50–79% [37]. The effects of intracameral anti-VEGF injection are rapid, and marked regression of NVI and NVA can be seen within a week of administration [31, 32, 38]. As with intravitreal administration, there is often recurrence of anterior segment neovascularization [32, 37–39]. In a retrospective case series by Wolf et al., eyes with NVG despite prior PRP were treated with a single intracameral anti-VEGF injection [39]. Resolution of NVI was noted in 92% of eyes at 1 week of follow-up. During 6 months of follow-up, NVI recurred in all eyes, with a median time to recurrence of 18 days (range 8–160 days), though the presence of NVI at 8 days may represent incomplete regression rather than NVI recurrence. A significant IOP-lowering effect was also observed at 1 week following treatment with a single intracameral anti-VEGF injection, but this analysis was not stratified by the status of the angle anatomy. More evidence is needed regarding whether anterior segment neovascularization recurs earlier after intracameral anti-VEGF injection compared to intravitreal anti-VEGF injection.

3.3 Subconjunctival Anti-VEGF Monotherapy

Subconjunctival administration of anti-VEGF in the setting of NVG has also been reported [40, 41]. In a consecutive case series, Ryoo et al. showed that a dose of 2.5–3.75 mg/0.1–0.15 mL bevacizumab injected near the limbus in two or three quadrants induced regression of iris and angle neovascularization and lowered IOP [41].

3.4 Topical Anti-VEGF Monotherapy

Topical administration of anti-VEGF in the setting of NVG has also been tried, but its efficacy appears limited. In a series by Waisbourd et al., eyes with NVG were treated with a 2-week course of topical bevacizumab (25 mg/mL) four times daily to assess whether topical anti-VEGF could be effective at regressing NVI [42]. Mean IOP reduction of 17.5% was observed, however only 38% patients had regression of NVI.

4 Indications for Repeat Anti-VEGF Administration

The aqueous half-life of a single intravitreal bevacizumab injection in non-vitrectomized human eyes is approximately 10 days [43], and the inhibitory effect may be transient [44]. As a result, there is typically recurrence of anterior segment neovascularization after the initial anti-VEGF treatment [13, 18, 20, 21, 28–30, 32, 35, 37, 38]. The cumulative proportion of eyes with recurrent anterior segment neovascularization appears to increase linearly with time [13]. There is currently no widely accepted consensus or standardized treatment guidelines regarding if and when to administer subsequent anti-VEGF in NVG eyes. Some perform repeat anti-VEGF injection for recurrent or persistent anterior segment neovascularization on clinical exam or fluorescein angiography [13, 20, 21, 30, 35, 36, 38, 45, 46]. Some perform repeat anti-VEGF injection for elevated IOP over 30 mmHg [13, 47]. Some use anti-VEGF as a temporizing measure before initiation of PRP or proceeding to IOP-lowering surgery and do not subsequently retreat [28–30, 32, 45–50]. Others treat with anti-VEGF on a scheduled rather as-needed basis [27]. The scheduled serial treatment strategy has the potential for sustained suppression of neovasculariza-

tion; however, further research is needed to develop an optimal treatment protocol.

5 Anti-VEGF as an Adjunct to Other Treatments

5.1 Anti-VEGF as an Adjunct to Panretinal Photocoagulation

Anti-VEGF can be used as an adjunct to PRP [30, 49–54]. Compared to PRP alone, the addition of anti-VEGF can lead to more rapid regression of NVI [50, 51]. In a retrospective case control study of 23 eyes, Ehlers et al. compared a same-day combination treatment of intravitreal anti-VEGF and PRP versus PRP alone in eyes with NVG [51]. There was no stratification by the status of the angle anatomy, open versus closed. Complete regression of NVI was observed more frequently in the combination treatment group than in the PRP only group, 100% versus 17% eyes. In addition, among eyes with NVI regression, the rate of regression was more rapid in the combination group than in the PRP only group (12 versus 127 days to complete regression, respectively). Regression of anterior segment neovascularization corresponded to a larger magnitude of IOP-lowering in the combination group. The combination group demonstrated an average IOP-lowering of 11 mmHg from initial treatment to the first follow-up at an average of 9.2 days, whereas the PRP only group had no change in IOP at the first follow-up at an average of 18.8 days. Similar results have been reported by other authors. In a retrospective consecutive case series, Vasudev et al. described 29 eyes with NVG treated with a single injection of intravitreal anti-VEGF followed by PRP 1 week later compared to PRP alone [50]. The baseline IOP was 32.8 mmHg in the combination group and 28.5 mmHg in the PRP alone group, and the two groups had similar extent of closed angles at baseline. Eyes in the intravitreal anti-VEGF group had more rapid NVI regression than eyes in the PRP alone group. More open angles were observed in the combination group than the control group at 6 months, and the difference persisted at 1 year of follow-up. The median IOP at the 6-month follow-up was lower in the combination group but there was no difference in IOP at the 12-month follow-up. There was no difference between the groups with respect to visual acuity outcomes. In a retrospective comparative case series of eyes with NVG treated with intravitreal anti-VEGF, Olmos et al. found that anti-VEGF delayed the need for IOP-lowering surgery, but PRP reduced rates of IOP-lowering surgery [55]. These studies suggest that utilizing anti-VEGF to promptly regress NVA in open-angle NVG can prevent progressive synechial angle closure and preserve open angles and potentially achieve better IOP control. Despite the advantages of adjunctive anti-VEGF, PRP remains a necessary definitive therapy in controlling the underlying retinal ischemia driving the neovascularization process and can reduce the need for IOP-lowering surgery. The role of PRP in managing NVG will be discussed in detail in the another chapter.

5.2   Anti-VEGF as an Adjunct to Trabeculectomy

Trabeculectomy may have limited success in the setting of NVG due to intraoperative or postoperative bleeding and excessive inflammation leading to scarring or encapsulation of the filtering bleb [8, 56]. Anti-VEGF medications can decrease fibroblast activity and have potential wound modulatory properties [56]. Studies exploring the use of anti-VEGF at time of trabeculectomy or bleb revision in the absence of NVG suggest a beneficial effect of anti-VEGF on bleb survival and IOP control [57]. In a histologic study of surgically excised trabecular meshwork tissue in eyes with NVG that underwent trabeculectomy, eyes treated with preoperative intravitreal anti-VEGF 2–7 days before trabeculectomy were found to have decreased edema, fibrin deposition, inflammation, and vascular congestion in the trabecular meshwork compared to eyes without preoperative anti-VEGF [58]. In patients with primary open-angle glaucoma without NVG, combination intravitreal anti-

VEGF and standard subconjunctival mitomycin C at time of trabeculectomy surgery resulted in more diffuse blebs with less vascularity compared to mitomycin C alone [59].

There is evidence that intravitreal anti-VEGF therapy as an adjunct to trabeculectomy decreases the risk of intraoperative and postoperative bleeding [45–48, 60–62]. However, anti-VEGF as an adjunct to trabeculectomy does not result in a more favorable long-term IOP, number of IOP-lowering medications, or rates of trabeculectomy revision [61–63]. In a retrospective interventional case series, Chen et al. compared eyes with NVG treated with trabeculectomy with adjunctive preoperative intravitreal anti-VEGF versus trabeculectomy alone [61]. Compared to the trabeculectomy alone group, the combination group had a higher frequency of NVI regression, improved visual acuity compared to their own baseline, fewer cases of progression to no light perception, and fewer intraoperative or postoperative complications, such as intraoperative bleeding, postoperative hyphema, hypotony, flat anterior chamber, or elevated IOP over 30 mmHg. However, there were no statistically significant differences in IOP at the final follow-up (179 ± 97 days for the anti-VEGF group, and 196 ± 108 days for the trabeculectomy alone group), number of IOP-lowering medications, or need for trabeculectomy revision. In another study, Takihara et al. compared eyes with NVG treated with trabeculectomy with adjunctive intravitreal anti-VEGF 1–4 days prior to surgery versus trabeculectomy alone [62]. Compared to the trabeculectomy alone group, the combination group had lower rates of hyphema and lower IOP at postoperative day 7 and day 10. By postoperative month 3, there were no differences in the IOP between the two groups. These studies suggest that anti-VEGF as a preoperative adjunct to trabeculectomy can decrease intraoperative and postoperative bleeding but does not necessarily improve long-term IOP control, which is limited by scarring of the filtering bleb in the setting of NVG. The role of trabeculectomy in managing NVG will be discussed in detail in another chapter.

5.3 Anti-VEGF as an Adjunct to Aqueous Shunt Surgery

Due to the relatively high failure rates of trabeculectomy in the setting of NVG, aqueous shunts are more frequently employed as the IOP-lowering surgery of choice for NVG. The valved Ahmed FP7 implant is commonly chosen because it provides immediate IOP lowering. There is evidence that intravitreal anti-VEGF as an adjunct to the Ahmed FP7 valved aqueous shunt decreases bleeding-associated complications. The incidence of hyphema, vitreous hemorrhage, and suprachoroidal hemorrhages are lower when anti-VEGF is combined with the Ahmed shunt [64–72]. In a systematic review including six studies involving 256 eyes [65–69, 73], Hwang et al. compared eyes with NVG treated with the Ahmed shunt with adjunctive intravitreal anti-VEGF versus the Ahmed alone. Compared to the Ahmed alone group, the combination group had a higher rate of achieving adequate IOP control at 1 year (66% versus 83%, respectively) [64]. The incidence of bleeding-associated complications, such as hyphema, vitreous hemorrhage, and suprachoroidal hemorrhages was lower in the combination group compared to the Ahmed alone group. Compared to the Ahmed alone group, the combination group also had a lower incidence of other adverse effects, such as hypotony, flat chamber, choroidal detachment/effusion, tube-associated complications, and corneal decompensation.

Although there is strong evidence that anti-VEGF as an adjunct to aqueous shunt surgery reduces complications, especially bleeding-associated complications, there is no consensus regarding the effect of adjunctive anti-VEGF on postoperative IOP outcomes [67, 69–71, 73–75]. In a prospective non-randomized trial, Tang et al. compared 43 NVG eyes treated with the Ahmed shunt and adjunctive intravitreal anti-VEGF 3 to 14 days prior to surgery versus the Ahmed alone [74]. Surgical success was defined as IOP 6–21 mmHg with or without topical medications and without complications or reoperation, and there was no statistically significant difference in the surgical success rate between the combination group and the Ahmed alone group at 12 months (72% versus 68%, respectively).

Other studies have suggested that intravitreal anti-VEGF as an adjunct to the Ahmed shunt in NVG may improve IOP control. In a prospective clinical trial, 50 eyes with NVG were randomized to undergo the Ahmed shunt with adjunctive subconjunctival bevacizumab 2.5 mg/0.1 mL at the time of surgery ($n = 25$) or Ahmed alone ($n = 25$) [76]. At the 6-month follow-up, the IOP was significantly lower in the combination group compared to the Ahmed alone group, but there was no difference at the 12-month follow-up. Surgical success was defined as IOP 5–21 mmHg with at least 20% reduction in IOP without glaucoma medications (complete success), or with no more than two medications (qualified success). The rates of complete, qualified, and cumulative success rate at 12 months, defined as sum of complete and qualified success, were higher in the combination group compared to the Ahmed alone group (20% versus 12%, 72% versus 56%, and 92% versus 68%, respectively). In another prospective trial, Mahdy et al. randomized 40 eyes with NVG to PRP followed by the Ahmed shunt with or without adjunctive intravitreal anti-VEGF [65]. Surgical success was defined as IOP < 21 mmHg (with or without IOP-lowering medications), and the success rate at 18 months was higher in the combination group compared to the Ahmed alone group (95% versus 50%, respectively). The combination group had lower IOP at all postoperative time points compared to the Ahmed alone group. The need for additional IOP-lowering surgery (second Ahmed shunt) was lower in the combination group compared to the Ahmed alone group (5% versus 50%, respectively). These results suggest that a combination of anti-VEGF, PRP, and aqueous shunt implantation may result in better IOP control and lower failure rates in the setting of NVG. The role of aqueous shunts in managing NVG will be discussed in detail in another chapter.

5.4 Anti-VEGF as an Adjunct to Micro-incisional Glaucoma Surgery (MIGS)

Micro-incisional glaucoma surgery (MIGS) is a new category of IOP-lowering surgery that has not been fully evaluated in the treatment of NVG. Our current understanding of surgical outcomes in NVG management primarily comes from the pre-anti-VEGF era. Since anti-VEGF treatments can regress anterior segment neovascularization and prevent progression to synechial closure in eyes with open angles, anti-VEGF combined with angle-based MIGS could be an effective strategy. More research is needed to evaluate the efficacy of combing anti-VEGF and MIGS procedures to salvage the conventional aqueous outflow pathway to maintain IOP control in NVG. The role of MIGS in managing NVG will be discussed in detail in another chapter.

6 Conclusion

In summary, intravitreal and intracameral anti-VEGF agents have been used as stand-alone or adjunctive treatments for NVG and have been shown to effectively and rapidly reduce anterior segment neovascularization. The effect of anti-VEGF on IOP lowering appears to depend on the angle status, with greater IOP-lowering effect reported in the earlier stages of NVG before the angle has become synechially closed. Anti-VEGF agents can be used as an adjunct to traditional glaucoma surgeries (trabeculectomy and aqueous shunt) to decrease the risk of intraoperative and postoperative bleeding-related complications, and there is some evidence to support that adjunctive anti-VEGF may also improve the final IOP outcome. As MIGS are being evaluated in various types of glaucoma, the ability of anti-VEGF agents to regress anterior segment neovascularization and maintain open-angle status may allow novel avenues in IOP control in NVG. Overall, anti-VEGF agents play an important role, in combination with PRP and traditional IOP-lowering surgery, in the management of NVG.

References

1. Aiello LP, et al. Vascular endothelial growth factor in ocular fluid of patients with diabetic retinopathy and other retinal disorders. New Engl J Med. 1994;331:1480–7.
2. Pe'er J, et al. Upregulated expression of vascular endothelial growth factor in proliferative diabetic retinopathy. Br J Ophthalmol. 1996;80:241.
3. Tolentino MJ, et al. Vascular endothelial growth factor is sufficient to produce iris neovascularization and neovascular glaucoma in a nonhuman primate. Arch Ophthalmol. 1996;114:964–70.
4. Adamis AP, et al. Increased vascular endothelial growth factor levels in the vitreous of eyes with proliferative diabetic retinopathy. Am J Ophthalmol. 1994;118:445–50.
5. Tripathi RC, Lixa J, Tripathi BJ, Chalam KV, Adamis AP. Increased level of vascular endothelial growth factor in aqueous humor of patients with neovascular glaucoma. Ophthalmology. 1998;105:232–7.
6. A randomized clinical trial of early panretinal photocoagulation for ischemic central vein occlusion. The Central Vein Occlusion Study Group N report. Ophthalmology. 1995;102:1434–44.
7. Rodrigues GB, et al. Neovascular glaucoma: a review. Int J Retin Vitreous. 2016;2:26.
8. Sivak-Callcott JA, O'Day DM, Gass JDM, Tsai JC. Evidence-based recommendations for the diagnosis and treatment of neovascular glaucoma 1 1 the authors do not have any proprietary or financial interest in any products or devices discussed in this study. Ophthalmology. 2001;108:1767–76.
9. Adamis AP, et al. Inhibition of vascular endothelial growth factor prevents retinal ischemia—associated iris neovascularization in a nonhuman primate. Arch Ophthalmol. 1996;114:66–71.
10. Park SC, Su D, Tello C. Anti-VEGF therapy for the treatment of glaucoma: a focus on ranibizumab and bevacizumab. Expert Opin Biol Ther. 2012;12:1641–7.
11. Apte RS, Chen DS, Ferrara N. VEGF in signaling and disease: beyond discovery and development. Cell. 2019;176:1248–64.
12. Ferrara N, Adamis AP. Ten Years of anti-vascular endothelial growth factor therapy. Nat Rev Drug Discov. 2016;15:385–403.
13. Moraczewski AL, Lee RK, Palmberg PF, Rosenfeld PJ, Feuer WJ. Outcomes of treatment of neovascular glaucoma with intravitreal bevacizumab. Br J Ophthalmol. 2009;93:589.
14. LUCENTIS®, (ranibizumab). Full prescribing information leaflet. Genetech, Inc; South San Francisco, CA, USA. 2017. (n.d.).
15. EYLEA®, (aflibercept). Full prescribing information leaflet. Regeneron Pharmaceuticals, Inc; Tarrytown, NY, USA. 2017. (n.d.).
16. BEOVU®, (brolucizumab). full prescribing information leaflet. Novartis Pharmaceuticals Corporation; East Hanover, NJ, USA. 2020. (n.d.).

17. Shazly TA, Latina MA. Neovascular glaucoma: etiology, diagnosis and prognosis. Semin Ophthalmol. 2009;24:113–21.

18. Wakabayashi T, et al. Intravitreal bevacizumab to treat iris neovascularization and neovascular glaucoma secondary to ischemic retinal diseases in 41 consecutive cases. Ophthalmology. 2008;115:1571–1580.e3.

19. Maturi RK, et al. Effect of intravitreous anti-vascular endothelial growth factor vs sham treatment for prevention of vision-threatening complications of diabetic retinopathy: the Protocol W Randomized Clinical Trial. JAMA Ophthalmol. 2021;139:701.

20. Avery RL, et al. Intravitreal bevacizumab (Avastin) in the treatment of proliferative diabetic retinopathy. Ophthalmology. 2006;113:1695-1705.e6.

21. Lüke J, Nassar K, Lüke M, Grisanti S. Ranibizumab as adjuvant in the treatment of rubeosis iridis and neovascular glaucoma—results from a prospective interventional case series. Graefe's Arch Clin Exp Ophthalmol. 2013;251:2403–13.

22. Dunavoelgyi R, Zehetmayer M, Simader C, Schmidt-Erfurth U. Rapid improvement of radiation-induced neovascular glaucoma and exudative retinal detachment after a single intravitreal ranibizumab injection. Clin Exp Ophthalmol. 2007;35:878–80.

23. Kahook MY, Schuman JS, Noecker RJ. Intravitreal bevacizumab in a patient with neovascular glaucoma. Ophthalmic Surg Lasers Imaging. 2006;37:144–6.

24. Yazdani S, Hendi K, Pakravan M, Mahdavi M, Yaseri M. Intravitreal bevacizumab for neovascular glaucoma. J Glaucoma. 2009;18:632–7.

25. Inatani M, et al. Efficacy and safety of intravitreal aflibercept injection in Japanese patients with neovascular glaucoma: outcomes from the VENERA Study. Adv Ther. 2020:1–10. https://doi.org/10.1007/s12325-020-01580-y.

26. Grisanti S, et al. Intracameral Bevacizumab for Iris Rubeosis. Am J Ophthalmol. 2006;142:158–60.

27. SooHoo JR, Seibold LK, Pantcheva MB, Kahook MY. Aflibercept and neovascular glaucoma. Clin Exp Ophthalmol. 2015;43:803–7.

28. Davidorf FH, Mouser JG, Derick RJ. Rapid improvement of Rubeosis iridis from a single bevacizumab (avastin) injection. Retina. 2006;26:354–6.

29. Iliev ME, Domig D, Wolf-Schnurrbursch U, Wolf S, Sarra G-M. Intravitreal bevacizumab (Avastin®) in the treatment of neovascular glaucoma. Am J Ophthalmol. 2006;142:1054–6.

30. Gheith ME, Siam GA, de Barros DSM, Garg SJ, Moster MR. Role of intravitreal bevacizumab in neovascular glaucoma. J Ocul Pharmacol Ther. 2007;23:487–91.

31. Ha JY, Lee TH, Sung MS, Park SW. Efficacy and safety of intracameral bevacizumab for treatment of neovascular glaucoma. Korean J Ophthalmol. 2017;31:538–47.

32. Duch S, Buchacra O, Milla E, Andreu D, Tellez J. Intracameral bevacizumab (Avastin) for neovascular glaucoma. J Glaucoma. 2009;18:140–3.

33. Nomoto H, et al. Pharmacokinetics of bevacizumab after topical, subconjunctival, and intravitreal administration in rabbits. Invest Ophthalmol Vis Sci. 2009;50:4807–13.

34. Bhagat PR, Agrawal KU, Tandel D. Study of the effect of injection bevacizumab through various routes in neovascular glaucoma. J Curr Glaucoma Pract. 2016;10:39–48.

35. Oshima Y, Sakaguchi H, Gomi F, Tano Y. Regression of iris neovascularization after intravitreal injection of bevacizumab in patients with proliferative diabetic retinopathy. Am J Ophthalmol. 2006;142:155–157.e1.

36. Saito Y, et al. Clinical factors related to recurrence of anterior segment neovascularization after treatment including intravitreal bevacizumab. Am J Ophthalmol. 2010;149:964-972.e1.

37. Grover S, Gupta S, Sharma R, Brar VS, Chalam KV. Intracameral bevacizumab effectively reduces aqueous vascular endothelial growth factor concentrations in neovascular glaucoma. Br J Ophthalmol. 2009;93:273.

38. Chalam KV, Gupta SK, Grover S, Brar VS, Agarwal S. Intracameral avastin dramatically resolves iris neovascularization and reverses neovascular glaucoma. Eur J Ophthalmol. 2007;18:255–62.

39. Wolf A, von Jagow B, Ulbig M, Haritoglou C. Intracameral injection of bevacizumab for the treatment of neovascular glaucoma. Ophthalmologica. 2011;226:51–6.

40. Mizote M, Baba T, Hirooka K, Yamaji H, Shiraga F. Vascular endothelial growth factor concentrations in aqueous humor before and after subconjunctival injection of bevacizumab for neovascular glaucoma. Jpn J Ophthalmol. 2010;54:242–4.

41. Ryoo NK, Lee EJ, Kim T-W. Regression of iris neovascularization after subconjunctival injection of bevacizumab. Korean J Ophthalmol. 2011;27:299–303.

42. Waisbourd M, et al. Topical bevacizumab for neovascular glaucoma: a pilot study. Pharmacology. 2014;93:108–12.

43. Krohne TU, Eter N, Holz FG, Meyer CH. Intraocular pharmacokinetics of bevacizumab after a single intravitreal injection in humans. Am J Ophthalmol. 2008;146:508–12.

44. Bakri SJ, Snyder MR, Reid JM, Pulido JS, Singh RJ. Pharmacokinetics of intravitreal bevacizumab (Avastin). Ophthalmology. 2007;114:855–9.

45. Kobayashi S, et al. Long-term outcomes after preoperative intravitreal injection of bevacizumab before trabeculectomy for neovascular glaucoma. J Glaucoma. 2016;25:281–4.

46. Elmekawey H, Khafagy A. Intracameral ranibizumab and subsequent mitomycin C augmented trabeculectomy in neovascular glaucoma. J Glaucoma. 2014;23:437–40.

47. Kitnarong N, Sriyakul C, Chinwattanakul S. A prospective study to evaluate intravitreous ranibizumab as adjunctive treatment for trabeculectomy in neovascular glaucoma. Ophthalmol Ther. 2015;4:33–41.

48. Fakhraie G, et al. Surgical outcomes of intravitreal bevacizumab and guarded filtration surgery in neovascular glaucoma. J Glaucoma. 2010;19:212–8.

49. Batioğlu F, Astam N, Özmert E. Rapid improvement of retinal and iris neovascularization after a single intravitreal bevacizumab injection in a patient with central retinal vein occlusion and neovascular glaucoma. Int Ophthalmol. 2008;28:59–61.

50. Vasudev D, Blair MP, Galasso J, Kapur R, Vajaranant T. Intravitreal Bevacizumab for Neovascular Glaucoma. J Ocul Pharmacol Ther. 2009;25:453–8.

51. Ehlers JP, et al. Combination intravitreal bevacizumab/panretinal photocoagulation versus panretinal photocoagulation alone in the treatment of neovascular glaucoma. Retina. 2008;28:696–702.

52. Wasik A, Song H-F, Grimes A, Engelke C, Thomas A. Bevacizumab in conjunction with panretinal photocoagulation for neovascular glaucoma. Optometry J Am Optom Assoc. 2009;80:243–8.

53. Douat J, et al. Utilisation du bevacizumab en injection intravitréenne dans le traitement du glaucome néovasculaire. À propos de 20 cas. J Français D'ophtalmologie. 2009;32:652–63.

54. Wittström E, Holmberg H, Hvarfner C, Andréasson S. Clinical and electrophysiologic outcome in patients with neovascular glaucoma treated with and without bevacizumab. Eur J Ophthalmol. 2011;22:563–74.

55. Olmos LC, et al. Long-term outcomes of neovascular glaucoma treated with and without intravitreal bevacizumab. Eye. 2016;30:463–72.

56. Wong J, Wang N, Miller JW, Schuman JS. Modulation of human fibroblast activity by selected angiogenesis inhibitors. Exp Eye Res. 1994;58:439–51.

57. Horsley MB, Kahook MY. Anti-VEGF therapy for glaucoma. Curr Opin Ophthalmol. 2010;21:112–7.

58. Yoshida N, et al. Intravitreal bevacizumab treatment for neovascular glaucoma: histopathological analysis of trabeculectomy specimens. Graefe's Arch Clin Exp Ophthalmol. 2011;249:1547.

59. Kahook MY. Bleb morphology and vascularity after trabeculectomy with intravitreal ranibizumab: a pilot study. Am J Ophthalmol. 2010;150:399-403.e1.

60. Cornish KS, Ramamurthi S, Saidkasimova S, Ramaesh K. Intravitreal bevacizumab and augmented trabeculectomy for neovascular glaucoma in young diabetic patients. Eye. 2009;23:979–81.

61. Chen C-H, et al. Adjunctive intravitreal bevacizumab-combined trabeculectomy versus trabeculectomy alone in the treatment of neovascular glaucoma. J Ocul Pharmacol Ther. 2010;26:111–8.

62. Takihara Y, et al. Combined intravitreal bevacizumab and trabeculectomy with mitomycin C versus trabeculectomy with mitomycin C alone for neovascular glaucoma. J Glaucoma. 2011;20:196–201.

63. Nakano S, Nakamuro T, Yokoyama K, Kiyosaki K, Kubota T. Prognostic factor analysis of intraocular pressure with neovascular glaucoma. J Ophthalmol. 2016;2016:1–9.

64. Hwang HB, Han JW, Yim HB, Lee NY. Beneficial effects of adjuvant intravitreal bevacizumab injection on outcomes of Ahmed glaucoma valve implantation in patients with neovascular glaucoma: systematic literature review. J Ocul Pharmacol Ther. 2015;31:198–203.

65. Mahdy RA, Nada WM, Fawzy KM, Alnashar HY, Almosalamy SM. Efficacy of intravitreal bevacizumab with panretinal photocoagulation followed by Ahmed valve implantation in neovascular glaucoma. J Glaucoma. 2013;22:768–72.

66. Eid TM, Radwan A, el-Manawy W, el-Hawary I. Intravitreal bevacizumab and aqueous shunting surgery for neovascular glaucoma: safety and efficacy. Can J Ophthalmol J Can D'ophtalmologie. 2009;44:451–6.

67. Arcieri ES, et al. Efficacy and safety of intravitreal bevacizumab in eyes with neovascular glaucoma undergoing ahmed glaucoma valve implantation: 2-year follow-up. Acta Ophthalmol. 2015;93:e1–6.

68. Sevim MS, Buttanri IB, Kugu S, Serin D, Sevim S. Effect of intravitreal bevacizumab injection before Ahmed glaucoma valve implantation in neovascular glaucoma. Ophthalmologica. 2013;229:94–100.

69. Zhou M, et al. Adjunctive with versus without intravitreal bevacizumab injection before Ahmed glaucoma valve implantation in the treatment of neovascular glaucoma. Chin Med J-peking. 2013;126:1412–7.

70. Sahyoun M, et al. Long-term results of Ahmed glaucoma valve in association with intravitreal bevacizumab in neovascular glaucoma. J Glaucoma. 2015;24:383–8.

71. Kang JY, Nam KY, Lee SJ, Lee SU. The effect of intravitreal bevacizumab injection before Ahmed valve implantation in patients with neovascular glaucoma. Int Ophthalmol. 2014;34:793–9.

72. Zhou M, Xu X, Zhang X, Sun X. Clinical outcomes of Ahmed glaucoma valve implantation with or without intravitreal bevacizumab pretreatment for neovascular glaucoma. J Glaucoma. 2016;25:551–7.

73. Ma KT, et al. Surgical results of Ahmed valve implantation with intraoperative bevacizumab injection in patients with neovascular glaucoma. J Glaucoma. 2012;21:331–6.

74. Tang M, et al. Efficacy of intravitreal ranibizumab combined with Ahmed glaucoma valve implantation for the treatment of neovascular glaucoma. BMC Ophthalmol. 2016;16:7.

75. Noor NA, Mustafa S, Artini W. Glaucoma drainage device implantation with adjunctive intravitreal bevacizumab in neovascular glaucoma: 3-year experience. Clin Ophthalmol. 2017;11:1417–22.

76. Miraftabi A, et al. Effect of subconjunctival bevacizumab injection on the outcome of Ahmed glaucoma valve implantation: a randomized control trial. Clin Exp Ophthalmol. 2018;46:750–6.

Medical IOP-Lowering Therapy for Neovascular Glaucoma

Pathik P. Amin and Mary Qiu

1 Introduction

The management of neovascular glaucoma (NVG) requires timely and aggressive intervention to control the intraocular pressure (IOP). Markedly elevated IOP can cause rapid and irreversible loss of visual function and lead to significant pain and discomfort. Visual prognosis improves with early detection and intervention.

Prompt medical therapy is meant to temporize the acute IOP elevation until a more definitive surgical intervention can be performed. In the earlier stages of NVG, when the iridocorneal angle is still open and has not yet become obstructed by peripheral anterior synechiae (PAS), the IOP may normalize with medical IOP-lowering therapy in conjunction with anti-neovascular treatments. However, in the later stages of NVG, when the angle has already become obstructed by PAS, medical IOP-lowering therapy and anti-neovascular treatments are often insufficient to normalize the IOP, and surgical intervention is often required to achieve IOP control. Even after IOP-lowering surgery has been performed, medications remain a mainstay of NVG treatment to control IOP long term. It is

imperative that there is concurrent intervention by the retina specialist to reduce the underlying neovascular drive and eliminate the angiogenic stimulus.

The clinical presentation and diagnosis of NVG are discussed in other chapters. This chapter will focus on the medical management of IOP in NVG.

2 Topical Administration of IOP-Lowering Agents

Regardless of the angle status or if IOP-lowering surgery will eventually be required, medical therapy to lower IOP is necessary to preserve optic nerve health, increase patient comfort, and improve the clarity of the media for anterior segment and fundus examination.

Topical medical therapy initially consists of fast-acting aqueous suppressants such as beta-blockers, alpha-adrenergic agonists, and carbonic anhydrase inhibitors (CAI) [1]. These agents have an onset of action within 1 hour of instillation. Table 1 describes important characteristics of IOP-lowering medications.

Beta-blockers target receptors on the nonpigmented ciliary epithelium to reduce the active transport of aqueous humor and therefore the rate of aqueous production [2]. The IOP-lowering effect of beta-blockers is a reduction of 20% to 25% from baseline when used twice per day [3].

P. P. Amin (✉) · M. Qiu
Department of Ophthalmology and Visual Science,
The University of Chicago Medicine,
Chicago, IL, USA
e-mail: ppamin@bsd.uchicago.edu;
maryqiu@bsd.uchicago.edu

© The Author(s), under exclusive license to Springer Nature Switzerland AG 2022
M. Qiu (ed.), *Neovascular Glaucoma*, Essentials in Ophthalmology,
https://doi.org/10.1007/978-3-031-11720-6_15

Table 1 Characteristics of IOP-lowering medications

Medication class	Route	Mechanism of action	Onset of action	Peak effect	Trough effect
Alpha-adrenergic agonists	Topical	Decrease aqueous humor production (short term ~1 month); increase uveoscleral outflow (long term)	<1 h	2–3 h	10–14 h
Beta-receptor antagonists	Topical	Decrease aqueous humor production	<1 h	1–2 h	12–24 h
Prostaglandin analogs	Topical	Increase uveoscleral outflow	6 h	12 h	≥24 h
Rho kinase inhibitors	Topical	Increase trabecular meshwork outflow; decrease episcleral venous pressure; decrease aqueous production	–	–	–
Carbonic anhydrase inhibitors (CAI)	Topical	Decrease aqueous humor production	<1 h	2–3 h	8–12 h
	Oral		1–2 h	2–4 h	8–12 h
	IV		5–10 min	15 min	4–5 h
Osmotics	Oral	Increase plasma osmolarity, shifting fluid from eye to blood circulation; decrease aqueous humor production	15–30 min	1–2 h	4–5 h
	IV			30–60 min	6 h

The onset of action occurs within 1 hour with peak effect at 1–2 hours after dosing. Topical beta-blockers can be categorized as nonselective and cardioselective agents. Nonselective beta-blocker agents include timolol, levobunolol, carteolol, and betaxolol. Timolol is the most commonly used and readily available of the group and is available in 0.25% and 0.5% concentrations. There is no difference in efficacy between the two concentrations [4]. The only cardioselective beta-blocker agent available is betaxolol, which has a high affinity for the beta-1 receptor type and therefore improves the cardiac and pulmonary risk profile. While topical beta-blockers are generally well-tolerated, nonselective agents are contraindicated in patients with chronic obstructive pulmonary disease, congestive heart failure, bradycardia, or atrioventricular heart block [5]. A cardioselective beta-blocker agent can be a useful alternative in these patients. However, betaxolol is less efficacious at lowering IOP compared to timolol [6], because beta-2 is the predominant beta-receptor in the eye [7]. Furthermore, the ocular hypotensive effective of topical therapy is reduced in patients with concurrent systemic beta-blocker therapy [8]. Nevertheless, timolol should still be used in an acute setting when the goal is rapid IOP reduction, as long as there are no contraindications.

Selective alpha-2 receptor agonists, such as brimonidine, initially cause a reduction of aqueous humor production through vasoconstriction in the ciliary body [9]. Potency through this initial pathway lasts for approximately 1 month, after which the predominate mechanism of action is via increased outflow through the uveoscleral pathway by ciliary muscle contraction [10]. Brimonidine and apraclonidine are both available at generic formulations. Generic brimonidine is currently available in 0.15% and 0.2% formulations, with the 0.2% formulation being more cost-effective. Brimonidine is also available in a brand name version, Alphagan-P, using purite instead of BAK as the preservative, is currently available in 0.10% and 0.15% formulations. The IOP-lowering effect of brimonidine is a reduction of 20% to 25% from baseline [11]. The onset of action occurs within 1 hour with peak effect at 2 to 3 hours after dosing [12]. While brimonidine is generally well-tolerated, there can be some ocular side effects such as conjunctival hyperemia, allergic conjunctivitis, and ocular pruritus [13]. In fact, hypersensitivity reactions that include follicular conjunctivitis can occur in up to 20% of patients [14]. Common systemic side effects include dry mouth, drowsiness, and fatigue. Apraclonidine is a mixed alpha-receptor agonist with a mild affinity for alpha-2 over alpha-1 receptors [15]. There is no difference in efficacy between brimonidine and apraclonidine [16]. However, the apraclonidine is more likely to produce adverse effects due to reduced alpha-receptor selectivity and increased likelihood of crossing the blood–brain barrier.

Carbonic anhydrase is an important enzyme in the ciliary processes of the eye that is involved in the regulation and production of aqueous humor. Dorzolamide and brinzolamide inhibit the production of this enzyme [17]. While both are available as generic formulations, dorzolamide is currently more cost-effective. The IOP-lowering effect of topical CAIs is a reduction of 15 to 20% from baseline, with no difference in efficacy between twice per day versus three times per day dosing [14, 18]. The onset of action occurs between 1 and 2 hours with peak effect at 2 hours after dosing [19]. Common side effects include blurred vision, tearing, stinging, and itching [20]. In patients with allergies to sulfonamide antibiotics, it may still be reasonable to initiate therapy with a topical CAI as there is little evidence to support that a sulfonamide antibiotic allergy also increases susceptibility to allergic reactions from all sulfonamide-based drugs [21]. However, these patients should be followed very carefully for the development of adverse reactions [22]. Little information is available regarding the systemic adverse effects of topical CAIs, but it is well-established that some amount of drug quickly enters the systemic circulation. Patients with chronic kidney disease should be educated on the rare but serious systemic adverse effects.

Prostaglandin analogs may ultimately be included in the long-term IOP management plan. These potent but slower-acting agents increase uveoscleral outflow by binding to receptors in the ciliary body to induce smooth muscle relaxation [23]. In addition, remodeling of the extracellular matrix within the ciliary body leads to reduced outflow resistance [24]. The IOP-lowering effect of prostaglandin analogs is a reduction of 25% to 35% from baseline with once per day dosing [25]. The onset of action occurs within 6 hours with peak effect at 12 hours after dosing [26]. Prostaglandin analogs include latanoprost, travoprost, bimatoprost, and tafluprost. Generic formulations are available for all except tafluprost. Tafluprost is only available under the brand name Zioptan, which is currently the only preservative-free formulation in this drug class. There are

almost no systemic side effects of topical prostaglandin analogs. Common ocular side effects include stinging upon instillation, conjunctival hyperemia, and hypertrichosis. Other ocular changes can include iris pigmentation changes, darkening of periocular skin, and increase in inflammation. In the acute phase, their effect can be equivocal as they also increase inflammatory makers and can lead to further breakdown of the blood–aqueous barrier. There is debate on whether prostaglandins lead to exacerbation of macula edema and uveitis. The current literature states that these agents may be used in non-surgical patients without significant concern [27, 28]. In addition, the presence of PAS does not hinder the IOP-lowering abilities of prostaglandins [29].

Rho kinase inhibitors (RKIs) are a novel class of IOP-lowering medication that primarily increase aqueous outflow through the trabecular meshwork, but also have secondary mechanisms of action that decrease episcleral venous pressure and reduce aqueous humor production [30]. The two most common RKIs are netarsudil and ripasudil, of which only netarsudil is approved for use in the USA [31]. Netarsudil is currently available as brand name Rhopressa. Since the conventional outflow pathway is often compromised in NVG due to a fibrovascular scaffolding and/or PAS obstructing the trabecular meshwork, netarsudil may have limited efficacy in this setting. However, there are no studies to date that have examined efficacy in the setting of NVG with PAS, and further longitudinal clinical data are needed.

Cholinergic agents such as pilocarpine increase aqueous outflow through the conventional pathway but decrease outflow through the uveoscleral pathway [32]. However, pilocarpine and other cholinergic agents are contraindicated as they have the potential to exacerbate inflammation, shallow the anterior chamber, and increase the level of synechial angle closure [33]. This paradoxical mechanism of action can occur in a setting of significant IOP elevation, where an ischemic iris sphincter does not constrict, but the ciliary muscle still contracts [34]. This leads to anterior displacement of the iris–lens structure whereby shallowing the anterior chamber [35].

Common differentials to acute elevation of IOP include primary angle-closure crisis, uveitis, and hyphema (unrelated to NVG), all of which have special considerations. Pilocarpine is indicated for primary angle-closure crisis but should be avoided in uveitis and traumatic hyphema as it may increase vascular permeability and exacerbate the formation of posterior synechiae [36]. Furthermore, its miotic effect can impair the ability to perform a thorough posterior segment evaluation, which is critical when evaluating patients with NVG.

3 Topical Administration of Other Agents (for Comfort)

Other topical medications can be used to reduce inflammation and relieve pain to improve ocular comfort. Cycloplegics, such as atropine 1%, can help reduce ciliary muscle spasm and prevent hyphema [37]. Patients with NVG also tend to present with concurrent inflammation, so it is prudent to prescribe topical corticosteroids such as prednisolone acetate 1% or difluprednate (Durezol) 0.05% [38]. Difluprednate is available in a generic formulation and requires less frequent dosing than prednisolone acetate, at a ratio of 1:2 [39]. These agents are not contraindicated in an acute setting, even with PAS formation or elevated IOP.

4 Oral Administration of IOP-Lowering Agents

Certain oral medications, especially CAIs, have been used for decades as ocular hypotensive agents. They are an effective way to rapidly lower IOP. However, a systemic route of administration leads to additional considerations as chances of adverse reactions increase.

Acetazolamide and methazolamide are oral CAIs that, in addition to their action on the cili-ary epithelium of the eye, act on the kidney to reduce bicarbonate reabsorption at the proximal tube and increase renal excretion of sodium, potassium, and water. This reduces aqueous humor production and helps lower IOP quickly [40]. Studies have shown IOP reductions ranging from 15% to 34% within hours of oral acetazolamide in patients with primary open-angle glaucoma and ocular hypertension [41, 42]. Oral and topical CAIs can produce a synergistic effect. When oral acetazolamide is added to topical dorzolamide, there is an additional 16% reduction in aqueous production [43, 44]. The most common side effects associated with oral acetazolamide include gastrointestinal upset, paresthesia of the extremities and face, malaise, fatigue, frequent urination, and drug-induced metabolic acidosis. These side effects are much more common with prolonged use of the medication. Methazolamide is less effective than acetazolamide but has fewer side effects and is well-tolerated by most patients. It may be better suited in chronic IOP management rather than in the setting of acutely elevated IOP.

The most common dosing for acetazolamide is 250 mg immediate release (IR) four times per day (or 500 mg sustained release (SR) sequels twice a day) and for methazolamide is 50 mg two times per day. For IV administration of acetazolamide, 500 mg IV may be administered with a repeat dose 2–4 hours later. Careful consideration is needed when prescribing acetazolamide in a setting of renal and hepatic disease, high-dose aspirin therapy, allergies, epilepsy, or pulmonary disease. Contraindications include sulfonamide allergies, history of kidney stones, renal failure, and liver cirrhosis [46]. Acetazolamide is a highly protein-bound drug, not metabolized, and is cleared from the body unchanged solely through renal excretion [47]. Therefore, dosing should be adjusted (see Table 2) to account for renal impairment and dialysis. Careful monitoring of neurologic disturbance in these patients is recommended. Dosage adjustments for mild hepatic disease at not necessary as the drug is not

Table 2 Dosage Adjustments for acetazolamide in patients with renal compromise

Kidney status	Dosage adjustment
CrCl > 50 mL/min	Full dose (250 mg PO QID, or 500 mg sequels PO BID)
CrCl 10–50 mL/min	Half dose (250 mg PO BID, or 500 mg sequels PO daily) [54]
CrCl < 10 mL/min	Do not administer [54]
Hemodialysis	Half dose (250 mg PO BID or 500 mg sequels PO daily). Coordinate monitoring with nephrologist.
Peritoneal dialysis	125 mg PO daily (do not use sequels) [45]

metabolized by the liver. Utilization of this drug in patients with a history of epilepsy should be done in coordination with neurology.

Hyperosmotic agents, such as a glycerol and mannitol, are also options for short term or emergent IOP lowering. These medications increase the osmolarity of the plasma and cause a shift of fluid from the eye to the blood circulation [48]. This effect is more pronounced at higher IOPs. The status of the blood–aqueous barrier, often diminished in the presence of ocular inflammation, may limit the efficacy of these agents [49]. A secondary mechanism of hyperosmotic agents is reduction of aqueous humor production through a central nervous system pathway involving osmoreceptors in the hypothalamus [50]. Intravenous agents produce a more rapid and greater reduction in IOP lowering than their orally administered counterparts.

Mannitol is the intravenous hyperosmotic agent of choice and an onset of action within 15–30 minutes with a duration of approximately 6 hours [51]. A mannitol dose of 1–2 g/kg over 30–60 minutes is recommended, with the option of repeating every 8 hours as necessary [52]. IV administration, while more potent, also leads to a higher risk of cellular dehydration and central nervous system complications causing disorientation and dementia. In addition, patients with abnormal cardiac status and renal compromise are at risk for increased pulmonary edema and congestive heart failure. IV mannitol is typically administered in the emergency room setting, with careful monitoring of vital signs and hemodynamic status.

Oral glycerol has an onset of action of 15 to 30 minutes, with a duration of 4–5 hours [53]. The recommended administration is a 50% solution in a dose of 1.5 gm/kg with a flavoring agent [55]. Due to poor ocular tissue penetration and confinement in the extracellular fluid space, multiple doses can be administered. Headaches, nausea, vomiting, and diuresis are the most common side effects. Intense diuresis can lead to urinary retention, especially in males in benign prostate hyperplasia, which requires catheterization. Due to the significant carbohydrate value, diabetic patients can develop ketoacidosis and other complications.

In most clinical situations, systemic CAI combined with aggressive topical medical therapy is sufficient to temporize the IOP. However, there may be certain situations where hyperosmotic agents may be critical. Most side effects stemming from hyperosmotics are dose-related, so the minimum amount needed to adequately reduce IOP should be administered, and the patient should be monitored very carefully afterward.

5 Conclusion

Neovascular glaucoma requires timely and aggressive medical and surgical therapy. IOP-lowering medications play a key role during the acute presentation to reduce the IOP, clear the cornea to improve the view for the eye exam, and improve patient comfort while surgical intervention, if needed, can be planned. After IOP-lowering surgery is performed, medications remain a mainstay of NVG treatment to control IOP long term.

A collaborative multidisciplinary approach between glaucoma and retina specialists addressing medical and surgical IOP lowering and the underlying angiogenic factors is crucial. Providers should plan an efficient workflow that can promptly address acute presentations of NVG. Ultimately, a timely, evidence-based approach can help optimize patient outcomes.

References

1. Löffler KU. Neovaskularisationsglaukom: aetiology, pathogenesis and treatment. Ophthalmologe. 2006;103(12):1057–64. https://doi.org/10.1007/s00347-006-14317.
2. Schmidl D, Schmetterer L, Garhöfer G, Popa-Cherecheanu A. Pharmacotherapy of glaucoma. J Ocul Pharmacol Ther. 2015;31(2):63–77. https://doi.org/10.1089/jop.2014.0067.
3. European Glaucoma Society. Terminology and guidelines for glaucoma. 3rd ed. Savona: Editrice DOGMA; 2008.
4. Campbell S, Hickey-Dwyer M, Harding S. Double-masked three-period crossover investigation of timolol in control of raised intraocular pressure. Eye. 1993;7:105–8. https://doi.org/10.1038/eye.1993.22.
5. Lama PJ. Systemic adverse effects of beta-adrenergic blockers: an evidence-based assessment. Am J Ophthalmol. 2002;134:749–60.
6. Allen RC, Hertzmark E, Walker AM, Epstein DL. A double-masked comparison of betaxolol vs timolol in the treatment of open-angle glaucoma. Am J Ophthalmol. 1986;101(5):535–41.
7. Trope GE, Clark B. Beta adrenergic receptors in pigmented ciliary processes. Br J Ophthalmol. 1982;66:788–92.
8. Schuman JS. Effects of systemic beta-blocker therapy on the efficacy and safety of topical brimonidine and timolol. Brimonidine study groups 1 and 2. Ophthalmology. 2000;107(6):1171–7.
9. Cantor LB. The evolving pharmacotherapeutic profile of brimonidine, an alpha 2-adrenergic agonist, after four years of continuous use. Expert Opin Pharmacother. 2000;1:815–34.
10. Cantor LB. Brimonidine in the treatment of glaucoma and ocular hypertension. Ther Clin Risk Manag. 2006;2(4):337–46. https://doi.org/10.2147/tcrm.2006.2.4.337.
11. Kampik A, Arias-Puente A, O'Brart DP, Vuori ML. European latanoprost study group. Intraocular pressure-lowering effects of latanoprost and brimonidine therapy in patients with open-angle glaucoma or ocular hypertension: a randomized observer-masked multicenter study. J Glaucoma. 2002;11:90–6.
12. Walters TR. Development and use of brimonidine in treating acute and chronic elevations of intraocular pressure: a review of safety, efficacy, dose response, and dosing studies. Surv Ophthalmol. 1996;41(Suppl 1):S19–26.
13. Arthur S, Cantor LB. Update on the role of alpha-agonists in glaucoma management. Exp Eye Res. 2011;93:271–83.
14. Lester M. Brinzolamide ophthalmic suspension: a review of its pharmacology and use in the treatment of open angle glaucoma and ocular hypertension. Clin Ophthalmol. 2008;2(3):517–23.
15. Gharagozloo NZ, Relf SJ, Brubaker RF. Aqueous flow is reduced by the alpha-adrenergic agonist, apraclonidine hydrochloride (ALO 2145). Ophthalmology. 1988;95:1217e1220.
16. Schadlu R, Maus TL, Nau CB, Brubaker RF. Comparison of the efficacy of apraclonidine and brimonidine as aqueous suppressants in humans. Arch Ophthalmol. 1998;116(11):1441–4. https://doi.org/10.1001/archopht.116.11.1441.
17. Balfour JA, Wilde MI. Dorzolamide. A review of its pharmacology and therapeutic potential in the management of glaucoma and ocular hypertension. Drugs Aging. 1997;10(5):384–403. https://doi.org/10.2165/00002512-199710050-00006.
18. Sugrue MF. Pharmacological and ocular hypotensive properties of topical carbonic anhydrase inhibitors. Prog Retin Eye Res. 2000;19(1):87–112.
19. Lippa EA, Carlson L-E, Ehinger B, et al. Dose response and duration of action of dorzolamide, a topical carbonic anhydrase inhibitor. Arch Ophthalmol. 1992;110:495–9.
20. Strahlman E, Tipping R, Vogel R, et al. A double-masked, randomized I-year study comparing dorzolamide (Trusopt), timolol, and betaxolol. Arch Ophthalmol. 1995;113:1009–16.
21. Stock JG. Sulfonamide hypersensitivity and acetazolamide. Arch Ophthalmol. 1990;108:634–5.
22. Guedes GB, Karan A, Mayer HR, Shields MB. Evaluation of adverse events in self-reported sulfa-allergic patients using topical carbonic anhydrase inhibitors. J Ocul Pharmacol Ther. 2013;29(5):456–61. https://doi.org/10.1089/jop.2012.0123. Epub 2013 Feb 27
23. Weinreb RN, Toris CB, Gabelt BT, Lindsey JD, Kaufman PL. Effects of prostaglandins on the aqueous humor outflow pathway. Surv Ophthalmol. 2002;47(suppl 1):S53–64.
24. Lindén C, Alm A. Prostaglandin analogues in the treatment of glaucoma. Drugs Aging. 1999;14(5):387–98. https://doi.org/10.2165/00002512-199914050-00006.
25. Toris CB, Gabelt BT, Kaufman PL. Update on the mechanism of action of topical prostaglandins for intraocular pressure reduction. Surv Ophthalmol. 2008;53(Suppl1):S107–20.
26. Larsson LI. Intraocular pressure over 24 hours after single-dose administration of latanoprost 0.005% in healthy volunteers. A randomized, double-masked, placebo controlled, cross-over single center study. Acta Ophthalmol Scand. 2001;79(6):567–71. https://doi.org/10.1034/j.1600-0420.2001.790604.x.
27. Reza Razeghinejad M. The effect of latanoprost on intraocular inflammation and macular Edema. Ocul Immunol Inflamm. 2019;27(2):181–8. https://doi.org/10.1080/09273948.2017.1372485.
28. Hu J, Vu JT, Hong B, Gottlieb C. Uveitis and cystoid macular oedema secondary to topical prostaglandin

analogue use in ocular hypertension and open angle glaucoma. Br J Ophthalmol. 2020;104(8):1040–4. https://doi.org/10.1136/bjophthalmol-2019-315280. Epub 2020 Jun 12. PMID: 32532763; PMCID: PMC7577108

29. Kumar S, Malik A, Singh M, Sood S. Efficacy of latanoprost in management of chronic angle closure glaucoma. Nepal J Ophthalmol. 2009;1(1):32–6.

30. Ren R, Li G, Le TD, Kopczynski C, Stamer WD, Gong H. Netarsudil increases outflow facility in human eyes through multiple mechanisms. Invest Ophthalmol Vis Sci. 2016;57(14):6197–209.

31. Choy M. Pharmaceutical Approval Update. P T. 2018;43(4):205–27.

32. Nilsson SF. The uveoscleral outflow routes. Eye (Lond). 1997;11(Pt 2):149–54. https://doi.org/10.1038/eye.1997.43.

33. Havens SJ, Gulati V. Neovascular Glaucoma. Dev Ophthalmol. 2016;55:196–204. https://doi.org/10.1159/000431196.

34. The Pilocarpine Paradox, Journal of Glaucoma: August 1996 – Volume 5 – Issue 4 – p 225–227.

35. Day AC, Nolan W, Malik AN, Viswanathan AC, Foster PJ. Pilocarpine induced acute angle closure. BMJ Case Rep. 2012:2012. https://doi.org/10.1136/bcr.01.2012.5694.

36. Mori M, Araie M, Sakurai M, et al. Effects of pilocarpine and tropicamide on blood-aqueous barrier permeability in man. Invest Ophthalmol Vis Sci. 1992;33(2):416–23.

37. Rodrigues GB, Abe RY, Zangalli C, et al. Neovascular glaucoma: a review. Int J Retina Vitreous. 2016;2:26. https://doi.org/10.1186/s40942-016-0051-x.

38. Rodgin SG. Neovascular glaucoma associated with uveitis. J Am Optom Assoc. 1987;58(1):499–503.

39. Sheppard JD, Toyos MM, Kempen JH, Kaur P, Foster CS. Difluprednate 0.05% versus prednisolone acetate 1% for endogenous anterior uveitis: a phase III, multicenter, randomized study. Invest Ophthalmol Vis Sci. 2014;55(5):2993–3002. Published 2014 May 6. https://doi.org/10.1167/iovs.13-12660.

40. Costagliola C, dell'Omo R, Romano MR, Rinaldi M, Zeppa L, Parmeggiani F. Pharmacotherapy of intraocular pressure—part II. Carbonic anhydrase inhibitors, prostaglandin analogues and prostamides. Expert Opin Pharmacother. 2009;10(17):2859–70. https://doi.org/10.1517/14656560903300129.

41. Macdonald MJ, Gore SM, Cullen PM, Phillips CI. Comparison of ocular hypotensive effects of acetazolamide and atenolol. Br J Ophthalmol. 1977;61(5):345–8.

42. Loiselle AR, de Kleine E, van Dijk P, Jansonius NM. Intraocular and intracranial pressure in glaucoma patients taking acetazolamide. PLoS One. 2020;15(6):e0234690. Published 2020 Jun 18. https://doi.org/10.1371/journal.pone.0234690.

43. Maus TL, Larsson LI, McLaren JW, Brubaker RF. Comparison of dorzolamide and acetazolamide as suppressors of aqueous humor flow in humans. Arch Ophthalmol. 1997;115(1):45–9. https://doi.org/10.1001/archopht.1997.01100150047008.

44. Centofanti M, et al. Comparative effects of intraocular pressure between systemic and topical carbonic anhydrase inhibitors: a clinical masked, cross-over study. Pharmacol Res. 1997;35(5):481–5.

45. Schwenk MH, Blaustein DA, Wagner JD. The pharmacokinetics of acetazolamide during CAPD. Adv Perit Dial. 1994;10:44–6.

46. Zaidi FH, Kinnear PE. Acetazolamide, alternate carbonic anhydrase inhibitors and hypoglycaemic agents: comparing enzymatic with diuresis induced metabolic acidosis following intraocular surgery in diabetes. Br J Ophthalmol. 2004;88(5):714–5.

47. Chapron DJ, Sweeny KR, Feig PU, Kramer PA. Influence of advanced age on the disposition of acetazolamide. Br J Clin Pharmacol. 1985;19:363–71.

48. Galin MA, Binkhorst RD, Kwitko ML. Ocular dehydration. Am J Ophthalmol. 1968;66:233.

49. Stamper R. Becker-Shaffer's diagnosis and therapy of the glaucomas. 8th ed; 2009. p. 431–4.

50. Krupin T, Podos SM, Becker B. Alteration of intraocular pressure after third ventricle injections of osmotic agents. Am J Ophthalmol. 1973;76:948.

51. Allen CH, Ward JD. An evidence-based approach to management of Increased Intracranial Pressure. Crit Care Clin. 1998;14(3):485–96.

52. Crouch ER Jr, Crouch ER. Management of traumatic hyphema: therapeutic options. J Pediatr Ophthalmol Strabismus. 1999;36(5):238–50. [PubMed 10505828]

53. Drance SM. Effect of oral glycerol on intraocular pressure in normal and glaucomatous eyes. Arch Ophthalmol. 1964;72(4):491–3. https://doi.org/10.1001/archopht.1964.00970020491009.

54. Nissenson AR, Richard NF. Clinical Dialysis. McGraw Hill Medical Pub Division, 2005.

55. Virno M, et al. Oral glycerol in ophthalmology: a valuable new method for the reduction of intraocular pressure. Am J Ophthalmol. 1963;55:1133.

Trabeculectomy for Neovascular Glaucoma

Kevin M. Halenda and Annapurna Singh

1 Introduction

There is currently no consensus regarding the optimal surgical approach for lowering intraocular pressure (IOP) in neovascular glaucoma (NVG). In general, IOP-lowering surgery is indicated when medical therapy fails to adequately control IOP. In the earlier stages of NVG, the IOP may be elevated in the setting of an anatomically open angle. In the more advanced stages of NVG, the IOP may be more profoundly elevated and less responsive to medical IOP-lowering therapy due to contracture of fibrovascular membranes and resultant peripheral anterior synechiae (PAS). Common surgical strategies for lowering IOP include bypassing the conventional outflow pathway with trabeculectomy or aqueous shunt surgery and/or reducing aqueous production with cyclophotocoagulation. This chapter will discuss the history, indications, and special considerations when performing trabeculectomy in the setting of NVG.

K. M. Halenda
West Virginia University Eye Institute,
Morgantown, WV, USA
e-mail: kevin.halenda1@hsc.wvu.edu

A. Singh (✉)
Cole Eye Institute, Cleveland Clinic Foundation,
Cleveland, OH, USA
e-mail: singha2@ccf.org

2 History

The trabeculectomy creates a fistula underneath a partial-thickness scleral flap to establish communication between the anterior chamber and the subconjunctival space. The name "trabeculectomy" may be a misnomer since the tissue excised underneath the scleral flap may not necessarily contain any trabecular meshwork. The trabeculectomy functions by bypassing the obstructed aqueous outflow at the iridocorneal angle and creating a subconjunctival filtering bleb. First described in its modern form by Cairns in the 1960s, the trabeculectomy has historically been considered the "gold standard" incisional procedure in surgical glaucoma management [1, 2].

3 Bleb Morphology

The presence of a functioning filtering bleb is indicative of a successful trabeculectomy. Many research studies define surgical "success" as IOP < 21 mm Hg, with or without IOP-lowering medications, which represents qualified and unqualified success, respectively. Treatment goals in the setting of NVG will be discussed in greater detail in another chapter. Wound healing is detrimental to the long-term success of a trabeculectomy since subconjunctival fibrosis increases resistance to aqueous outflow and impedes percolation of aqueous into the filtering bleb. Furthermore, occlusion of the internal ostium of the sclerostomy by fibrotic tissue can result in trabeculectomy failure. There are four prototypical bleb morphologies as follows: polycystic, diffuse, flat, and encapsulated; the latter two are typically dysfunctional or nonfunctional [3].

4   Wound Healing after Trabeculectomy

The primary mediators of wound healing in the subconjunctival space are fibroblasts originating from the Tenon's capsule [3]. Traditionally, the use of frequent topical corticosteroids during the postoperative period has been used to suppress wound healing and promote bleb function. The off-label adjuvant use of antifibrotic agents such as 5-flurouracil (5-FU) and mitomycin C (MMC) is common practice with modern trabeculectomy surgery to reduce wound healing and promote successful outcomes, though these advantages must be weighed against their significant accompanying risks, including local tissue toxicity and an increased risk of complications such as hypotony and delayed-onset bleb leaks [4]. More recently, the widespread use of intraocular antivascular endothelial growth factor (anti-VEGF) agents has been introduced as adjunctive therapy to IOP-lowering surgery as a potentially more targeted therapy which can both modulate fibrosis and regress the anterior segment neovascularization associated with NVG [5].

5   Surgical Techniques

5.1   Standard Trabeculectomy

NVG has long been recognized as an especially challenging form of glaucoma to manage with traditional filtering surgeries given the high failure rates in this type of glaucoma. Case series reporting results of filtering operations without antifibrotic agents for patients with NVG are small and often include historical filtering techniques such as full-thickness filters and posterior lip sclerectomies in aphakic patients [6, 7]. One case series reported surgical success in 7/12 (58%) of NVG eyes treated with a standard trabeculectomy during a mean follow-up period of 15.7 months [6]. A large retrospective case series of 534 eyes (including 5 with NVG) undergoing trabeculectomy without antifibrotic agents reported a failure rate of 80% among the NVG eyes [8].

5.2   Trabeculectomy with Mitomycin C

Mitomycin C (MMC), an antibiotic molecule originally isolated from *Streptomyces caespitosus*, has multiple properties rendering it useful in medical applications, including the induction of apoptosis in fibroblasts, inhibition of angiogenesis, and cytotoxicity [4]. The use of MMC as an antifibrotic agent during trabeculectomy to modulate postoperative subconjunctival scarring was first described by Chen in the early 1980s [9, 10]. MMC may be applied intraoperatively to the scleral bed during trabeculectomy via saturated cellulose sponges or subconjunctival injection and is typically used in the concentration range of 0.1–0.5 mg/mL with variable application durations [11].

While the use of intraoperative MMC to augment trabeculectomy is essentially standard practice in the modern era, there are limited data focusing on MMC-augmented trabeculectomy specifically in the setting of NVG. MMC-augmented trabeculectomy for NVG has been reported to have a success rate of 60–70% at approximately 1-year follow-up, although the presence of neovascularization of the iris (NVI) and angle, technique of MMC application, and success criteria vary by study [12–14]. Hyung et al. reported a much lower success rate of only 29% of NVG eyes undergoing trabeculectomy with MMC at 1 year; however, only 7/24 (29%) eyes underwent preoperative panretinal photocoagulation (PRP) and 100% of the eyes had evident NVI [15]. Indeed, studies on trabeculectomy in the setting of NVG which included preoperative PRP or cryotherapy to ablate the ischemic retina and regress anterior segment neovascularization have reported higher success rates between 67% and 71% at 1 year [12, 14]. A trend of declining success rates over time has been consistently demonstrated [12–15]. Success rates have been reported to be approximately 52–63% with 1.5- to 3-year follow-up [12–14, 16]. A large retrospective study with longer follow-up reported the success rate of MMC-augmented trabeculectomy in 101 NVG eyes to be 51.7% at 5 years [13].

5.3 Trabeculectomy with 5-Flurouracil

5-fluorouracil (5-FU) is a pyrimidine analog capable of inhibiting fibroblast proliferation which was similarly introduced for adjunctive use in trabeculectomy in the early 1980s [17]. The adjunctive use of 5-FU for enhancing the function of trabeculectomy can be both intraoperative and postoperative as a series of subconjunctival injections [18], because a single application of 5-FU is much less efficacious than MMC [4].

As with MMC-augmented trabeculectomy, there are limited data available regarding 5-FU-augmented filtering surgery in the setting of NVG. The earliest case series from the 1980s investigated a variety of filtering procedures augmented with 5-FU and reported success rates of 60–70% at approximately 1 year in NVG eyes [19–21]. In studies where most eyes received preoperative PRP, success rates have been reported to be between 65% and 69% at approximately 1 year [19, 21]. With longer follow-up duration, the success rate declines. One study with mean follow-up of nearly 3 years (35.8 months) reported 55% success [16]. A case series of 34 NVG eyes in 1995 reported a success rate of 28% at 5 years and a median survival of 38.7 months [22].

5.4 Comparison of Trabeculectomy with Mitomycin C Versus 5-Fluorouracil

There is evidence to support an advantage of MMC over 5-FU for filtration surgery regarding IOP-lowering and failure rates [23], including among high-risk eyes [24–26]. However, few studies have directly compared adjunctive 5-FU and MMC for trabeculectomy in the setting of NVG. A randomized trial published in 1997 compared a single intraoperative application of MMC (0.4 mg/mL × 5 min) to a series of ten 5 mg subconjunctival 5-FU injections among eyes with high-risk glaucoma including 3 NVG eyes (2 treated with MMC, 1 treated with 5-FU) [27]. This trial reported that at 12-month follow-up, there was no significant difference between the overall success rate of the MMC group (100.0%) and the 5-FU group (84.6%), and all 3 NVG eyes in the study were surgical successes. Notably, complication rates were similar between the two groups, with the exception of corneal epithelial defects, which occurred at a significantly higher rate among the 5-FU group (53%) than the MMC group (12%) [27]. Another more recent randomized trial published in 2007 of 40 NVG eyes compared a single application of 0.2 mg/mL MMC for 2 minutes to a series of ten 5 mg postoperative subconjunctival 5-FU injections [16]. No significant difference was observed in the overall success rate, which was approximately 55% in both cohorts. The 5-FU group had higher rates of complications including hyphema and corneal epithelial defects compared to the MMC group. The rate of progression to NLP vision was also higher in the 5-FU group (44%) compared to the MMC group (9%), although this was confounded by longer follow-up in the 5-FU cohort (35.8 months) than in the MMC cohort (18.6 months) [16]. Overall, based on limited evidence, trabeculectomy augmented with MMC or 5-FU in the setting of NVG has comparable success, although there is greater risk of corneal complications when 5-FU is used. Augmenting a trabeculectomy with MMC remains more popular than 5-FU, as evidenced by a 2016 American Glaucoma Society (AGS) survey of practice patterns [28].

5.5 Trabeculectomy with Antivascular Endothelial Growth Factor (VEGF)

In addition to being a driving factor of ocular neovascularization in the setting of ischemic retinopathy [29], VEGF is an important mediator of wound healing via its promotion of angiogenesis during the proliferative phase [4]. Inhibition of VEGF is possible with several commercially available drugs, among the most widely used being bevacizumab (Avastin, Genentech, San Francisco, CA, USA), aflibercept (Eylea, Regeneron, Tarrytown, NY, USA), and ranibizumab (Lucentis, Genentech, San Francisco, CA, USA) [30]. VEGF is known to be present in higher concentrations in the aqueous humor of eyes with glaucoma [31], especially in the case of NVG [32], and exhibits increased expression in ocular tissues during the postoperative period [33]. VEGF has also been shown to stimulate fibroblast activity in vitro, and its inhibition has been shown to decrease collagen deposition, reduce conjunctival vascularity, and enhance bleb function in an animal trabeculectomy model [33]. Histopathologic correlation comparing trabecular tissue specimens in NVG eyes undergoing trabeculectomy with and without preoperative intravitreal bevacizumab (2–7 days prior to trabeculectomy) has demonstrated relatively reduced inflammatory infiltrate, edema, hemorrhage, and fibrin in the trabecular meshwork in treated eyes [34]. As such, there has also been interest since the early-mid 2000s in the off-label use of anti-VEGF (subconjunctival, intracameral, or intravitreal delivery) as a possibly safer and more targeted method to achieve adjunctive antifibrosis in the setting of trabeculectomy, particularly for NVG [5].

5.6 Trabeculectomy with Subconjunctival Anti-VEGF

Subconjunctival anti-VEGF in the setting of trabeculectomy was described in 2006 as a possible method to rescue failing blebs [35] and in 2008 as a possible prophylaxis against bleb failure in the setting of subsequent intraocular surgery [36]. Subconjunctival anti-VEGF may reduce local bleb vascularity [36–39], although this effect is transient [39]. Additionally, this strategy has not been extensively studied in the setting of NVG, where the presence and/or recurrence of anterior segment neovascularization threatens the long-term function of the bleb. A prospective trial published in 2011 compared outcomes of 55 eyes (33 with NVG) undergoing trabeculectomy with adjunctive subconjunctival bevacizumab versus placebo; in this study, there was no significant difference in success rate or bleb morphology at 1 year, although the anti-VEGF cohort did demonstrate significantly reduced bleb vascularity compared with the placebo cohort. Additionally, while a subanalysis of NVG eyes showed that the success rate was higher at 1 year among the eyes receiving subconjunctival anti-VEGF during trabeculectomy (72.2% vs 66.0%), this difference did not reach statistical significance [38]. Randomized trials comparing adjunctive subconjunctival anti-VEGF with MMC or 5-FU [40–43] and MMC augmentation with or without subconjunctival anti-VEGF [39, 44] show comparable success rates, although these trials exclude NVG since it is risk factor for bleb failure. A single case series published in 2010 with limited follow-up reported that 2 NVG eyes treated with trabeculectomy with MMC and subconjunctival bevacizumab maintained IOP <16 mm Hg with a localized avascular bleb at 6 months [45]. It is unknown whether a single intraoperative subconjunctival anti-VEGF injection dramatically influences the long-term longevity of a bleb in NVG, and serial regimens have not been investigated for this purpose.

5.7 Trabeculectomy with Intracameral Anti-VEGF

Although intracameral anti-VEGF is known to regress anterior segment neovascularization [46], few studies have explored intracameral anti-VEGF as a strategy to enhance trabeculectomy function in the setting of NVG. A small case series published in 2009 describes outcomes in four NVG eyes undergoing trabeculectomy with adjunctive intracameral anti-VEGF; in this series, all four eyes received preoperative scatter PRP and a single intraoperative intracameral bevacizumab injection; all eyes maintained IOP between 10 and 14 mmHg without IOP-lowering medications at a mean follow-up of 12.8 months [47]. Another case series published in 2014 describes outcomes of 15 NVG eyes undergoing MMC-augmented trabeculectomy with adjunctive preoperative intracameral ranibizumab. All eyes in this series received preoperative PRP, and intracameral ranibizumab was administered to completely regress NVI (2 eyes required a second injection) followed by a MMC-augmented trabeculectomy within 4 weeks of the first injection [48]. At 6 months, 14/15 eyes (93.3%) achieved success [48]. A randomized controlled trial published in 2009 compared outcomes in 19 NVG eyes undergoing MMC-augmented trabeculectomy with two different doses of adjunctive preoperative intracameral bevacizumab (9 patients received 1.25 mg bevacizumab and 10 patients received 2.5 mg bevacizumab); in this trial, there was no difference in IOP or NVI regression at 6 months between the groups receiving different doses of intracameral bevacizumab, though the pooled group that received intracameral bevacizumab demonstrated a significantly lower failure rate at 6 months compared to a retrospective control group that underwent standard MMC-augmented trabeculectomy without adjunctive intracameral bevacizumab by the same surgeon (failure rate 5% versus 31%, respectively) [49].

5.8 Trabeculectomy with Intravitreal Anti-VEGF

In addition to being useful for treating macular edema and/or retinal neovascularization, intravitreal anti-VEGF has been described as a strategy to enhance trabeculectomy function in the setting of NVG [50]. Numerous case series have explored the utility of preoperative intravitreal anti-VEGF injections for this purpose (Table 1). Preoperative intravitreal anti-VEGF has been reported to rapidly regress anterior segment neovascularization and lower the risk of intraoperative and postoperative bleeding [51–53]. Several case series published between 2010 and 2015 have reported the success rates of MMC-augmented trabeculectomy with adjunctive preoperative intravitreal anti-VEGF in cohorts of 15 to 30 NVG eyes to be approximately 60–90% at 6–9 months of short-term follow-up [54–56]. Case series with ≥1 year of follow-up have reported success rates of MMC-augmented trabeculectomy with adjunctive preoperative intravitreal anti-VEGF to be approximately 70–80%. Another case series published in 2016 describes 3-year outcomes in 12 NVG eyes undergoing MMC-augmented trabeculectomy with adjunctive intravitreal anti-VEGF; in this series, the success rate at both 1 and 3 years was 83.3% (10/12 eyes) [57]. Additionally, two retrospective studies have compared MMC-augmented trabeculectomy with and without adjunctive intravitreal anti-VEGF [58, 59]. A retrospective comparative case series published by Saito et al. in 2010 compared outcomes in 52 NVG eyes undergoing MMC-augmented trabeculectomy with (n = 20) or without (n = 32) adjunctive preoperative anti-VEGF; in this study, the group receiving adjunctive intravitreal anti-VEGF had a significantly higher success rate of 95% at 6 months compared to 75% at 6 months in the control group [59]. Another retrospective comparative case series published by Takihara et al. in 2011 compared outcomes in 57 NVG eyes undergoing MMC-augmented trabeculec-

Table 1 Adjunctive use of preoperative intravitreal anti-VEGF combined with trabeculectomy with MMC

Author (year)	Study type	Study period	# NVG eyes	Anti-VEGF	Pre-op PRP	Antimetabolite	Follow-up period	Success rate
Jonas (2007)	Interventional case series	Unreported	1	B*	Focal laser	5-FU 0.2 mL (25 mg/mL) intra-op	4 weeks	100%
Kitnarong (2008)	Interventional case series	Unreported	6	B	Yes	MMC, unknown concentration	Mean 24.7 weeks	83.30%
Cornish (2009)	Interventional case series	Unreported	2	B	Yes	MMC 0.2 mg/mL	6–7 months	100%
Alkawas (2010)	Interventional case series	03/2006–04/2008	17	B	Yes	MMC 0.4 mg/mL × 3 min	6 months	88.20%
Chen (2010)	Comparative case series	01/2005–12/2007	42 (14 IVB, 28 control)	B	Yes	MMC 0.2 mg/mL × 2 min; variable use	Mean 179 ± 97 days IVB, 196 ± 108 days control	78% IVB, 64% Control (p > 0.05)
Fakhraie (2010)	Interventional case series	11/2006–03/2007	27	B	Yes	MMC 0.2 mg/mL × 4 min	Mean 8.7 months	61%
Saito (2010)	Comparative case series	01/2003–05/2008	52 (20 IVB, 32 control)	B	Yes	MMC 0.4 mg/mL × 4 min	6 months	95% IVB, 75% Control (p < 0.05)
Takihara (2011)	Comparative case series	06/2005–05/2007	57 (24 IVB, 33 control)	B	Yes	MMC 0.4 mg/mL × 4 min	360 days	65.2% IVB, 65.3% Control (p > 0.05)
Kitnarong (2015)	Interventional case series	12/2008–12/2009	15	R	Yes	MMC 0.4 mg/mL × 1–3 min	Mean 39 weeks	86.70%
Kobayashi (2016)	Interventional case series	04/2009–04/2010	12	B	Yes	MMC 0.4 mg/mL × 5 min	Mean 43.0 ± 7.0 months	83.30%

B: bevacizumab (1.25 mg), B*: bevacizumab (1.5 mg), R: ranibizumab (0.5 mg)

tomy with ($n = 24$) or without (n = 33) adjunctive preoperative anti-VEGF; in this study, the group receiving adjunctive intravitreal anti-VEGF had surgical success rates of 87.5%, 79.2%, and 65.2% at 4, 8, and 12 months, respectively, whereas the control group had surgical success rates of 75.0%, 71.9%, and 65.3%, respectively [58]. In both studies, the rates of bleeding-associated complications were lower in the group that received adjunctive preoperative intravitreal anti-VEGF. In summary, adjunctive preoperative intravitreal anti-VEGF before MMC-augmented trabeculectomy lowers the rate of bleeding-associated complications and may enhanced IOP-lowering in the short term, but the results may not be sustained. Limitations of these studies include variable surgical success criteria and lack of standardization in the treatment of the underlying retinal pathology that led to the NVG [58, 59].

5.9 Trabeculectomy with Ex-PRESS Shunt

Trabeculectomy with the Ex-PRESS shunt (Alcon Laboratories, Fort Worth, TX) has been described in the setting of NVG. The technique for performing a trabeculectomy with the Ex-PRESS shunt replaces the sclerostomy with the implantation of a stainless steel and magnetic resonance imaging-compatible nonvalved device underneath a scleral flap. Two models are available as follows: The P50 has a 50 μm lumen, and the P200 has a 200 μm lumen. Trabeculectomy with the Ex-PRESS shunt may be associated with less hypotony-related complications compared to a standard trabeculectomy since the Ex-PRESS lumen is smaller in diameter than a typical sclerostomy; furthermore, inserting the Ex-PRESS may be less inflammatory since an iridectomy is not required [60]. Avoiding an iridectomy is theoretically advantageous in the setting of NVG since iris tissue with incompletely regressed NVI is especially prone to bleeding, and postoperative hyphema has been reported to be a risk factor for trabeculectomy failure in the setting of NVG [61].

A few studies have examined outcomes of trabeculectomy with Ex-PRESS shunt in the setting of NVG with mixed results. Yu et al. described a case series of four patients who underwent an MMC-augmented trabeculectomy with Ex-PRESS shunt, of which three required bleb revision and subsequent shunt repositioning to achieve IOP ≤ 21 mmHg at last follow-up (mean follow-up 20.8 months) [62]. In contrast, Hanna et al. reported success at last visit in 5/5 eyes treated with MMC-augmented trabeculectomy with Ex-PRESS shunt and adjunctive preoperative intravitreal bevacizumab during follow-up between 12 and 15 months, though 2 patients received the P50 and 3 received the P200 device [63]. The only retrospective comparative study comparing outcomes of NVG eyes undergoing MMC-augmented trabeculectomy with and without Ex-PRESS shunt reported a significantly lower success rate (IOP ≤ 21 mmHg with or without topical medication) in the Ex-PRESS shunt group compared to the trabeculectomy group (31.8% versus 69.3%, respectively), although postoperative complications including hyphema and bleb leaks were significantly lower in the Ex-PRESS shunt group [64].

6 Complications of Trabeculectomy in NVG

Early and late complications of trabeculectomy include hypotony, bleb leak, shallow anterior chamber, hyphema, cataract, vitreous hemorrhage, hypotony maculopathy, choroidal effusion, suprachoroidal hemorrhage, blebitis, and endophthalmitis [65]. Bleeding-associated complications after trabeculectomy are more common in NVG eyes than eyes with other types of glaucoma. Since NVG eyes have anterior segment neovascularization which may or may not be fully regressed by the time of IOP-lowering surgery, postoperative hyphema rates have been reported to be as high as 58% in NVG eyes undergoing trabeculectomy [13, 55, 61]. In NVG eyes, vision loss may be profound, is often multifactorial, and may be related to glaucomatous optic neuropathy and/or progression of the underlying retinal pathology [6, 66, 67].

7 Risk Factors for Trabeculectomy Failure in NVG

NVG has long been recognized as a significant risk factor for trabeculectomy failure [8]. Several risk factors associated with trabeculectomy failure in NVG have been identified. A retrospective case series of 49 NVG eyes reported that postoperative hyphema was associated with a higher failure rate at 24 months compared to eyes without postoperative hyphema [61]. The trabeculectomy failures may be related to the hyphema itself, or the hyphema may be a proxy for inadequately regressed anterior and posterior segment neovascularization, so it may be prudent to aggressively treat the underlying neovascular drive both before and after the trabeculectomy to enhance the likelihood that the trabeculectomy will have enduring success. Others have reported previous history of vitrectomy to be a risk factor for trabeculectomy failure in the setting of NVG, which is hypothesized to be due to theoretically higher levels of interleukin-6 (IL-6) and other inflammatory cytokines in postvitrectomy eyes [12]. The largest retrospective analysis examining prognostic factors in 101 NVG eyes in a Japanese population also identified younger age (<50 years) and previous vitrectomy as independent predictors of trabeculectomy failure [13]. A subanalysis of patients with history of vitrectomy in this study identified the presence of an unrepaired retinal detachment or proliferative membrane, but not time from vitrectomy to trabeculectomy, as significant predictors of trabeculectomy failure in the setting of NVG [13]. One study investigating prognostic factors for trabeculectomy failure among vitrectomized eyes also independently identified NVG as a risk factor for trabeculectomy failure [68].

8 Trabeculectomy Versus Aqueous Shunt

Aqueous shunts were initially utilized in eyes with refractory glaucoma after failed trabeculectomy. Since NVG is a known risk factor for trabeculectomy failure, aqueous shunts are currently more popular than trabeculectomy as the primary IOP-lowering surgery in the setting of NVG [28]. The use of both valved and nonvalved aqueous shunts has been described in the setting of NVG [69–74]. MMC-augmented trabeculectomy may have comparable efficacy and safety compared to aqueous shunts in the setting of NVG. In 2004, Im et al. published a retrospective study of 66 NVG eyes comparing the success rates of MMC-augmented trabeculectomy versus Ahmed glaucoma valve (AGV) surgery; the success rate at 1 year was 78.2% in the trabeculectomy group and 88.5% in the AGV group [75]. In another retrospective comparative study of 40 NVG eyes comparing MMC-augmented trabeculectomy to the AGV, surgical success for the trabeculectomy group was 65% at 1 year and 55% at 2 years, and surgical success for the AGV group was 70% at 1 year and 60% at 2 years [76]. Engin et al. described success rates of AGV versus modified trabeculectomy (trabeculectomy combined with cyclectomy, without antimetabolite augmentation); the success rate at 1 year was 50% in the AGV group and 72% in the modified trabeculectomy group, and there were no significant differences in postoperative IOP, preservation of VA, or complications [77]. Liu et al. compared MMC-augmented trabeculectomy with adjunctive intravitreal ranibizumab to standard AGV (without antimetabolite and without anti-VEGF) in a prospective, interventional case series and reported significantly lower IOP at 6 months as well as fewer early and late postoperative complications in the MMC-augmented trabeculectomy group compared to the AGV group. The trabeculectomy group achieved success more frequently than the AGV group (94% versus 68%, respectively) [66]. A recent prospective, randomized trial published in 2021 by Tokumo et al. compared the nonvalved Baerveldt glaucoma implant (BGI) to trabeculectomy in 50 NVG eyes that had undergone PRP but not intravitreal anti-VEGF; this study reported no significant difference in IOP control or success rates at 1 year; the success rate in the BGI group was 59.1%, and the success rate in the trabeculectomy group was 61.6%, though there were more late complications in the BGI group compared to the trabeculectomy group (13 versus 4, respectively) [78]. MMC-augmented trabeculectomy has similar efficacy to an aqueous shunt in NVG and may be a more practical option in resource-limited areas. However, early success is highly dependent on complete regression of anterior segment neovascularization, which is best achieved with the synergistic combination of preoperative intravitreal anti-VEGF and PRP. Aqueous shunts in the setting of NVG will be discussed in detail in another chapter.

9   Conclusion

NVG remains a challenging type of glaucoma to treat due to anterior segment neovascularization and proliferation of fibrovascular tissue in the iridocorneal angle which may recur even after an initially successful trabeculectomy. Historically, long-term success rates for trabeculectomy in the setting of NVG have been relatively poor. However, in the modern era, augmentation with MMC and adjunctive anti-VEGF has improved trabeculectomy success rates in the setting of NVG. Preoperative anti-VEGF regresses anterior segment neovascularization and reduces bleeding complications, which leads to improved bleb function, at least in the short term. However, for a trabeculectomy in the setting of NVG to have durable long-term success, prompt and aggressive treatment of the underlying neovascular drive is paramount to prevent recurrence of the anterior segment neovascularization which threatens the function of the bleb. Other surgical IOP-lowering strategies in the setting of NVG will be discussed in other chapters, and further research is needed to determine the most optimal multidisciplinary NVG treatment algorithm to both control IOP and address the underlying ischemic etiology.

References

1. Cairns JE. Trabeculectomy. Preliminary report of a new method. Am J Ophthalmol. 1968;66(4):673–9.
2. Koike KJ, Chang PT. Trabeculectomy: a brief history and review of current trends. Int Ophthalmol Clin. 2018;58(3):117–33.
3. Skuta GL, Parrish RK 2nd. Wound healing in glaucoma filtering surgery. Surv Ophthalmol. 1987;32(3):149–70.
4. Seibold LK, Sherwood MB, Kahook MY. Wound modulation after filtration surgery. Surv Ophthalmol. 2012;57(6):530–50.
5. Slabaugh M, Salim S. Use of anti-VEGF agents in glaucoma surgery. J Ophthalmol. 2017;2017:1645269.
6. Allen RC, Bellows AR, Hutchinson BT, Murphy SD. Filtration surgery in the treatment of neovascular glaucoma. Ophthalmology. 1982;89(10):1181–7.
7. Herschler J, Agness D. A modified filtering operation for neovascular glaucoma. Arch Ophthalmol. 1979;97(12):2339–41.
8. Mietz H, Raschka B, Krieglstein GK. Risk factors for failures of trabeculectomies performed without antimetabolites. Br J Ophthalmol. 1999;83(7):814–21.
9. Chen CW, editor. Enhanced intraocular pressure controlling effectiveness of trabeculectomy by local application of mitomycin C1983.
10. Chen CW, Huang HT, Bair JS, Lee CC. Trabeculectomy with simultaneous topical application of mitomycin-C in refractory glaucoma. J Ocul Pharmacol. 1990;6(3):175–82.
11. Fan Gaskin JC, Nguyen DQ, Soon Ang G, O'Connor J, Crowston JG. Wound healing modulation in glaucoma filtration surgery-conventional practices and new perspectives: the role of antifibrotic agents (part I). J Curr Glaucoma Pract. 2014;8(2):37–45.
12. Kiuchi Y, Sugimoto R, Nakae K, Saito Y, Ito S. Trabeculectomy with mitomycin C for treatment of neovascular glaucoma in diabetic patients. Ophthalmologica. 2006;220(6):383–8.
13. Takihara Y, Inatani M, Fukushima M, Iwao K, Iwao M, Tanihara H. Trabeculectomy with mitomycin C for neovascular glaucoma: prognostic factors for surgical failure. Am J Ophthalmol. 2009;147(5):912–8. 8.e1
14. Mandal AK, Majji AB, Mandal SP, Das T, Jalali S, Gothwal VK, et al. Mitomycin-C-augmented trabeculectomy for neovascular glaucoma. A preliminary report. Indian J Ophthalmol. 2002;50(4):287–93.
15. Hyung SM, Kim SK. Mid-term effects of trabeculectomy with mitomycin C in neovascular glaucoma patients. Korean J Ophthalmol. 2001;15(2):98–106.
16. Sisto D, Vetrugno M, Trabucco T, Cantatore F, Ruggeri G, Sborgia C. The role of antimetabolites in filtration surgery for neovascular glaucoma: intermediate-term follow-up. Acta Ophthalmol Scand. 2007;85(3):267–71.
17. Gressel MG, Parrish RK 2nd, Folberg R. 5-fluorouracil and glaucoma filtering surgery: I. an animal model. Ophthalmology. 1984;91(4):378–83.
18. Palanca-Capistrano AM, Hall J, Cantor LB, Morgan L, Hoop J, WuDunn D. Long-term outcomes of intraoperative 5-fluorouracil versus intraoperative mitomycin C in primary trabeculectomy surgery. Ophthalmology. 2009;116(2):185–90.
19. Heuer DK, Parrish RK 2nd, Gressel MG, Hodapp E, Palmberg PF, Anderson DR. 5-fluorouracil

and glaucoma filtering surgery. II. A pilot study. Ophthalmology. 1984;91(4):384–94.

20. Weinreb RN. Adjusting the dose of 5-fluorouracil after filtration surgery to minimize side effects. Ophthalmology. 1987;94(5):564–70.

21. Rockwood EJ, Parrish RK 2nd, Heuer DK, Skuta GL, Hodapp E, Palmberg PF, et al. Glaucoma filtering surgery with 5-fluorouracil. Ophthalmology. 1987;94(9):1071–8.

22. Tsai JC, Feuer WJ, Parrish RK 2nd, Grajewski AL. 5-fluorouracil filtering surgery and neovascular glaucoma. Long-term follow-up of the original pilot study. Ophthalmology. 1995;102(6):887–92. discussion 92–3.

23. Cabourne E, Clarke JC, Schlottmann PG, Evans JR. Mitomycin C versus 5-Fluorouracil for wound healing in glaucoma surgery. Cochrane Database Syst Rev. 2015;11:Cd006259.

24. Katz GJ, Higginbotham EJ, Lichter PR, Skuta GL, Musch DC, Bergstrom TJ, et al. Mitomycin C versus 5-fluorouracil in high-risk glaucoma filtering surgery. Extended follow-up. Ophthalmology. 1995;102(9):1263–9.

25. Akarsu C, Onol M, Hasanreisoglu B. Postoperative 5-fluorouracil versus intraoperative mitomycin C in high-risk glaucoma filtering surgery: extended follow up. Clin Exp Ophthalmol. 2003;31(3):199–205.

26. Anand N, Dawda VK. A comparative study of mitomycin C and 5-fluorouracil trabeculectomy in West Africa. Middle East Afr J Ophthalmol. 2012;19(1):147–52.

27. Kitazawa Y, Kawase K, Matsushita H, Minobe M. Trabeculectomy with mitomycin. A comparative study with fluorouracil. Arch Ophthalmol. 1991;109(12):1693–8.

28. Vinod K, Gedde SJ, Feuer WJ, Panarelli JF, Chang TC, Chen PP, et al. Practice preferences for glaucoma surgery: a Survey of the American Glaucoma Society. J Glaucoma. 2017;26(8):687–93.

29. Campochiaro PA. Ocular neovascularization. J Mol Med (Berl). 2013;91(3):311–21.

30. Pożarowska D, Pożarowski P. The era of anti-vascular endothelial growth factor (VEGF) drugs in ophthalmology, VEGF and anti-VEGF therapy. Central-European J Immunol. 2016;41(3):311–6.

31. Hu DN, Ritch R, Liebmann J, Liu Y, Cheng B, Hu MS. Vascular endothelial growth factor is increased in aqueous humor of glaucomatous eyes. J Glaucoma. 2002;11(5):406–10.

32. Tripathi RC, Li J, Tripathi BJ, Chalam KV, Adamis AP. Increased level of vascular endothelial growth factor in aqueous humor of patients with neovascular glaucoma. Ophthalmology. 1998;105(2):232–7.

33. Li Z, Van Bergen T, Van de Veire S, Van de Vel I, Moreau H, Dewerchin M, et al. Inhibition of vascular endothelial growth factor reduces scar formation after glaucoma filtration surgery. Invest Ophthalmol Vis Sci. 2009;50(11):5217–25.

34. Yoshida N, Hisatomi T, Ikeda Y, Kohno R, Murakami Y, Imaki H, et al. Intravitreal bevacizumab treatment for neovascular glaucoma: histopathological analysis of trabeculectomy specimens. Graefes Arch Clin Exp Ophthalmol. 2011;249(10):1547–52.

35. Kahook MY, Schuman JS, Noecker RJ. Needle bleb revision of encapsulated filtering bleb with bevacizumab. Ophthalmic Surg Lasers Imaging. 2006;37(2):148–50.

36. Coote MA, Ruddle JB, Qin Q, Crowston JG. Vascular changes after intra-bleb injection of bevacizumab. J Glaucoma. 2008;17(7):517–8.

37. Kapetansky FM, Pappa KS, Krasnow MA, Baker ND, Francis CD. Subconjunctival injection(s) of bevacizumab for failing filtering blebs. Invest Ophthalmol Vis Sci. 2008;49(13):4149.

38. Ghanem A. Trabeculectomy with or without intraoperative sub-conjunctival injection of bevacizumab in treating refractory glaucoma. J Clin Exp Ophthalmol. 2011;02

39. Kiddee W, Orapiriyakul L, Kittigoonpaisan K, Tantisarasart T, Wangsupadilok B. Efficacy of adjunctive subconjunctival bevacizumab on the outcomes of primary trabeculectomy with mitomycin C: a prospective randomized placebo-controlled trial. J Glaucoma. 2015;24(8):600–6.

40. Nilforushan N, Yadgari M, Kish SK, Nassiri N. Subconjunctival bevacizumab versus mitomycin C adjunctive to trabeculectomy. Am J Ophthalmol. 2012;153(2):352–7.e1.

41. Akkan JU, Cilsim S. Role of subconjunctival bevacizumab as an adjuvant to primary trabeculectomy: a prospective randomized comparative 1-year follow-up study. J Glaucoma. 2015;24(1):1–8.

42. Pro MJ, Freidl KB, Neylan CJ, Sawchyn AK, Wizov SS, Moster MR. Ranibizumab versus mitomycin C in primary trabeculectomy—a pilot study. Curr Eye Res 2015;40(5):510–5.

43. Jurkowska-Dudzińska J, Kosior-Jarecka E, Zarnowski T. Comparison of the use of 5-fluorouracil and bevacizumab in primary trabeculectomy: results at 1 year. Clin Exp Ophthalmol. 2012;40(4):e135–42.

44. Muhsen S, Compan J, Lai T, Kranemann C, Birt C. Postoperative adjunctive bevacizumab versus placebo in primary trabeculectomy surgery for glaucoma. Int J Ophthalmol. 2019;12(10):1567–74.

45. Choi JY, Choi J, Kim YD. Subconjunctival bevacizumab as an adjunct to trabeculectomy in eyes with refractory glaucoma: a case series. Korean J Ophthalmol. 2010;24(1):47–52.

46. Chalam KV, Gupta SK, Grover S, Brar VS, Agarwal S. Intracameral Avastin dramatically resolves iris neovascularization and reverses neovascular glaucoma. Eur J Ophthalmol. 2008;18(2):255–62.

47. de Moraes CGV, Facio AC, Costa JH, Malta RFS. Intracameral bevacizumab and mitomycin C trabeculectomy for eyes with neovascular glaucoma: a case series. J Ocul Biol Dis Infor. 2009;2(1):40–6.

48. Elmekawey H, Khafagy A. Intracameral ranibizumab and subsequent mitomycin C augmented trabeculectomy in neovascular glaucoma. J Glaucoma. 2014;23(7):437–40.

49. Gupta V, Jha R, Rao A, Kong G, Sihota R. The effect of different doses of intracameral bevacizumab on surgical outcomes of trabeculectomy for neovascular glaucoma. Eur J Ophthalmol. 2009;19(3):435–41.

50. Jonas JB, Spandau UH, Schlichtenbrede F. Intravitreal bevacizumab for filtering surgery. Ophthalmic Res. 2007;39(2):121–2.

51. Chen CH, Lai IC, Wu PC, Chen YJ, Chen YH, Lee JJ, et al. Adjunctive intravitreal bevacizumab-combined trabeculectomy versus trabeculectomy alone in the treatment of neovascular glaucoma. J Ocul Pharmacol Ther. 2010;26(1):111–8.

52. Kitnarong N, Chindasub P, Metheetrairut A. Surgical outcome of intravitreal bevacizumab and filtration surgery in neovascular glaucoma. Adv Ther. 2008;25(5):438–43.

53. Cornish KS, Ramamurthi S, Saidkasimova S, Ramaesh K. Intravitreal bevacizumab and augmented trabeculectomy for neovascular glaucoma in young diabetic patients. Eye (Lond). 2009;23(4):979–81.

54. Kitnarong N, Sriyakul C, Chinwattanakul S. A prospective study to evaluate Intravitreous ranibizumab as adjunctive treatment for trabeculectomy in neovascular glaucoma. Ophthalmol Ther. 2015;4(1):33–41.

55. Alkawas AA, Shahien EA, Hussein AM. Management of neovascular glaucoma with panretinal photocoagulation, intravitreal bevacizumab, and subsequent trabeculectomy with mitomycin C. J Glaucoma. 2010;19(9):622–6.

56. Fakhraie G, Katz LJ, Prasad A, Eslami Y, Sabour S, Zarei R, et al. Surgical outcomes of intravitreal bevacizumab and guarded filtration surgery in neovascular glaucoma. J Glaucoma. 2010;19(3):212–8.

57. Kobayashi S, Inoue M, Yamane S, Sakamaki K, Arakawa A, Kadonosono K. Long-term outcomes after preoperative intravitreal injection of bevacizumab before trabeculectomy for neovascular glaucoma. J Glaucoma. 2016;25(3):281–4.

58. Takihara Y, Inatani M, Kawaji T, Fukushima M, Iwao K, Iwao M, et al. Combined intravitreal bevacizumab and trabeculectomy with mitomycin C versus trabeculectomy with mitomycin C alone for neovascular glaucoma. J Glaucoma. 2011;20(3):196–201.

59. Saito Y, Higashide T, Takeda H, Ohkubo S, Sugiyama K. Beneficial effects of preoperative intravitreal bevacizumab on trabeculectomy outcomes in neovascular glaucoma. Acta Ophthalmol. 2010;88(1):96–102.

60. Sarkisian SR. The ex-press mini glaucoma shunt: technique and experience. Middle East Afr J Ophthalmol. 2009;16(3):134–7.

61. Nakatake S, Yoshida S, Nakao S, Arita R, Yasuda M, Kita T, et al. Hyphema is a risk factor for failure of trabeculectomy in neovascular glaucoma: a retrospective analysis. BMC Ophthalmol. 2014;14(1):55.

62. Yu T-C, Tseng G-L, Chen C-C, Liou S-W. Surgical treatment of neovascular glaucoma with ex-PRESS glaucoma shunt: case report. Medicine. 2017;96(35).

63. Hanna R, Tiosano B, Graffi S, Gaton D. Clinical efficacy and safety of the EX-PRESS filtration device in patients with advanced neovascular glaucoma and proliferative diabetic retinopathy. Case Rep Ophthalmol. 2018;9(1):67–75.

64. Kawabata K, Shobayashi K, Iwao K, Takahashi E, Tanihara H, Inoue T. Efficacy and safety of Ex-PRESS® mini shunt surgery versus trabeculectomy for neovascular glaucoma: a retrospective comparative study. BMC Ophthalmol. 2019;19(1):75.

65. Watson PG, Jakeman C, Ozturk M, Barnett MF, Barnett F, Khaw KT. The complications of trabeculectomy (a 20-year follow-up). Eye. 1990;4(3):425–38.

66. Liu L, Xu Y, Huang Z, Wang X. Intravitreal ranibizumab injection combined trabeculectomy versus Ahmed valve surgery in the treatment of neovascular glaucoma: assessment of efficacy and complications. BMC Ophthalmol. 2016;16:65.

67. Fernández-Vigo J, Castro J, Cordido M, Fernández-Sabugal J. Treatment of diabetic neovascular glaucoma by panretinal ablation and trabeculectomy. Acta Ophthalmol. 1988;66(6):612–6.

68. Inoue T, Inatani M, Takihara Y, Awai-Kasaoka N, Ogata-Iwao M, Tanihara H. Prognostic risk factors for failure of trabeculectomy with mitomycin C after vitrectomy. Jpn J Ophthalmol. 2012;56(5):464–9.

69. Netland PA. The Ahmed glaucoma valve in neovascular glaucoma (an AOS thesis). Trans Am Ophthalmol Soc. 2009;107:325–42.

70. Every SG, Molteno ACB, Bevin TH, Herbison P. Long-term results of Molteno implant insertion in cases of neovascular glaucoma. Arch Ophthalmol. 2006;124(3):355–60.

71. Sidoti PA, Dunphy TR, Baerveldt G, LaBree L, Minckler DS, Lee PP, et al. Experience with the Baerveldt glaucoma implant in treating neovascular glaucoma. Ophthalmology. 1995;102(7):1107–18.

72. Mermoud A, Salmon JF, Alexander P, Straker C, Murray AD. Molteno tube implantation for neovascular glaucoma. Long-term results and factors influencing the outcome. Ophthalmology. 1993;100(6):897–902.

73. Yalvac IS, Eksioglu U, Satana B, Duman S. Long-term results of Ahmed glaucoma valve and Molteno implant in neovascular glaucoma. Eye (Lond). 2007;21(1):65–70.

74. Krupin T, Kaufman P, Mandell AI, Terry SA, Ritch R, Podos SM, et al. Long-term results of valve implants in filtering surgery for eyes with neovascular glaucoma. Am J Ophthalmol. 1983;95(6):775–82.

75. Im YW, Lym HS, Park CK, Moon JI. Comparison of mitomycin C trabeculectomy and Ahmed valve implant surgery for neovascular glaucoma. J Korean Ophthalmol Soc. 2004;45(9):1515–21.

76. Shen CC, Salim S, Du H, Netland PA. Trabeculectomy versus Ahmed glaucoma valve implantation in neovascular glaucoma. Clin Ophthalmol. 2011;5:281–6.

77. Engin KN, Yılmazlı C, Engin G, Bilgiç L. Results of combined cyclectomy/trabeculectomy procedure compared with Ahmed glaucoma valve implant in neovascular glaucoma cases. ISRN Ophthalmol. 2011;2011:680827.

78. Tokumo K, Komatsu K, Yuasa Y, Murakami Y, Okumichi H, Hirooka K, et al. Treatment outcomes in the neovascular glaucoma tube versus trabeculectomy study. Graefes Arch Clin Exp Ophthalmol. 2021;

Aqueous Shunt for Neovascular Glaucoma

Wesam S. Shalaby, Dilru C. Amarasekera, and Aakriti Garg Shukla

1 Introduction

The angiogenic and inflammatory nature of neovascular glaucoma (NVG) presents unique challenges in surgical management. In NVG, retinal or other ocular ischemia leads to the formation of proangiogenic factors such as vascular endothelial growth factor (VEGF) [1], which stimulates the proliferation of fibrovascular tissue that obstructs aqueous outflow through trabecular meshwork resulting in elevated intraocular pressure (IOP) [2]. In the earlier stages, the iridocorneal angle is still open and the IOP can sometimes be controlled with a combination of antineovascular treatments and medical IOP-lowering ther-

apy. However, in the later stages, the fibrovascular tissue contracts and peripheral anterior synechiae (PAS) develop, resulting in secondary synechial angle closure and profoundly elevated IOP that is often refractory to medical IOP-lowering therapy. Uncontrolled IOP in the setting of NVG can result in devastating vision loss, and surgical intervention is often required to achieve adequate IOP control.

The underlying principle behind traditional glaucoma surgery is to bypass the obstructed trabecular meshwork and divert aqueous out of the eye via a surgically created outflow pathway. Trabeculectomy, the historical "gold standard" IOP-lowering surgery that was discussed in detail in another chapter, has relatively poor success rates in NVG eyes. Aqueous shunts are typically considered the first-line traditional glaucoma surgery in the setting of NVG, because they are less susceptible to conjunctival scarring that contributes to trabeculectomy failure. Aqueous shunts are tubes that are attached to valved or nonvalved endplates of varying size. The tube forms a fistula between the anterior chamber, ciliary sulcus, or vitreous cavity and an equatorial capsule overlying the endplate. The presence of a synthetic tube theoretically maintains a patent sclerostomy, providing an ostomy for aqueous flow that is less likely to become permanently plugged due to hemorrhage, inflammatory factors, etc., than the sclerostomy punch of trabeculectomy [3, 4]. Additionally, the aqueous shunt endplate main-

The original version of the chapter has been revised. A correction to this chapter can be found at https://doi.org/10.1007/978-3-031-11720-6_21

W. S. Shalaby
Bernard and Shirlee Brown Glaucoma Research Laboratory, Department of Ophthalmology, Columbia University Irving Medical Center, New York, NY, USA

Tanta Medical School, Tanta University, Tanta, Gharbia, Egypt

D. C. Amarasekera · A. G. Shukla (✉)
Bernard and Shirlee Brown Glaucoma Research Laboratory, Department of Ophthalmology, Columbia University Irving Medical Center, New York, NY, USA
e-mail: ag2965@cumc.columbia.edu

M. Qiu (ed.), *Neovascular Glaucoma*, Essentials in Ophthalmology, https://doi.org/10.1007/978-3-031-11720-6_17

tains the subconjunctival and/or sub-Tenon's space where the aqueous is filtered. This is in contrast to trabeculectomy, in which the conjunctiva and/or Tenon's capsule can scar directly onto the sclera, resulting in bleb failure. Angiogenesis facilitates migration of fibroblasts into the conjunctiva, leading to collagen deposition and scarring of the trabeculectomy bleb, even in the setting of antifibrotic agents such as 5-fluorouracil and mitomycin C [5, 6]. Another strategy for IOP lowering in NVG eyes is to reduce aqueous production with transscleral cyclophotocoagulation (CPC) [7, 8], which will be explored in another chapter.

This chapter discusses the mechanisms, surgical techniques, outcomes, and complications of various types of aqueous shunt surgery in NVG. We also describe outcomes of combined retinal treatment and aqueous shunt surgery and secondary treatment options if aqueous shunt failure occurs.

2 Valved and Nonvalved Aqueous Shunts in Neovascular Glaucoma

Aqueous shunts are commonly used in the management of glaucoma cases where a trabeculectomy is likely to fail, such as NVG [3, 9–11]. The use of aqueous shunts has become increasingly popular, with a 231% increase between 1994 and 2003 and a further 54% increase between 2003 and 2012 based on United States Medicare data [12]. Likewise, an observational cohort study using Medicare data from 2017 found that trabeculectomies and aqueous shunts made up nearly equal proportions of glaucoma surgery overall (13.1% and 11.4%, respectively) [13]. Additionally, a survey of glaucoma surgeons in 2016 revealed that aqueous shunts were preferred in seven out of eight clinical settings. This demonstrated a significant shift toward aqueous shunts in contrast to a similar previous survey from 1996, which found that trabeculectomy was preferred in eight out of eight clinical settings [14].

All commercially available aqueous shunts share a common design based on the original Molteno implant (Molteno Ophthalmic Limited, Dunedin, New Zealand) [15]. This design consists of a silicone tube that is inserted into the eye which shunts aqueous to an equatorial endplate, leading to a fornix-based capsule. A feature common to all aqueous shunts is construction of the endplate from materials that are resistant to fibroblast adherence. The silicone tube may be inserted into the anterior chamber (Fig. 1a), ciliary sulcus (Fig. 1b), or vitreous cavity (Fig. 1c), and the tube insertion location is based on individual eye characteristics. Typically, the endplate is placed over the equatorial sclera in the superotemporal quadrant as a primary location and the inferonasal quadrant as a secondary location. The various aqueous shunt types differ in size and material composition of the endplate, as well as the presence or absence of a valve [16]. The first attempt at developing an aqueous shunt was reported in 1907, when Rollet implanted a horse-hair thread connecting the anterior chamber to the subconjunctival space near the limbus [17]. This resulted in postoperative hypotony, and modifications including the placement of an external ligature were implemented to prevent complications. Of aqueous shunts currently used, the first was developed in 1973 by Molteno [15], and soon thereafter, Krupin added a valve mechanism in 1976 [18]. The advantages of an aque-

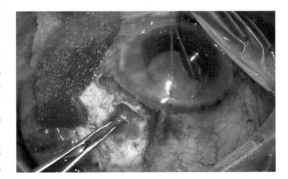

Fig. 1 Aqueous shunt insertion into the anterior chamber. The tube is inserted through a sclerotomy created using a 23-gauge needle in the superotemporal quadrant

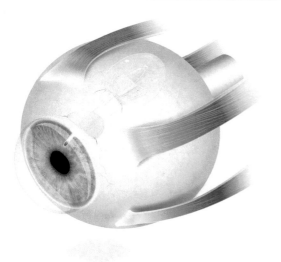

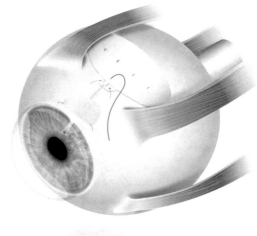

Fig. 2 Ahmed glaucoma valve

Fig. 3 Baerveldt glaucoma implant

ous shunt over trabeculectomy include the following: (1) the presence of a permanent sclerostomy (the tube); (2) aqueous drainage to the equatorial region where the potential for conjunctival scarring may be less than the anterior conjunctiva at the limbus; (3) a predetermined capsular area (the endplate).

Currently, the most commonly used aqueous shunts are the Ahmed glaucoma valve (AGV, New World Medical, Los Ranchos, CA, USA) (Fig. 2) and the Baerveldt glaucoma implant (BGI, Advanced Medical Optics, Santa Ana, CA, USA) (Fig. 3) [19, 20]. While both the AGV and BGI share a tube and endplate design, they differ in two important aspects. Firstly, the AGV has a flow restricting valve on its endplate that limits aqueous outflow when the IOP becomes low; the valve limits early hypotony-related complications without the need for external tube ligation. Secondly, the surface area of the BGI

(350 mm^2) is almost double that of the AGV (184 mm^2); the larger endplate of the BGI has been shown to result in lower IOP long term [21]. Additionally, the AGV's higher long-term IOPs may be related to the exposure of the filtering area to postoperative inflammatory material in the aqueous, which may produce more vigorous scarring of the fibrous capsule surrounding the endplate [20, 22]. The BGI has been found to have a higher complication rate than the AGV, due in part to the absence of a valve mechanism. In the United States, the AGV is currently the only commercially available valved aqueous shunt, though there are several nonvalved aqueous shunts commercially available including the BGI, Molteno, Schocket (self-assembled), and Ahmed ClearPath (New World Medical, Los Ranchos, CA, USA). Figure 4 includes images of the most common commercially available aqueous shunts.

Fig. 4 Most common
commercially available
aqueous shunts
implants: (1) single-
plate Molteno, (2)
double-plate Molteno,
(3) Krupin slit valve, (4)
Ahmed glaucoma valve,
(5) 350 mm² Baerveldt
glaucoma implant, (6)
250 mm² Baerveldt
glaucoma implant

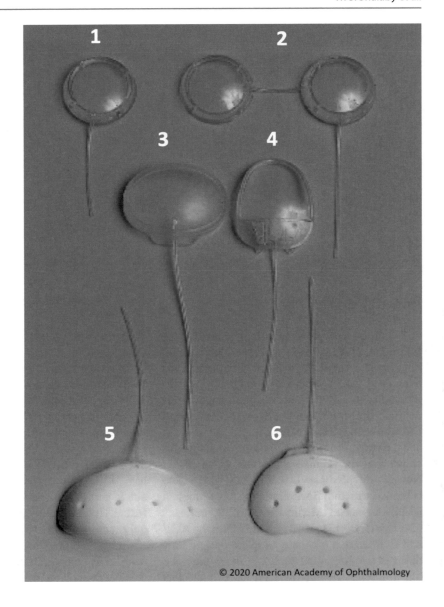

3   Nonvalved Aqueous Shunts

3.1   Molteno

3.1.1   Molteno Device and Procedure

The Molteno implant was designed by Anthony
Molteno in 1973 [15]. By 2004, the tube biomaterial was modified from polypropylene to silicone.

The device has a silicone tube attached to a round
polypropylene endplate. The most commonly used
version of this aqueous shunt, the Molteno 3
implant, is a flexible, larger, single-plate device and
is available in three plate sizes, 185 mm², 245 mm²,
and a pediatric size 80 mm². The double-plate
implant continues to be available and is composed
of two plates connected by a 10 mm silicone tube.

3.1.2 Molteno Outcomes

In a case series published in 1977, Molteno et al. reported outcomes of 12 NVG eyes that underwent a Molteno implant [23]. In this study, IOP improved in 11 of 12 eyes (with or without IOP-lowering medications) at 3–6 months postoperatively. Early complications included variable degrees of hyphema (12/12 eyes), which may be related to the presence of active neovascularization of the angle at the time of tube placement and iris incarcerating tube lumen (3/12 eyes), which was cleared surgically in one case and required a second implant in two cases. The authors noted that cases that resulted in iris incarceration were early on in their case series and may have been due to a lack of surgeon experience. Late complications included prolonged hypotony requiring implant removal (1/12 eyes) and late IOP rise requiring second aqueous shunt (1/12 eyes).

Following this initial case series of Molteno implant outcomes in the setting of NVG, several other studies have reported success rates ranging from 22% to 67% [22, 24–27]. Minckler et al. evaluated 90 patients with refractory glaucoma (18 with NVG) who underwent single-plate Molteno shunt implantation [22]. The reported success rate (success defined as IOP ≤ 21 mmHg with at least 6 months' follow-up) among the NVG cases was 47% [22]. The 5-year results demonstrated further decline in success to 22% in NVG eyes [24]. Similarly, Freedman et al. reported a success rate (success defined as IOP ≤ 21 mm Hg with or without adjunctive medical therapy) of 67% with Molteno shunts in NVG patients after mean follow-up duration of 30 months, suggesting modest success with this device in the setting of NVG [27]. Likewise, Ancker et al. reported a success rate (success defined as IOP <20 mm Hg without medications) of 67% in NVG eyes that had undergone the Molteno implant through an average follow-up duration of 15.5 months [25]. The authors reported that tube occlusion, recurrent hyphema, and inadequate postoperative management were the primary reasons for failure. Mills and colleagues evaluated the long-term outcome of the Molteno implant through a median follow-up duration of 44 months (range, 6–107 months) on

20 NVG eyes and found a success rate of 50% [26]. In this study, success was defined as a postoperative IOP of ≤ 22 mmHg with (qualified success) or without (complete success) glaucoma medications and no additional glaucoma surgery, phthisis, or loss of light perception. A more recent prospective study of 145 NVG eyes followed up for a mean of 3.3 years demonstrated that success (as defined as IOP of 21 mmHg or less) at 1, 2, and 5 years was 72%, 60%, and 40%, respectively; failure to control IOP was significantly correlated with persistent iris neovascularization [28].

The Molteno implant is not commonly used for NVG eyes as it necessitates a ligature suture, as with all nonvalved aqueous shunts. This feature prevents immediate lowering of IOP, which most NVG eyes require. While perioperative panretinal photocoagulation (PRP) was not found to have a significant impact on outcomes [28] and the role of anti-VEGF injections has not been studied in the setting of Molteno implant, these retinal interventions would be logical adjuvant treatments as they are associated with improved outcomes with other aqueous shunts in the setting of NVG.

3.2 Schocket Implant

3.2.1 Schocket Device and Procedure

In 1982, Stanley Schocket reported on the Schocket procedure, which he described as an anterior chamber aqueous shunt linked to an encircling band device. This device was specifically for eyes with prior scleral buckle for retinal detachment, which can be a risk factor for glaucoma development [29–31]. While the scleral buckle is an important tool in the treatment of retinal detachment, it requires significant conjunctival dissection during its implantation and limits subsequent surgical IOP-lowering options. The proposed mechanism for the Schocket procedure is based on the theory that increased episcleral venous pressure inhibits aqueous humor drainage after encircling band surgery and uveoscleral outflow is obstructed by the band. The Schocket procedure shunts aqueous to the capsule of an encircling silicone band (#20), which is secured to the globe, and creates a surface area of 300 mm². Aqueous occupies the space between the band and its encapsulating fibrous tissue for 360 degrees and then diffuses into the orbit, creating a pathway connecting the anterior chamber with periocular lymphatics and venous system [29].

Omi et al. [32] modified Schocket's original technique [29] by using a silicone band encircling the equator for 90 degrees, instead of the 360-degree band originally described by Schocket. This group also used a larger silicone band (#31) which is 0.5 mm wider than the original Schocket band (#20). Additionally, the silicone tube was protected with a scleral graft, instead of Schocket's use of scleral delamination. Finally, Omi et al. [32] and others [22] ligated the tube with an absorbable suture similar to the ligating suture used for other nonvalved aqueous shunts, to reduce the risk of postoperative hypotony and anterior chamber shallowing.

3.2.2 Schocket Outcomes

In 1982, Schocket et al. described the original surgical technique and outcomes in 19 NVG eyes with follow-up ranging from 5 to 26 months [29]. At the end of the follow-up period, 18 of 19 eyes (95%) had IOP ≤20 mmHg. The mean preoperative IOP was 54.1 mmHg, and the mean postoperative IOP was 16.2 mmHg at the final follow-up visit with minimal need for IOP-lowering medications (only 3 patients required 1–2 medications). Common postoperative complications included prolonged flat anterior chamber (74%), hyphema (21%), and acceleration of cataract formation (25%). Preoperative panretinal cryotherapy or PRP was performed according to the presence or absence of media opacity, respectively, to reduce the risk of hyphema [29]. These results were comparable to other aqueous shunts used in the setting of NVG at that time (initial data on the Krupin and Molteno implants) [33–35]. Schocket et al. postulated that the success of the Schocket procedure depends on the formation of a fibrous capsule around the silicone band to provide resistance to aqueous outflow and avoid hypotony-related complications [33, 34]. Success

rates (success defined as IOP ≤21 mmHg) with other procedures in the setting of NVG have ranged between 59% and 72% [23, 36–38], while Schocket et al's small study with long-term follow-up had a 96% success rate [39].

Using the modified Schocket technique as described above [39], 55 eyes with various forms of refractory glaucoma (12/55 eyes were NVG) were evaluated for average follow-up duration of 10.3 ± 5.4 months. IOP remained <21 mmHg in 50 eyes (90.9%), 13 of which (26.0%) were on no IOP-lowering medications. Complications were reported in 13 eyes (23.6%) and were most commonly tube occlusion by iris (5.4%), tube occlusion by vitreous (3.6%) and choroidal effusion (3.6%), and tube retraction (3.6%); treatment was successful in 11 eyes [39]. While the modified Schocket procedure appears to provide favorable outcomes with a possible enhanced safety profile as compared to the original procedure, it may not be an option in all eyes. Adequate filtration may not result in cases in which incomplete conjunctival scarring is present around the encircling device or when encircling bands are posteriorly located or are thin and narrow.

The Schocket procedure is not a common management choice for NVG eyes, as it requires the presence of an encircling scleral buckle and its modified approach requires a ligature suture, which does not lend itself to the immediate IOP lowering that most NVG eyes require. As with other IOP-lowering treatments in the setting of NVG, adjuvant anti-VEGF and/or PRP is expected to be associated with better outcomes. Published reports on the Schocket procedure were prior to the anti-VEGF era, and outcomes with adjuvant anti-VEGF treatment have not yet been reported.

3.3 Baerveldt Glaucoma Implant

3.3.1 Baerveldt Device and Procedure

In 1992, George Baerveldt pioneered a nonvalved silicone implant with an even larger surface area than existing devices with the introduction of endplates sized at 250 mm² and

350 mm² [40, 41]. As with all nonvalved aqueous shunts, the BGI requires tube ligation with a dissolvable suture to prevent early hypotony until a fibrous capsule forms around the endplate to provide resistance to aqueous outflow. As a result, IOP lowering with a BGI is not immediate, and there are numerous strategies such as fenestrations, wicks, and orphan trabeculectomy to enhance early IOP lowering with nonvalved aqueous shunts. Winged nonvalved aqueous shunts including BGI require implantation under the rectus muscles; this is especially important in the larger 350 mm² version of the implant.

3.3.2 Baerveldt Outcomes

The Ahmed Baerveldt Comparison (ABC) study compared the AGV versus BGI in various types of refractory glaucoma including NVG. During the ABC's 5 years of follow-up, the BGI was found to be more effective in providing long-term IOP control than the AGV and was associated with less dependence on IOP-lowering medications, albeit a higher complication rate mostly related to early postoperative hypotony [19].

In a case series published in 1995, Sidoti et al. reported outcomes of 36 NVG eyes that underwent BGIs (18 BGI 350 mm², 16 BGI 500 mm², 2 BGI 200 mm²) [3]. Success, which was defined as final IOP ≤21 mmHg without additional IOP-lowering surgery or devastating complication, was 79% and 56% at 12 and 18 months, respectively. Visual acuity remained stable or improved in 10/36 (31%) patients. Postoperative complications included flat anterior chamber, serous choroidal detachment, and obstruction of the tube tip with fibrovascular tissue, each of which occurred in 4/36 (11%) patients; unfortunately, 11/36 (31%) patients lost light perception due to glaucomatous optic neuropathy or the underlying ischemic retinal disease. There were no significant differences between the groups receiving the 350 and 500 mm² implants with respect to success rates, percentage of postoperative IOP reduction, or complication rates, suggesting an upper limit of endplate size as it relates to effectiveness and safety. A more recent retrospective comparative study by Shalaby and colleagues in

2020 evaluated the outcomes of AGV versus BGI in 152 NVG eyes [42]. BGI achieved significant IOP and medication reduction at month 6 and the final visit (29.6 ± 25.8 months). Surgical failure defined as IOP >21 mmHg with IOP-lowering medications or < 5 mmHg at two consecutive visits, loss of light perception vision, or additional IOP-lowering surgery occurred in 25.9% of BGI eyes by 6 months. At the final visit, 14.8% of BGI eyes progressed to no light perception, which was comparable to the AGV outcomes.

The aforementioned studies suggest that BGIs may be a suitable surgical option for IOP lowering in the setting of NVG. Because the tube is ligated, additional maneuvers including tube fenestrations, concurrent procedures, and an aggressive medication regimen are necessary to enhance early IOP lowering. Extra precautions in the form of activity limitation should be taken at the time of expected tube opening, which is about 6 weeks from the procedure. Throughout the postoperative course, excellent control of the underlying neovascular drive with anti-VEGF and/or PRP is necessary to optimize outcomes. Additional research in this area is needed to balance the potential benefits and risks of NVG management with BGI.

3.4 Ahmed ClearPath

3.4.1 ClearPath Device and Procedure

In 2019, the Ahmed ClearPath implant (New World Medical, Los Ranchos, CA, USA) was introduced as a new nonvalved aqueous shunt [43]. The Ahmed ClearPath (Fig. 5) features a flexible, contoured plate that conforms to the eye's curvature. Two sizes are available as follows: The 350 mm² requires implantation of the wings under the rectus muscles, and the 250 mm² is a smaller single quadrant implant that can be positioned between two rectus muscles without manipulating them. The anchoring eyelets are positioned more anteriorly on the ClearPath than other aqueous shunts to enhance ease of suturing the endplate to the sclera [43]. The device is similar in mechanism to the BGI,

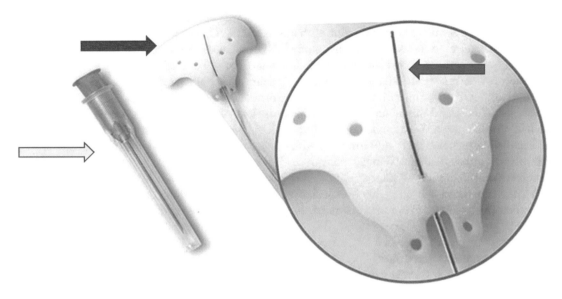

Fig. 5 Ahmed ClearPath implant. The flexible contoured plate that conforms to the eye's curvature (red arrow), a 23-gauge needle for tube insertion (yellow arrow), and prethreaded ripcord suture (blue arrow)

with some features that may streamline the surgical procedure.

3.4.2 ClearPath Outcomes

The outcomes of the Ahmed ClearPath implant in the setting of NVG are yet to be published but are expected to be similar to those of the BGI given their common features.

---

4 Valved Aqueous Shunts

4.1 Krupin Eye Valve

4.1.1 Krupin Device and Procedure

In 1976, Theodore Krupin designed a pressure-sensitive unidirectional valve to provide filtration restriction through a passive mechanism. The Krupin slit valve (Hood Laboratories, Pembroke, Massachusetts, USA) is composed of a silicone tube with an outer diameter of 0.64 mm and several horizontal and vertical slits that act as pressure-sensitive and unidirectional valves. The tube is sutured within the groove of a silicone implant. The 180-degree implant is placed beneath 3 rectus muscles [18]. The device is

designed to open when IOP is >11 mmHg and close when IOP is <9 mmHg [18]. The original Krupin valve is currently not available. Two modified versions of the Krupin shunt, a valved (flow-restrictive mechanism) and a nonvalved implant, were approved by the US Food and Drug Administration (FDA) for the treatment of refractory glaucoma. Both the smaller, valved version (209 mm^2), and the larger, nonvalved implant (365 mm^2) are currently being tested for safety and efficacy in pilot studies.

4.1.2 Krupin Outcomes

Limited studies published between 1980 and 1996 of Krupin outcomes in NVG reveal modest surgical success of 36–77% over variable follow-up periods [33, 36, 44, 45]. In one report, 68% of eyes (40 NVG eyes) had a postoperative IOP ≤24 mm Hg and 50% of eyes were on no IOP-lowering medication during the mean follow-up period of 13.8 months. Failure was primarily attributed to scarring of the external capsule [33] and reported early complications included shallow or flat anterior chamber (53.6%), hypotony (57.1%), high IOP (25%), serous choroidal effusion (25%), fibrinous uveitis (17.9%), tube occlusion by fibrin (17.9%), and choroidal hemorrhage (7.1%). Late complications included external conjunctival fibrosis (42.9%), tube occlusion by fibrovascular tissue (17.9%), cataract (7.1%), bullous keratopathy (7.1%), exposure of the silicone valve (7.1%), and phthisis bulbi (7.1%) [36].

4.2 Ahmed Glaucoma Valve

4.2.1 AGV Device and Procedure

The AGV was developed by Mateen Ahmed in 1993 and provides a regulated valve mechanism to limit aqueous humor outflow [46, 47]. This device consists of 3 parts as follows: (1) a plate with a surface area of 184 mm^2 composed of silicone, polypropylene, or porous polyethylene; (2) a silicone drainage tube; and (3) a silicone valve mechanism overlying the plate. The AGV valve mechanism consists of thin silicone elastomer membranes, which are 8 mm long and 7 mm wide and create a Venturi-shaped chamber. The membranes are designed to open and close in response to IOP variations to maintain IOP in the range of 8–12 mmHg, theoretically allowing for immediate IOP reduction while preventing hypotony-associated complications. However, the AGV may be associated with a higher rate of long-term failure as compared to the BGI, the other most common aqueous shunt [48, 49].

Since the IOP is often profoundly elevated in NVG, the AGV is a commonly utilized aqueous shunt in the setting of NVG because it provides immediate IOP lowering. However, eventual encapsulation of the AGV endplate by a thick fibrotic capsule and/or occlusion of the valve mechanism by a fibrous stalk of tissue can lead AGV failure. The fibrous capsule around the AGV forms around 4–6 weeks. A thicker and more congested capsule surrounding the AGV plate may contribute to the increased likelihood of the hypertensive phase, which may be the result of early contact of aqueous inflammatory mediators with overlying tissues. These inflammatory mediators may be greater in NVG, leading to a thicker fibrous capsule surrounding the AGV endplate. Another possibility may be higher aqueous hydrostatic pressure within the drainage area, which could compress, compact, and stiffen the capsule. It has been shown that early aqueous suppressant treatment may improve AGV implantation outcomes in terms of IOP reduction, success rate, and hypertensive phase frequency [50]. Alternatively, using a thin layer of cotton soaked with mitomycin C to encompass the valve plate may decrease the incidence of encapsulated cyst following AGV implantation [51]. Additionally, the use of adjunctive sub-Tenon's injection of triamcinolone acetonide with AGV has been shown to blunt peak IOP levels and improve visual outcomes, but has not been shown to lower the incidence of the hypertensive phase [52].

4.2.2 Ahmed Valve Outcomes

In a retrospective case series published in 2019, Xie et al. reported the outcomes of 66 NVG eyes that underwent AGV [10]. Approximately 60% of eyes had prior PRP, and 47% had prior intravitreal anti-VEGF. IOP was significantly lower at all postoperative visits compared to the baseline, and the surgical success (defined as IOP between 6 mmHg and 21 mmHg with or without IOP-lowering medications) was 66.7% at 12 months. Multivariate regression analysis revealed that younger age, PRP, and absence of postoperative complications were significant factors influencing the surgical success rate ($P < 0.05$ for all) [10]. Another retrospective case–control study published by Netland et al. in 2009 included 38 NVG eyes and 38 non-NVG control eyes that underwent AGV, with average follow-up duration of 18 months [9]. All NVG eyes were treated with PRP or endolaser immediately before or after surgery; anti-VEGF was not used. Surgical success (defined as IOP between 6 mmHg and 21 mmHg without additional IOP-lowering surgery and without loss of light perception) was lower for the NVG group compared to the control group at all time points (73.1%, 61.9%, and 20.6% at 1 year, 2 years, and 5 years for NVG eyes compared to 89.2%, 81.8%, and 81.8% at 1 year, 2 years, and 5 years for control eyes). Additionally, regression analysis revealed that NVG was a risk factor for surgical failure [9].

Studies on AGV outcomes with adjunctive intravitreal anti-VEGF have been more encouraging. A prospective, nonrandomized study published by Eid et al. in 2009 included 20 NVG eyes that received intravitreal anti-VEGF 1–2 weeks prior to AGV with (10 eyes) or without PRP (10 eyes) and 10 historical control NVG eyes that underwent PRP (without anti-VEGF) before AGV [53]. This analysis reported that surgical success (defined as IOP ≤25 mmHg with or without IOP-lowering medications without devastating complications, loss of light perception, or the need for additional IOP-lowering surgery) and complications were comparable between the two groups at a minimum follow-up of 1 year [53]. Furthermore, a meta-analysis conducted by Zhou et al. comparing AGV outcomes with and without intravitreal anti-VEGF found that the anti-VEGF group had numerically greater (but not statistically significant) IOP-lowering efficacy (P = 0.152) [54]. Additionally, while the anti-VEGF group had higher rate of complete surgical success and lower frequency of hyphema, both groups had comparable reduction of IOP-lowering medications [54]. Likewise, other studies have also reported that adjunctive anti-VEGF reduces intraocular bleeding (including hyphema, vitreous hemorrhage, and suprachoroidal hemorrhage) after AGV [55–58].

Another consideration for aqueous shunt efficacy is its biomaterial, which may affect capsule formation around the plate, especially in inflammatory settings such as NVG. A prospective randomized study published in 2018 by Lubiński et al. compared NVG eyes undergoing polypropylene (23 eyes) versus silicone (27 eyes) AGVs [59]. This analysis reported that surgical success was higher in silicone AGVs than propylene AGVs (66.7% versus 27.3%; P < 0.007) through 2 years of follow-up. Additionally, the total number of complications in both groups was similar, except for a higher occurrence of fibrous capsule scarring in the polypropylene valve group (18% versus 35%, P < 0.04). Such results suggest that silicone AGV may be more effective in the setting of NVG.

5   Complications of Aqueous Shunts for Neovascular Glaucoma

The complications of valved and nonvalved aqueous shunts have been well described [19, 20, 48, 60, 61], and there are special considerations in the setting of NVG. Given the presence of iris and angle neovascularization, intraoperative and postoperative hyphema are more commonly seen in NVG eyes compared to eyes with other types of glaucoma (15.8% versus 2.6%), where anti-VEGF is not used [9]. In a meta-analysis evaluating the outcomes of AGV in NVG, hyphema and flat anterior chamber were found to be the most common complications and concomitant intravitreal anti-VEGF was shown to significantly reduce postoperative hyphema [54].

The rate of tube exposure would also be expected to be higher among NVG eyes. Vasculopathies are associated with changes in the conjunctival vasculature similar to those found in the retinal vasculature, suggesting that there is poor conjunctival perfusion which may theoretically result in less tissue modulation and poorer tissue strength [62]. In a case–control study, Koval et al. investigated the potential risk factors for aqueous shunt exposure and reported that Hispanic ethnicity (P = 0.012), NVG (P = 0.006), previous trabeculectomy (P = 0.007), and combined surgery (including cataract surgery, corneal transplant, vitrectomy) (P = 0.038) were the strongest predictors for tube exposure [63]. In this study, the most common underlying etiology of NVG was diabetes [63]. Theoretically, prolonged topical steroid use may be a potential risk factor for tube exposure. Eyes with NVG are more likely to be on topical steroids for anterior segment inflammation or macular edema. In such cases, intravitreal injection of steroids may be safer than prolonged topical steroid use to lower the risk of tube exposure. A study by Chaku et al. identified younger age and preoperative inflammation as risk factors for tube exposure [64]. Interestingly, the study also revealed a statistically significant association between topical steroid use and tube exposure.

Major vision loss is a devastating outcome after any ophthalmic surgery and is unfortunately common in the setting of NVG. The ABC [19] and the Ahmed versus Baerveldt (AVB) [20] studies were multicenter randomized prospective clinical trials that compared the outcomes of AGV and BGI in uncontrolled glaucoma over 5 years. Notably, 24 of 25 eyes in the ABC and 7 of 14 eyes in the AVB that progressed to no light perception vision had NVG, reflecting this condition's poor visual outcomes. The ABC demonstrated that the cumulative proportion of NVG eyes that progressed to no light perception vision in the AGV group was 28.3%, which was significantly lower than the 51.1% of NVG eyes that progressed to no light perception vision in the BGI group ($P = 0.03$) [19]. However, in Shalaby et al's study, there was no statistically significant difference in progression to no light perception vision between the AGV and BGI groups (18.7% versus 14.8%; $P = 0.53$), despite the larger sample size compared to the ABC's NVG subgroup ($n = 152$ versus $n = 80$) [42]. Using univariate and multivariate regression analysis, the authors also showed that poor preoperative visual acuity, bilaterality of the underlying retinal pathology, and failure to undergo early PRP were associated with progression to no light perception vision. These findings suggest that the underlying ischemic pathology in NVG may influence the visual outcomes more so than worsening glaucomatous optic neuropathy, choice of IOP-lowering treatment, and demographics [42].

Furthermore, a study by Netland et al. which included 76 AGV eyes demonstrated that although IOP control and complications were similar between the NVG and non-NVG groups, visual outcomes were worse in the NVG group, with 23.7% of NVG eyes progressing to no light perception vision ($P = 0.002$), compared to no patients in the control group [9]. Additionally, the majority of eyes that progressed to no light perception did not have elevated IOP during the postoperative period, suggesting a potential ischemic mechanism for visual decline rather than elevated IOP. This study and others highlight the importance of close monitoring and treatment of

anterior and posterior segment neovascularization in these patients, since IOP elevation is only one of many variables that may be associated with poor outcomes in NVG eyes.

Hypotony and its related events (shallow or flat anterior chamber, choroidal effusion, and hypotony-related maculopathy) are well-known complications of aqueous shunts, especially non-valved shunts [19, 20, 61]. Leaving viscoelastic in the anterior chamber at the end of surgery is recommended if the preoperative IOP is very high, which is often the case in NVG. Other management strategies to prevent or reverse hypotony include the prophylactic insertion of a thick ripcord suture to keep the tube lumen partially occluded after the ligature suture dissolves, religating the tube, plugging the tube *ab interno*, or removing the tube.

6   Suppressing the Underlying Neovascular Drive

The two main treatment goals for NVG are as follows: (1) adequate IOP control with medical or surgical therapy to prevent progressive glaucomatous optic neuropathy and (2) adequate treatment of the underlying etiology with antineovascular treatments [65–68]. PRP and anti-VEGF are each discussed in detail in other chapters. Treating the underlying source of the neovascularization before aqueous shunt surgery may reduce the incidence of surgical complications such as intraoperative or postoperative hyphema, which can lead to vision loss, acute IOP elevation, and long-term aqueous shunt failure. After the aqueous shunt has been implanted to control IOP, it is critical that the patient has close follow-up with the retina service to adequately treat the underlying disease until quiescence is achieved. Furthermore, detailed anterior segment exams looking for recurrent iris or angle neovascularization remain important, even after the IOP has been controlled with an aqueous shunt, because anterior segment neovascularization is a sign that the posterior segment neovascular drive is not adequately controlled.

There is evidence that the success rate of aqueous shunt surgery is higher in the setting of adjunctive anti-VEGF compared to adjunctive PRP alone [42, 53]. A prospective nonrandomized study comparing the efficacy of intravitreal anti-VEGF versus PRP prior to aqueous shunt implantation in NVG found a surgical success rate of 90% with anti-VEGF and PRP, 80% with anti-VEGF alone, and 70% with PRP alone prior to aqueous shunt surgery [53]. Similar results were observed in a retrospective case–control study comparing combined PRP and anti-VEGF versus PRP alone in 23 NVG eyes, which demonstrated that combined treatment resulted in a more rapid decrease in IOP and increased frequency and rapidity of neovascularization regression [69]. The study by Shalaby et al. reported that PRP was highly significant as a protective factor against progression to no light perception vision ($P < 0.001$) after AGV or BGI in the setting of NVG [42].

7   Placement of Aqueous Shunts in the Ciliary Sulcus

The placement of aqueous shunts in the ciliary sulcus may have some advantages over traditional placement in the anterior chamber in the setting of NVG. Broad high PAS with a consequently shallow anterior chamber and hyper-deep sulcus are typical features of NVG and can introduce challenges in anterior chamber tube placement. Tube-cornea touch can result due to an excessively anterior tube placement in the setting of PAS, potentially accelerating corneal decompensation. Additionally, tube-iris touch can cause persistent postoperative iritis and/or cystoid macular edema. Additionally, cutting or chafing the PAS and/or iris root at the time of tube insertion can lead to hyphema. Sulcus tube placement avoids these potential challenges. Additionally, while sulcus tube placement is similar in concept to pars plana aqueous shunts in that it reduces potential corneal complications, it does not require a pars plana vitrectomy (PPV) if there is sufficient capsular remnant separating the vitreous from the sulcus space. However, a potential limitation is that tube placement in the sulcus and the vitreous cavity can take place only in the presence of pseudophakia and aphakia. Although there are limited studies on sulcus tube placement in NVG, available reports describe favorable outcomes. A retrospective review of 23 NVG eyes with AGV insertion into the sulcus with a mean follow-up duration of 9 months (range 3–24 months) reported a success rate of 78.6% (defined as IOP < 21 mmHg and 20% reduction in IOP, without further surgery for complications of IOP lowering, without loss of light perception) [70]. Other case reports of AGV insertion into the sulcus in the setting of NVG have reported similar success [71, 72].

8   Combined Aqueous Shunt and Retinal Surgery

Pars plana aqueous shunt placement is another alternative to traditional anterior chamber placement that can be considered when anterior chamber complications are anticipated based on anatomical considerations (e.g., high PAS and shallow peripheral anterior chamber), in the presence of corneal disease, or when a PPV is needed for another indication (i.e., vitreous hemorrhage, tractional retinal detachment). A concurrent or prior PPV is required to prevent vitreous occlusion of a pars plana tube. A thorough peripheral vitreous shave under scleral depression is critical, since it has been reported that 10% of eyes with a pars plana tube ultimately require return to the operating room because of tube occlusion [11, 73].

The literature contains several studies on the efficacy of various types of aqueous shunts combined with PPV for NVG. Although the visual potential of eyes with NVG is often poor, 67% of eyes that underwent PPV with pars plana AGV experienced significant improvement in visual acuity postoperatively (average of 2 lines) [74]. Approximately 35% of patients who underwent a PPV with pars plana Molteno or BGI experienced a similar gain in visual acuity [11, 74]. Additionally, Kolomeyer et al. described characteristics and outcomes of PPV and pars plana BGI in 89

NVG eyes with an average follow-up of 20 months [11]. Anti-VEGF injections were administered to 58% of the eyes preoperatively, at the discretion of the surgeon. Surgical success, defined as IOP between 6 mmHg and 21 mmHg with or without IOP-lowering medications, was achieved in 67% of eyes, and the postoperative IOP and number of IOP-lowering medications were significantly lower than the preoperative values. The most common complications included transient ocular hypertension (92%), transient hypotony (22%), hyphema (21%), corneal edema (19%), and vitreous hemorrhage (16%). The frequency of transient hypotony, vitreous hemorrhage, and rubeosis was significantly higher in 20-gauge when compared to 23- or 25-gauge PPV eyes. Nine eyes (10%) required return to the operating room, including 4 eyes for retinal detachment (unspecified whether the detachments were related to the tube or to the underlying disease) and 3 eyes for elevated IOP due to tube occlusion. Three eyes developed endophthalmitis, 14 eyes progressed to no light perception vision, and two progressed to phthisis [11]. Similar case series of PPV and pars plana AGV in NVG eyes demonstrated significant IOP lowering with few complications [74, 75].

9 Secondary Treatment Options if Aqueous Shunt Failure Occurs

Large randomized clinical trials have demonstrated that aqueous shunt failure occurs in 30% to 49% of all cases (regardless of glaucoma type) by 5 years of follow-up and that this proportion is as high as 66–71% in the setting of NVG [48, 76]. Supplemental medical IOP-lowering therapy is often first-line treatment and is often necessary in NVG, as nearly all patients (98.2%) required IOP-lowering medications by the 5-year time point in the ABC study [48]. For failed aqueous shunts that are refractory to medical therapy, IOP-lowering interventions include aqueous shunt revision (i.e., excision of a portion of the capsule overlying the endplate), second aqueous

shunt implantation, or CPC. In a study comparing aqueous shunt revision versus second aqueous shunt, 4 of 6 NVG eyes in the revision group and 2 of 2 NVG eyes in the second aqueous shunt group had IOP >21 mmHg despite maximal medical therapy at the last follow-up visit [77]. In this study, second shunt surgery was preferred over revision in the setting of an elevated capsule overlying the endplate. The two eyes with IOP <21 mmHg after revision underwent either an AGV or Molteno.

CPC has historically been associated with vision loss in the setting of NVG. Small case series of CPC after previously failed aqueous shunts in the setting of NVG demonstrated that 2 of 4 and 3 of 4 NVG eyes progressed to no light perception vision [78, 79]. Modifications in CPC delivery and technique as well as the introduction of micropulse CPC may lead to improved outcomes in this setting.

10 Conclusion

Aqueous shunts continue to be the first-line surgery for NVG. Valved aqueous shunts are commonly used since they allow for immediate IOP lowering which is often needed in the setting of acute NVG. On the other hand, nonvalved aqueous shunts are less commonly used in this setting, since IOP lowering does not typically occur until after the ligature suture dissolves. More aggressive medical and surgical strategies for early IOP lowering might expand the arena for nonvalved aqueous shunts to be used more commonly in the setting of NVG. Regardless of the type of aqueous shunt that is used, performing PRP and/or anti-VEGF injections to control retinal ischemia is vital in the perioperative period, as is close coordinated follow-up with retina and glaucoma specialists.

References

1. Brown GC, Magargal LE, Schachat A, Shah H. Neovascular glaucoma. Etiologic considerations. Ophthalmology. 1984;91(4):315–20.
2. Sivak-Callcott JA, O'Day DM, Gass JD, Tsai JC. Evidence-based recommendations for the diag-

nosis and treatment of neovascular glaucoma. Ophthalmology. 2001;108(10):1767–76. quiz1777, 1800

3. Sidoti PA, Dunphy TR, Baerveldt G, et al. Experience with the Baerveldt glaucoma implant in treating neovascular glaucoma. Ophthalmology. 1995;102(7):1107–18.

4. Seibold LK, Sherwood MB, Kahook MY. Wound modulation after filtration surgery. Surv Ophthalmol. 2012;57(6):530–50.

5. Hyung SM, Kim SK. Mid-term effects of trabeculectomy with mitomycin C in neovascular glaucoma patients. Korean J Ophthalmol. 2001;15(2):98–106.

6. Tsai JC, Feuer WJ, Parrish RK, Grajewski AL. 5-Fluorouracil filtering surgery and neovascular glaucoma. Long-term follow-up of the original pilot study. Ophthalmology. 1995;102(6):887–92. discussion 892–883.

7. Delgado MF, Dickens CJ, Iwach AG, et al. Long-term results of noncontact neodymium:yttrium-aluminum-garnet cyclophotocoagulation in neovascular glaucoma. Ophthalmology. 2003;110(5):895–9.

8. Eid TE, Katz LJ, Spaeth GL, Augsburger JJ. Tube-shunt surgery versus neodymium:YAG cyclophotocoagulation in the management of neovascular glaucoma. Ophthalmology. 1997;104(10):1692–700.

9. Netland PA. The Ahmed glaucoma valve in neovascular glaucoma (an AOS thesis). Trans Am Ophthalmol Soc. 2009;107:325–42.

10. Xie Z, Liu H, Du M, et al. Efficacy of Ahmed glaucoma valve implantation on neovascular glaucoma. Int J Med Sci. 2019;16(10):1371–6.

11. Kolomeyer AM, Seery CW, Emami-Naeimi P, Zarbin MA, Fechtner RD, Bhagat N. Combined pars plana vitrectomy and pars plana Baerveldt tube placement in eyes with neovascular glaucoma. Retina. 2015;35(1):17–28.

12. Arora KS, Robin AL, Corcoran KJ, Corcoran SL, Ramulu PY. Use of various glaucoma surgeries and procedures in Medicare beneficiaries from 1994 to 2012. Ophthalmology. 2015;122(8):1615–24.

13. Ma AK, Lee JH, Warren JL, Teng CC. GlaucoMap—distribution of glaucoma surgical procedures in the United States. Clin Ophthalmol. 2020;14:2551–60.

14. Vinod K, Gedde SJ, Feuer WJ, et al. Practice preferences for glaucoma surgery: a Survey of the American Glaucoma Society. J Glaucoma. 2017;26(8):687–93.

15. Molteno AC, Straughan JL, Ancker E. Long tube implants in the management of glaucoma. S Afr Med J. 1976;50(27):1062–6.

16. Patel S, Pasquale LR. Glaucoma drainage devices: a review of the past, present, and future. Semin Ophthalmol. 2010;25(5-6):265–70.

17. Le RM. drainage au irin de la chambre anterieure contre l'hypertonie et al douleur. Rev Gen Ophthalmol. 1906;25:481.

18. Krupin T, Podos SM, Becker B, Newkirk JB. Valve implants in filtering surgery. Am J Ophthalmol. 1976;81(2):232–5.

19. Budenz DL, Barton K, Gedde SJ, et al. Five-year treatment outcomes in the Ahmed Baerveldt comparison study. Ophthalmology. 2015;122(2):308–16.

20. Christakis PG, Kalenak JW, Tsai JC, et al. The Ahmed versus Baerveldt study: five-year treatment outcomes. Ophthalmology. 2016;123(10):2093–102.

21. Gedde SJ, Panarelli JF, Banitt MR, Lee RK. Evidenced-based comparison of aqueous shunts. Curr Opin Ophthalmol. 2013;24(2):87–95.

22. Minckler DS, Heuer DK, Hasty B, Baerveldt G, Cutting RC, Barlow WE. Clinical experience with the single-plate Molteno implant in complicated glaucomas. Ophthalmology. 1988;95(9):1181–8.

23. Molteno AC, Van Rooyen MM, Bartholomew RS. Implants for draining neovascular glaucoma. Br J Ophthalmol. 1977;61(2):120–5.

24. Lloyd MA, Sedlak T, Heuer DK, et al. Clinical experience with the single-plate Molteno implant in complicated glaucomas. Update of a pilot study. Ophthalmology. 1992;99(5):679–87.

25. Ancker E, Molteno AC. Molteno drainage implant for neovascular glaucoma. Trans Ophthalmol Soc U K. 1982;102(Pt 1):122–4.

26. Mills RP, Reynolds A, Emond MJ, Barlow WE, Leen MM. Long-term survival of Molteno glaucoma drainage devices. Ophthalmology. 1996;103(2):299–305.

27. Freedman J, Rubin B. Molteno implants as a treatment for refractory glaucoma in black patients. Arch Ophthalmol. 1991;109(10):1417–20.

28. Every SG, Molteno AC, Bevin TH, Herbison P. Long-term results of Molteno implant insertion in cases of neovascular glaucoma. Arch Ophthalmol. 2006;124(3):355–60.

29. Schocket SS, Lakhanpal V, Richards RD. Anterior chamber tube shunt to an encircling band in the treatment of neovascular glaucoma. Ophthalmology. 1982;89(10):1188–94.

30. Gedde SJ. Management of glaucoma after retinal detachment surgery. Curr Opin Ophthalmol. 2002;13(2):103–9.

31. Kornmann HL, Gedde SJ. Glaucoma management after vitreoretinal surgeries. Curr Opin Ophthalmol. 2016;27(2):125–31.

32. Omi CA, De Almeida GV, Cohen R, Mandia C Jr, Kwitko S. Modified Schocket implant for refractory glaucoma. Experience of 55 cases. Ophthalmology. 1991;98(2):211–4.

33. Krupin T, Kaufman P, Mandell A, et al. Filtering valve implant surgery for eyes wtih neovascular glaucoma. Am J Ophthalmol. 1980;89(3):338–43.

34. Folberg R, Hargett NA, Weaver JE, McLean IW. Filtering valve implant for neovascular glaucoma in proliferative diabetic retinopathy. Ophthalmology. 1982;89(3):286–9.

35. Molteno AC, Ancker E, Van Biljon G. Surgical technique for advanced juvenile glaucoma. Arch Ophthalmol. 1984;102(1):51–7.

36. Krupin T, Kaufman P, Mandell AI, et al. Long-term results of valve implants in filtering surgery for

eyes with neovascular glaucoma. Am J Ophthalmol. 1983;95(6):775–82.

37. Herschler J, Agness D. A modified filtering operation for neovascular glaucoma. Arch Ophthalmol. 1979;97(12):2339–41.

38. Sinclair SH, Aaberg TM, Meredith TA. A pars plana filtering procedure combined with lensectomy and vitrectomy for neovascular for neovascular glaucoma. Am J Ophthalmol. 1982;93(2):185–91.

39. Schocket SS, Nirankari VS, Lakhanpal V, Richards RD, Lerner BC. Anterior chamber tube shunt to an encircling band in the treatment of neovascular glaucoma and other refractory glaucomas. A long-term study. Ophthalmology. 1985;92(4):553–62.

40. Lloyd MA, Baerveldt G, Heuer DK, Minckler DS, Martone JF. Initial clinical experience with the Baerveldt implant in complicated glaucomas. Ophthalmology. 1994;101(4):640–50.

41. Siegner SW, Netland PA, Urban RC Jr, et al. Clinical experience with the Baerveldt glaucoma drainage implant. Ophthalmology. 1995;102(9):1298–307.

42. Shalaby WS, Myers JS, Razeghinejad R, Katz LJ, Pro M, Dale E, Fudemberg SJ, Mantravadi AV, Shukla AG. Outcomes of valved and nonvalved tube Shunts in neovascular glaucoma. Ophthalmol Glaucoma. 2021;4(2):182–192. https://doi.org/10.1016/j.ogla.2020.09.010. Epub 2020 Sep 18. PMID: 32956898.

43. New World Medical. Ahmed ClearPath®. https://www.newworldmedical.com/ahmed-clearpath/. Published 2019. Accessed 2021.

44. Krupin T, Ritch R, Camras CB, et al. A long Krupin-Denver valve implant attached to a 180 degrees scleral explant for glaucoma surgery. Ophthalmology. 1988;95(9):1174–80.

45. Mastropasqua L, Carpineto P, Ciancaglini M, Zuppardi E. Long-term results of Krupin-Denver valve implants in filtering surgery for neovascular glaucoma. Ophthalmologica. 1996;210(4):203–6.

46. Coleman AL, Hill R, Wilson MR, et al. Initial clinical experience with the Ahmed glaucoma valve implant. Am J Ophthalmol. 1995;120(1):23–31.

47. Coleman AL, Wilson MR, Tam M, et al. Initial clinical experience with the Ahmed glaucoma valve implant—correction. Am J Ophthalmol. 1995;120(5):684.

48. Christakis PG, Zhang D, Budenz DL, et al. Five-year pooled data analysis of the Ahmed Baerveldt Comparison Study and the Ahmed versus Baerveldt Study. Am J Ophthalmol. 2017;176:118–26.

49. Tsai JC, Johnson CC, Kammer JA, Dietrich MS. The Ahmed shunt versus the Baerveldt shunt for refractory glaucoma II: longer-term outcomes from a single surgeon. Ophthalmology. 2006;113(6):913–7.

50. Pakravan M, Rad SS, Yazdani S, Ghahari E, Yaseri M. Effect of early treatment with aqueous suppressants on Ahmed glaucoma valve implantation outcomes. Ophthalmology. 2014;121(9):1693–8.

51. Zhou M, Wang W, Huang W, Zhang X. Use of mitomycin C to reduce the incidence of encapsulated cysts following Ahmed glaucoma valve implantation in refractory glaucoma patients: a new technique. BMC Ophthalmol. 2014;14:107.

52. Yazdani S, Doozandeh A, Pakravan M, Ownagh V, Yaseri M. Adjunctive triamcinolone acetonide for Ahmed glaucoma valve implantation: a randomized clinical trial. Eur J Ophthalmol. 2017;27(4):411–6.

53. Eid TM, Radwan A, el-Manawy W, el-Hawary I. Intravitreal bevacizumab and aqueous shunting surgery for neovascular glaucoma: safety and efficacy. Can J Ophthalmol. 2009;44(4):451–6.

54. Zhou M, Xu X, Zhang X, Sun X. Clinical outcomes of Ahmed glaucoma valve implantation with or without intravitreal bevacizumab pretreatment for neovascular glaucoma: a systematic review and meta-analysis. J Glaucoma. 2016;25(7):551–7.

55. Hwang HB, Han JW, Yim HB, Lee NY. Beneficial effects of adjuvant intravitreal bevacizumab injection on outcomes of Ahmed glaucoma valve implantation in patients with neovascular glaucoma: systematic literature review. J Ocul Pharmacol Ther. 2015;31(4):198–203.

56. Mahdy RA, Nada WM, Fawzy KM, Alnashar HY, Almosalamy SM. Efficacy of intravitreal bevacizumab with panretinal photocoagulation followed by Ahmed valve implantation in neovascular glaucoma. J Glaucoma. 2013;22(9):768–72.

57. Arcieri ES, Paula JS, Jorge R, et al. Efficacy and safety of intravitreal bevacizumab in eyes with neovascular glaucoma undergoing Ahmed glaucoma valve implantation: 2-year follow-up. Acta Ophthalmol. 2015;93(1):e1–6.

58. Sahyoun M, Azar G, Khoueir Z, et al. Long-term results of Ahmed glaucoma valve in association with intravitreal bevacizumab in neovascular glaucoma. J Glaucoma. 2015;24(5):383–8.

59. Lubinski W, Krzystolik K, Goslawski W, Kuprjanowicz L, Mularczyk M. Comparison of polypropylene and silicone Ahmed(R) glaucoma valves in the treatment of neovascular glaucoma: a 2-year follow-up. Adv Clin Exp Med. 2018;27(1):15–20.

60. Gedde SJ, Feuer WJ, Lim KS, et al. Treatment outcomes in the primary tube versus trabeculectomy study after 3 years of follow-up. Ophthalmology. 2020;127(3):333–45.

61. Gedde SJ, Herndon LW, Brandt JD, et al. Postoperative complications in the tube versus trabeculectomy (TVT) study during five years of follow-up. Am J Ophthalmol. 2012;153(5):804–814 e801.

62. Owen CG, Newsom RS, Rudnicka AR, Ellis TJ, Woodward EG. Vascular response of the bulbar conjunctiva to diabetes and elevated blood pressure. Ophthalmology. 2005;112(10):1801–8.

63. Koval MS, El Sayyad FF, Bell NP, et al. Risk factors for tube shunt exposure: a matched case-control study. J Ophthalmol. 2013;2013:196215.

64. Chaku M, Netland PA, Ishida K, Rhee DJ. Risk factors for tube exposure as a late complication of glaucoma drainage implant surgery. Clin Ophthalmol. 2016;10:547–53.

65. Preliminary report on effects of photocoagulation therapy. The Diabetic Retinopathy Study Research Group. Am J Ophthalmol. 1976;81(4):383–96.

66. Hayreh SS, Klugman MR, Podhajsky P, Servais GE, Perkins ES. Argon laser panretinal photocoagulation in ischemic central retinal vein occlusion. A 10-year prospective study. Graefes Arch Clin Exp Ophthalmol. 1990;228(4):281–96.

67. Mason JO 3rd, Albert MA Jr, Mays A, Vail R. Regression of neovascular iris vessels by intravitreal injection of bevacizumab. Retina. 2006;26(7):839–41.

68. Kim LA, D'Amore PA. A brief history of anti-VEGF for the treatment of ocular angiogenesis. Am J Pathol. 2012;181(2):376–9.

69. Ehlers JP, Spirn MJ, Lam A, Sivalingam A, Samuel MA, Tasman W. Combination intravitreal bevacizumab/panretinal photocoagulation versus panretinal photocoagulation alone in the treatment of neovascular glaucoma. Retina. 2008;28(5):696–702.

70. Eslami Y, Mohammadi M, Fakhraie G, Zarei R, Moghimi S. Ahmed glaucoma valve implantation with tube insertion through the ciliary sulcus in pseudophakic/aphakic eyes. J Glaucoma. 2014;23(2):115–8.

71. Moon K, Kim YC, Kim KS. Ciliary sulcus Ahmed valve implantation. Korean J Ophthalmol. 2007;21(2):127–30.

72. Rush R. Ciliary sulcus Ahmed glaucoma valve tube placement in neovascular glaucoma. Ophthalmic Surg Lasers Imaging. 2009;40(5):489–92.

73. Luttrull JK, Avery RL, Baerveldt G, Easley KA. Initial experience with pneumatically stented Baerveldt implant modified for pars plana insertion for complicated glaucoma. Ophthalmology. 2000;107(1):143–9. discussion 149–150.

74. Wallsh JO, Gallemore RP, Taban M, Hu C, Sharareh B. Pars plana Ahmed valve and vitrectomy in patients with glaucoma associated with posterior segment disease. Retina. 2013;33(10):2059–68.

75. Faghihi H, Hajizadeh F, Mohammadi SF, Kadkhoda A, Peyman GA, Riazi-Esfahani M. Pars plana Ahmed valve implant and vitrectomy in the management of neovascular glaucoma. Ophthalmic Surg Lasers Imaging. 2007;38(4):292–300.

76. Gedde SJ, Schiffman JC, Feuer WJ, et al. Treatment outcomes in the tube versus trabeculectomy (TVT) study after five years of follow-up. Am J Ophthalmol. 2012;153(5):789–803 e782.

77. Shah AA, WuDunn D, Cantor LB. Shunt revision versus additional tube shunt implantation after failed tube shunt surgery in refractory glaucoma. Am J Ophthalmol. 2000;129(4):455–60.

78. Ness PJ, Khaimi MA, Feldman RM, et al. Intermediate term safety and efficacy of transscleral cyclophotocoagulation after tube shunt failure. J Glaucoma. 2012;21(2):83–8.

79. Semchyshyn TM, Tsai JC, Joos KM. Supplemental transscleral diode laser cyclophotocoagulation after aqueous shunt placement in refractory glaucoma. Ophthalmology. 2002;109(6):1078–84.

Cyclophotocoagulation for Neovascular Glaucoma

Michael A. Krause and Jonathan Eisengart

1　Historical Perspective

Patients with acute NVG can present challenges in intraocular pressure (IOP) management. Medical management is often insufficient to adequately lower IOP, especially if the angle has already progressed to synechial angle closure. Traditional outflow surgeries (e.g., trabeculectomy and aqueous shunts) often are fraught in acute NVG as well. In NVG eyes with active anterior segment neovascularization, trabeculectomy and aqueous shunts may be complicated by intraoperative and postoperative hyphema, especially in the era before anti-vascular endothelial growth factor (anti-VEGF). The hyphema can originate from decompression and rupture of delicate neovascular vessels or by directly incising these vessels during the tube insertion, sclerostomy, and/or iridectomy steps of aqueous shunts and/or trabeculectomy. Furthermore, broad high peripheral anterior synechiae (PAS) in the angle can further complicate tube insertion into the anterior chamber. Even when intraoperative and postoperative complications are avoided, long-term success rates for both trabeculectomy and aqueous shunts in the setting of NVG can be poor [1, 2]. Because of these challenges, other techniques were sought that could lower IOP in patients with NVG and other refractory glaucomas.

Ciliary body ablation to reduce aqueous production and thereby lower IOP was first described in 1936 [3]. Over the next several decades, various methods of cyclodestruction were described, including cyclodiathermy, cyclocryotherapy, and ultrasound ablation. These early techniques were often accompanied by serious complications, including severe pain, inflammation, hypotony, hemorrhage, vision loss, and scleral ectasia [4–6]. Because of these complications, ciliary body ablation was not widely adopted.

Laser for cycloablation was described in 1961 by Weekers et al, who utilized xenon arc photocoagulation in a transscleral approach. The authors found that although this technique was capable reducing IOP, lower energy resulted in a temporary effect, whereas higher energy resulted in better long-term efficacy but with serious adverse effects [7]. In 1972, Beckman et al reported the use of a ruby laser for transscleral cyclophotocoagulation (TSCPC) in 13 eyes with refractory glaucoma (6 with NVG) and found 85% of eyes achieved at least 30% IOP reduction at 6 months, and 53% of eyes had IOP between 5 and 22 mmHg at 24 months [8, 9]. Neodymium:yttrium−aluminum−garnet (Nd-YAG) laser for ciliary ablation was reported by the same group in 1973 and was reported to be more effective than ruby laser therapy [10]. In 1992, the use of semiconductor diode laser

M. A. Krause · J. Eisengart (✉)
Cole Eye Institute, Cleveland Clinic Foundation,
Cleveland, OH, USA

TSCPC was first reported by Hennis and Stewart in 14 eyes (3 with NVG), with successful IOP lowering in 71% at 6 months [11].

Micropulse TSCPC (MP-TSCPC), whereby the laser energy is delivered via a modified probe in short repetitive pulses with rest periods in between the pulses, was first introduced in 2010 by Tan et al in a study of 40 eyes with refractory glaucoma [12]. They reported a success rate (defined as IOP < 21 mmHg or a reduction of 30% from baseline) of 80% at 1 year with no hypotony or loss of visual acuity. The role of MP-TSCPC in the management of NVG is still being elucidated.

2   Current Perspective

Traditionally, CPC has been reserved for refractory glaucomas with poor visual prognosis due to potential complications, including pain, prolonged inflammation, hyphema, vitreous hemorrhage, hypotony, vision loss, and sympathetic ophthalmia (though this complication is exceedingly rare) [13, 14]. As surgeons have gained more familiarity with diode CPC, there is evidence that these procedures may result in fewer complications than previously thought, as prior reports were generally limited to sick eyes with poor visual prognosis. A 2001 prospective study in Ghana investigated TSCPC as primary surgical treatment [15]. The authors enrolled 92 patients with primary open-angle glaucoma. One eye was selected for treatment with CPC, and the other eye received standard treatment (topical medication or trabeculectomy). Seventy-nine patients completed at least 3 months of follow-up (mean 13.2 months). The authors reported no significant difference in visual acuity change between eyes treated with TSCPC and eyes treated with standard treatment (23% and 20%, respectively). A 2004 retrospective study reported long-term follow-up on 21 patients with good visual acuity (VA) (20/80 or better) who were treated with TSCPC (the majority of patients had OAG; no patients were diagnosed with NVG) [16]. At mean follow-up of 40.7 months, 81% of patients had VA within one line of pre-laser VA. A 2007 retrospec-

tive study analyzed 74 eyes (50% with NVG, 31% with primary open-angle glaucoma, and 8% with chronic angle-closure glaucoma) that underwent diode TSCPC with 1 year of follow-up [17]. VA was reported for eyes with primary open-angle glaucoma and chronic angle-closure glaucoma and did not change significantly from preoperative baseline. The reported success rate (defined as a 30% reduction in IOP with or without topical glaucoma medications) was 82.4% for all eyes and 75.7% for eyes with NVG. There were no reported cases of hypotony or phthisis. A 2010 retrospective study reported on 49 eyes (only 1 with NVG) with good preoperative VA (20/60 or better) who had undergone diode TSCPC [18]. At 5 years, 30.6% of eyes had lost two or more lines of VA, with the main reason for VA loss being progression of glaucoma. Successful IOP control (defined as IOP <22 mmHg and >6 mmHg without oral acetazolamide or other glaucoma surgery) was reported in 79.6% of eyes, and there were no reported cases of hypotony. Together, these studies provide evidence that CPC can be used in eyes with good visual potential and that the risk of severe adverse effects is likely lower than previously reported.

There is also evidence that CPC may be comparable to traditional glaucoma surgeries for IOP control in eyes with NVG. A 2009 retrospective study compared TSCPC with Ahmed glaucoma valve implantation in patients with NVG [19]. At 24 months, the success rate (defined as IOP >5 mmHg and <21 mmHg without loss of light perception) was 63.6 and 59.3% for CPC and Ahmed glaucoma valve, respectively. In 2018, Choy et al. published a randomized comparative trial of diode TSCPC versus Ahmed glaucoma valve in patients with NVG with no history of prior glaucoma surgery [20]. Twenty eyes with at least 6 months of follow-up were enrolled. The success rate (defined as IOP < 22 mmHg with or without medication and no hypotony-related maculopathy or choroidal detachment) was reported to be 86% for both treatments. VA was stable or improved in 72% of TSCPC eyes and 49% of Ahmed glaucoma valve eyes. A 2020 retrospective study compared 12 eyes with NVG that underwent trabeculectomy with Ex-PRESS shunt with 18 eyes with NVG that underwent TSCPC [21]. At one year, outcomes were reported to be similar for the two procedures. Preoperative IOP was 28.2 and 27.6 mmHg and IOP at 1 year was 15.36 and 15.44 mmHg for the Ex-PRESS group and the TSCPC group, respectively. Preoperative VA was similar between the two groups and worsened at 1 year in 8.3% and 11.1% of the Ex-PRESS group and the TSCPC group, respectively. CPC offers a viable alternative to traditional filtering surgery in patients with NVG, with comparable (or superior) success rates. However, there are no randomized control trials with standardized treatment regimens, which would further elucidate the role of CPC as compared to traditional filtering surgery in the treatment of NVG.

Consider the potential advantages of diode CPC over an aqueous shunt:

1. The IOP-lowering effect of CPC is not impacted by anterior segment neovascularization or hyphema. While hyphema can acutely obstruct a tube or the internal sclerostomy of a trabeculectomy, the success of CPC is unaffected by hyphema, which makes CPC particularly advantageous in situations where there is active anterior segment neovascularization and/or hyphema. Similarly, there is evidence that CPC is effective in eyes with silicone oil filling the posterior segment [22].

2. CPC can be performed in phakic eyes with shallow anterior chambers. Tubes can be difficult to position in the anterior chamber if there is broad high PAS or an intumescent lens. While posterior segment tube placement is possible in these situations, this would require more complex surgery including a complete pars plana vitrectomy. Trabeculectomy can be performed in eyes with peripherally shallow chambers due to PAS, but success rates of trabeculectomy is the setting of NVG is relatively poor. Conversely, CPC can be performed regardless of the anterior chamber and angle anatomy. While CPC does have a risk of progressive cataract in phakic eyes, it is unclear if the CPC poses a higher risk for cataract progression than aqueous shunts and trabeculectomies.

3. CPC can rapidly lower IOP, with most patients experiencing a significant reduction as soon as postoperative day 1 [23]. Rapid IOP reduction is important to clear the corneal edema for panretinal photocoagulation and to allow safe injection of anti-VEGF agents.

4. Because CPC is nonincisional and does not carry the risk of causing or worsening hyphema, it can be performed safely *before* or *concurrently with* anti-VEGF injection; conversely, because aqueous shunts can become obstructed by hyphema and blood clot from bleeding neovascularization, anti-VEGF should be given prior to surgery to regress anterior segment neovascularization.

5. CPC can be rapidly implemented, even in very sick patients. There is minimal case preparation, no sterile field is required, and the procedure length is only several minutes.

6. CPC in some cases can temporize an urgent and untenable situation and lower the IOP (even if only temporarily) until the underlying source of neovascularization can be addressed and the eye can be stabilized until a more definitive IOP-lowering procedure can be performed at a later time.

7. CPC has a much easier postoperative recovery than an aqueous shunt. Because CPC is nonincisional and the risk of hypotony-associated complications (such as suprachoroidal hemorrhage) is exceedingly rare, there are no postoperative restrictions against bending, lifting, exercising, or getting water in the eye, and there is no eye shield to wear.

MP-TSCPC is also being investigated as a primary IOP-lowering intervention in the setting of NVG. In a retrospective study, Breshears et al reported on 15 eyes with NVG treated with MP-TSCPC as a primary procedure [24]. Success (criteria not defined) was achieved for eight eyes. There were no reported complications. Helmy reported results of 50 eyes treated with ranibizumab followed by MP-TSCPC 1 week to 1 month later [25]. He reported success (defined as IOP >6 and <21 without oral acetazolamide, or 30% reduced from baseline) in 88% of eyes. There were no reported complications, and no eyes lost vision.

3   Case Study

A hypothetical patient illustrates the potential utility of CPC in acute NVG. A 64-year-old man with a history of hypertension, tobacco use, and untreated proliferative diabetic retinopathy presents urgently for pain and vision loss of the right eye. His pain started 1 week ago when he was hospitalized for an unrelated condition. His vision is counting fingers, and IOP is 55 mmHg. There is significant microcystic corneal edema, florid iris neovascularization, no layered hyphema, and a stable 1-piece posterior chamber intraocular lens in the capsular bag. The gonioscopic view of the angle is limited by corneal edema, so it is not possible to visualize whether there is angle neovascularization and/or peripheral anterior synechiae. The view to the posterior segment is also limited by corneal edema and poor pupillary dilation, but a B-scan reveals moderate vitreous hemorrhage and no retinal detachment. Initiation of maximal medical therapy (including oral acetazolamide) lowers the IOP to 40 mmHg. The corneal edema has cleared just enough to perform gonioscopy and visualize florid angle neovascularization with 360° of synechial angle closure.

How would you proceed? Your retina colleague has offered to administer an anti-VEGF injection but is somewhat reluctant given the concern for causing a hyphema and IOP spike. Furthermore, anti-VEGF injection and regression of anterior segment neovascularization would not be expected to further lower the IOP since the angle is already synechially closed [26, 27]. Given the florid anterior segment neovascularization, you are concerned about proceeding with an aqueous shunt due to the high risk of intraoperative and postoperative bleeding, in the absence of adequate pretreatment with anti-VEGF.

This relatively common situation is a good opportunity to utilize prompt CPC to rapidly lower IOP without performing an incisional procedure. The authors will typically proceed with a limited CPC (180°–225°—see surgical technique below) and with agreement from the retina doctors, give the first dose of intravitreal anti-VEGF intraoperatively. Administering anti-VEGF treatment in conjunction with CPC has not been shown to affect the success of laser treatment [28]. CPC in the acute setting may provide long-term IOP control. Alternatively, even if the IOP-lowering effect is only transient, there will typically be sufficient time for the retina specialists to treat the ischemia and induce regression of anterior segment neovascularization, and an aqueous shunt can be performed later under more controlled and safer circumstances.

4   Surgical Technique and Postoperative Management

Diode laser is the preferred modality for cyclophotocoagulation, due to its portability, cost, and efficiency [13]. Light energy is generated from a semiconductor solid-state diode laser system, such as Iridex Cyclo G6 (Iridex, Mountain View, CA). Light is emitted at 810 nm and is absorbed by the melanin in the pigmented ciliary epithelium, resulting in coagulation of the ciliary body epithelium and stroma [13, 29].

This procedure requires retrobulbar or general anesthesia. The authors will wait until the anesthetist delivers intravenous sedation. A retrobulbar block and the laser treatment can often be accomplished in several minutes before the patient wakes up; the anesthetist can supplement sedation as needed. Some patients may be able to tolerate this procedure in clinic with retrobulbar anesthesia but without intravenous sedation. One recommendation is to administer some of the retrobulbar anesthetic topically onto the ocular surface to lessen discomfort from the laser probe tip. For monocular patients or those on anticoagulation, some practitioners may be more comfortable with general anesthesia instead of a retrobulbar block. However, the authors will still administer a retrobulbar block in these situations, with a preference for a shorter-acting anesthetic in monocular patients, so they can regain vision shortly after the procedure.

Laser is delivered via the G-probe, which is designed to aim the laser ~1.2 mm posterior to the corneoscleral limbus. However, there is significant variation in ciliary body position relative the corneoscleral limbus, not only from person to person, but also from quadrant to quadrant in the same eye. Therefore, the authors prefer to use transillumination to identify the ciliary body to facilitate positioning the G-probe appropriately. A bright light source, such as a fiberoptic light pipe or a muscle light, is held at the limbus about 180° away from the intended area of treatment. A shadow of the ciliary body should be easily visible, and the red aiming beam of the G-probe or treatment laser is aimed onto the anterior edge of this shadow. This is particularly helpful in eyes with unusual anatomy or distorted limbal architecture. While a G-probe with a built-in transilluminator light is available, the authors have found it less useful since scatter from the bright light source makes the ciliary body shadow hard to identify in the immediate vicinity of the probe.

Traditionally, initial CPC settings are power 2000mW and a duration 2 seconds per spot [30]. Power is increased in 100 mW increments to a maximum of 2500 mW or until an audible "pop" is heard, at which point power is decreased by 100 mW. Power may be adjusted up or down according the occurrence of an audible "pop" as the probe is advanced around the limbus. Some surgeons prefer a longer laser duration at a lower power, 1250 mW for 4 seconds, believing it is less inflammatory [31]. A total of 8 laser spots are performed in each quadrant, sparing the 3 o'clock and 9 o'clock positions where the long posterior ciliary nerve is located. The extent of treatment is guided by the level of IOP elevation, visual potential, and any additional IOP-lowering surgeries the eye has already undergone or is planned in the future. Ischemic NVG eyes are at higher risk of phthisis than nonischemic glaucomatous eyes [14, 32], so the authors tend to limit the treatment to 180°–225°. In an eye with good visual potential, treatment limited to 180° may be indicated followed by an aqueous shunt in the future if needed. When choosing an aqueous shunt in an eye with prior CPC, consider that there may be an increased risk of postoperative hypotony due to impaired aqueous production; more evidence is needed to determine the optimal aqueous shunt choice in eyes with prior CPC. In an eye with poor visual potential and very high IOP where the primary goal is to relieve pain, a

larger extent of treatment, perhaps even as much as 270°, is indicated. Eyes with prior failed aqueous shunts may benefit from *lesser* CPC treatment, as the combination of a tube and CPC can be quite potent in IOP reduction; more evidence is needed to determine the optimal CPC settings in eyes with prior aqueous shunts.

An alternative CPC setting (commonly utilized by Dr Mary Qiu) is to place 16–24 spots across the entire 360°: 8–12 spots superiorly, 8–12 spots inferiorly, sparing the 3 o'clock and 9 o'clock positions, and not more than 24 spots total. The initial power setting is 1250 mW, and duration is 4 seconds; the power is increased in 50 mW increments to a maximum of 1500 mW or until an audible "pop" is heard, at which point the power is decreased by 50 mW to 100 mW for the remainder of the spots.

Aggressive use of perioperative steroid is imperative to control inflammation after CPC. A common regimen is peribulbar dexamethasone 10 mg administered deep through the inferior fornix at the end of CPC. It is also optional to ask the anesthetist to administer an intravenous dose of methylprednisolone 125 mg. In eyes at high risk for macular edema, which includes all NVG eyes, the authors have found intravitreal preservative-free triamcinolone acetonide 1% (IVTA) 2 mg at the end of CPC to be particularly efficacious. IVTA instead of subconjunctival dexamethasone often achieves potent and rapid control of inflammation as well as treat or prevent macular edema. Furthermore, since the potential for steroid-induced IOP elevation is mediated by trabecular meshwork dysfunction, and these NVG eyes typically have synechially closed angles (or a neovascular membrane over the angle), the authors postulate that NVG eyes may not develop additional steroid-induced IOP elevation. IVTA should not be used if the status of the posterior segment and absence of retinal detachment cannot be verified. The homegoing topical eye drop regimen is prednisolone acetate 1% every 2 hours while awake (or 4 times per day if IVTA is administered) and atropine sulfate 1% two times per day. The atropine can usually be stopped after 1 or 2 weeks. The prednisolone is slowly tapered over the course of the next 6–8 weeks, modified as needed according to the clinical exam during postoperative visits.

If a retrobulbar block is used, a soft patch (no shield) is placed on the eye after the CPC is completed to keep the eyelid closed until the retrobulbar anesthetic wears off. The next morning, the patient removes and discards the patch and begins the postoperative drops. If the CPC was performed under deep sedation or general anesthesia without a retrobulbar block, or with a short-acting retrobulbar block, then no patch is needed, and the patient can begin the postoperative drops shortly after surgery. Often, several IOP-lowering medications can be discontinued immediately (including a prostaglandin analog and the oral carbonic anhydrase inhibitor, if applicable, due to the risk of inflammation/macular edema and systemic side effects, respectively), although this guideline can be modified on a case-by-case basis given the clinical context. Postoperative visits are typically conducted at 1 week and 1 month, with additional visits as needed to carefully monitor the IOP and determine whether additional IOP-lowering procedures are needed. Prompt additional visits with the retina specialist should be scheduled for the patient to address the underlying source of neovascularization. The patient may need to be seen more frequently depending on the clinical course. Multidisciplinary coordinated care is critical to optimizing the outcome for NVG patients.

5   Complications of CPC in Neovascular Glaucoma

Complications of CPC include pain, vision loss, hypotony, corneal edema [33, 34], pigment dispersion [35], atonic pupil [15], lens subluxation [36], and necrotizing scleritis [37]. Sympathetic ophthalmia is a very rare complication following CPC (0.001–0.07%) [38–40]. The complication rates may be higher in eyes with NVG given the ischemic damage already suffered by these eyes. It should also be noted that early studies of CPC were restricted to eyes with end-stage disease, which may confound reported complication rates.

The rate of vision loss after CPC in eyes with NVG has been reported to be up to 40%, with more recent studies reporting lower rates. Indeed, the risk of vision loss may actually be less with CPC than with aqueous tube shunt or trabeculectomy. A 2016 Chinese retrospective study of 149 eyes with NVG reported 18.2% of patients treated with CPC had a decrease in VA, as opposed to 54.8% who underwent aqueous tube shunt, and 70.0% who underwent trabeculectomy [41]. They reported less robust IOP lowering following CPC as compared to aqueous tube shunt, but many fewer serious complications in the CPC group.

The degree of vision loss following CPC may depend on the baseline VA (worse baseline VA at higher risk) and on surgical history of the eye (prior pars plana vitrectomy or filtering surgery at higher risk). A 2004 retrospective study of outcomes of NVG patients treated with CPC found that 40% of patients lost vision [42]. However, among patients with baseline VA 20/200 or better, 50% maintained baseline VA, and none worsened beyond 20/200. Among patients who progressed to no-light-perception vision, all had a history of more complicated disease necessitating pars plana vitrectomy prior to CPC. Eyes with a history of prior failed aqueous tube shunt may also be at higher risk for vision loss, with some studies reporting 50–75% of NVG eyes progressing to no-light-perception vision (a major caveat being that NVG eyes represented a small proportion of these studies, and it is unclear what baseline VA these eyes had) [43, 44].

Reported rates of hypotony and phthisis following CPC in eyes with NVG vary. Earlier studies were generally restricted to eyes with poor prognosis and used more aggressive laser settings than we currently recommend. These studies reported a rate of hypotony up to 25%, with up to 8% of eyes becoming phthisical [42, 45, 46]. A more recent study reported a rate of hypotony less than 5% in eyes with NVG treated with CPC.

Rates of prolonged inflammation, hyphema, and vitreous hemorrhage following CPC in eyes with NVG are not commonly reported. A 2003 retrospective study reported uveitis in 1.9%, hyphema in 0.4%, and vitreous hemorrhage in

0.4% of NVG patients after CPC [46]. More data are needed regarding the true incidence of these complications. In our experience, post-CPC inflammation occurs which can be managed by aggressive postoperative steroid treatment, including IVTA. If inflammation is particularly robust, oral steroids may be helpful.

In eyes with NVG, vision loss, hypotony, and phthisis are the best characterized complications following CPC. Poor baseline VA and surgical history (pars plana vitrectomy or aqueous shunt) appear to be risk factors for these complications. While CPC does have some risks, the overall risk of complications may be lower than with aqueous tube shunt or trabeculectomy. CPC is capable of quickly lowering IOP and should be considered as first-line treatment of acute NVG especially when the angle is synechially closed at the time of the acute presentation.

6 Conclusion

In the authors' opinion, CPC should be the first-line IOP-lowering intervention for patients with acute NVG, active anterior segment neovascularization, and synechial angle closure, even in eyes with "good" visual potential. Due to the synechial angle closure, anti-VEGF and regression of anterior segment neovascularization would not be expected to improve aqueous outflow and lower IOP, in contrast to an NVG eye with NVA and an open angle. If there is active anterior segment neovascularization which has not yet been regressed with anti-VEGF, aqueous shunt surgery is prone to significant bleeding complications. In these eyes, prompt CPC has the potential to immediately lower IOP without incurring these bleeding risks, can be rapidly implemented with minimal equipment required, and can allow time for anti-neovascular treatments (anti-VEGF and PRP) to regress the active anterior segment neovascularization if additional IOP-lowering procedures are needed in the future. While the risks of CPC are well understood, they can be mitigated with judicious application of the laser and appropriately aggressive postoperative steroid treatment.

More research is needed to elucidate optimal CPC candidates, laser parameters, and treatment algorithms including use of concurrent anti-VEGF and/or IVTA, subsequent aqueous shunt after prior CPC, and coordination of a multidisciplinary treatment protocol with retina specialists. Furthermore, the potential role of MP-CPC in NVG has not been investigated, including whether MP-CPC is equally effective or offers and improved safety profile for these NVG eyes.

References

1. Tsai JC, Feuer WJ, Parrish RK, Grajewski AL. 5-fluorouracil filtering surgery and neovascular glaucoma: long-term follow-up of the original pilot study. Ophthalmology. 1995;102:887–93.
2. Yalvac IS, Eksioglu U, Satana B, Duman S. Long-term results of Ahmed glaucoma valve and Molteno implant in neovascular glaucoma. Eye. 2007;21:65–70.
3. Vogt A. Versuche zur intraokularen druckherabsetzung mittelst diathermiescha¨digung des corpus ciliare (Zyklodiather-miestichelung). Klin Monatsbl Augenheilkd. 1936;97:672–3.
4. Bietti G. Surgical intervention on the ciliary body. J Am Med Assoc. 1950;142:889.
5. Coleman DJ, Lizzi FL, Driller J, Rosado AL, Chang S, Iwamoto T, Rosenthal D. Therapeutic ultrasound in the treatment of glaucoma. Ophthalmology. 1985;92:339–46.
6. Coleman DJ, Lizzi FL, Driller J, et al. Therapeutic ultrasound in the treatment of glaucoma. Ophthalmology. 1985;92:347–53.
7. Weekers R, Lavergne G, Watillon M, Gilson M, Legros AM. Effects of photocoagulation of ciliary body upon ocular tension. Am J Ophthalmol. 1961;52:156–63.
8. Beckman H, Kinoshita A, Rota AN, Sugar HS. Transscleral ruby laser irradiation of the ciliary body in the treatment of intractable glaucoma. Trans Am Acad Ophthalmol Otolaryngol. 1972;76:423–36.
9. Beckman H, Waeltermann J. Transscleral ruby laser cyclocoagulation. Am J Ophthalmol. 1984;98:788–95.
10. Beckman H, Sugar HS. Neodymium laser cyclocoagulation. Arch Ophthalmol. 1973;90:27–8.
11. Hennis HL, Stewart WC. Semiconductor diode laser transscleral cyclophotocoagulation in patients with glaucoma. Am J Ophthalmol. 1992;113:81–5.
12. Tan AM, Chockalingam M, Aquino MC, Lim ZIL, See JLS, Chew PT. Micropulse transscleral diode laser cyclophotocoagulation in the treatment of refractory glaucoma. Clin Exp Ophthalmol. 2010;38:266–72.
13. Pastor SA, Singh K, Lee DA, Juzych MS, Lin SC, Netland PA, Nguyen NTA. Cyclophotocoagulation: a report by the American Academy of Ophthalmology. Ophthalmology. 2001;108:2130–8.

14. Ishida K. Update on results and complications of cyclophotocoagulation. Curr Opin Ophthalmol. 2013;24:102–10.

15. Egbert PR, Fiadoyor S, Budenz DL, Dadzie P, Byrd S. Diode laser transscleral cyclophotocoagulation as a primary surgical treatment for primary open-angle glaucoma. Arch Ophthalmol (Chicago, Ill 1960). 2001;119:345–50.

16. Wilensky JT, Kammer J. Long-term visual outcome of transscleral laser cyclotherapy in eyes with ambulatory vision. Ophthalmology. 2004;111:1389–92.

17. Ansari E, Gandhewar J. Long-term efficacy and visual acuity following transscleral diode laser photocoagulation in cases of refractory and non-refractory glaucoma. Eye. 2007;21:936–40.

18. Rotchford AP, Jayasawal R, Madhusudhan S, Ho S, King AJ, Vernon SA. Transscleral diode laser cycloablation in patients with good vision. Br J Ophthalmol. 2010;94:1180–3.

19. Yildirim N, Yalvac IS, Sahin A, Ozer A, Bozca T. A comparative study between diode laser cyclophotocoagulation and the Ahmed glaucoma valve implant in neovascular glaucoma. J Glaucoma. 2009;18:192–6.

20. Choy BNK, Lai JSM, Yeung JCC, Chan JCH. Randomized comparative trial of diode laser transscleral cyclophotocoagulation versus Ahmed glaucoma valve for neovascular glaucoma in Chinese—A pilot study. Clin Ophthalmol. 2018;12:2545–52.

21. Wagdy FM, Zaky AG. Comparison between the express implant and transscleral diode laser in neovascular glaucoma. J Ophthalmol. 2020;2020:3781249. https://doi.org/10.1155/2020/3781249.

22. Ghazi-Nouri SMS, Vakalis AN, Bloom PA, Bunce C, Charteris DG. Long-term results of the management of silicone oil-induced raised intraocular pressure by diode laser cycloablation. Eye. 2005;19:765–9.

23. Uppal S, Stead RE, Patil BB, Henry E, Moodie J, Vernon SA, King AJ. Short-term effect of diode laser cyclophotocoagulation on intraocular pressure: A prospective study. Clin Exp Ophthalmol. 2015;43:796–802.

24. Breshears B, Patrianakos TD, Giovingo M. Three-year retrospective study of treatment with micropulse cyclophotocoagulation as a primary procedure for neovascular glaucoma. Investig Ophthalmol Vis Sci. 2019;60:704.

25. Helmy H. Micropulse diode treatment in refractory neovascular glaucoma, high-energy level combined with adjunctive Ranibizumab. Egypt Retin J. 2020;7:41–9.

26. Lüke J, Nassar K, Lüke M, Grisanti S. Ranibizumab as adjuvant in the treatment of rubeosis iridis and neovascular glaucoma—results from a prospective interventional case series. Graefes Arch Clin Exp Ophthalmol. 2013;251:2403–13.

27. Wakabayashi T, Oshima Y, Sakaguchi H, Ikuno Y, Miki A, Gomi F, Otori Y, Kamei M, Kusaka S, Tano Y. Intravitreal bevacizumab to treat iris neovascularization and neovascular glaucoma secondary to ischemic retinal diseases in 41 consecutive cases. Ophthalmology. 2008;115(1571–80):1580.e1–3.

28. Fong AW, Lee GA, O'Rourke P, Thomas R. Management of neovascular glaucoma with transscleral cyclophotocoagulation with diode laser alone versus combination transscleral cyclophotocoagulation with diode laser and intravitreal bevacizumab. Clin Exp Ophthalmol. 2011;39:318–23.

29. Pratesi R. Diode lasers in photomedicine. IEEE J Quantum Electron. 1984;20:1433–9.

30. Spencer AF, Vernon SA. "Cyclodiode": results of a standard protocol. Br J Ophthalmol. 1999;83:311–6.

31. Khodeiry MM, Sheheitli H, Sayed MS, Persad PJ, Feuer WJ, Lee RK. Treatment outcomes of slow coagulation transscleral cyclophotocoagulation in pseudophakic patients with medically uncontrolled glaucoma. Am J Ophthalmol. 2021;229:90–9.

32. Ramli N, Htoon HM, Ho CL, Aung T, Perera S. Risk factors for hypotony after transscleral diode cyclophotocoagulation. J Glaucoma. 2012;21:169–73.

33. Kumar H, Gupta S, Agarwal A. Corneal edema following diode laser cyclophotocoagulation in an eye with secondary glaucoma. Indian J Ophthalmol. 2008;56:317–8.

34. Chan PP, Lam MCW, Baig N. Case report—acute corneal subepithelial hydrops (ACSH) during micropulse transscleral cyclophotocoagulation (MPTSC). BMC Ophthalmol. 2020;20:409.

35. Hossain P, Ghosh G, Vernon SA. Assessing the "cyclodiode G-probe" using a grey scale test: reproducibility and differences between probes. Eye (Lond). 2003;17:167–76.

36. Rao VJ, Dayan M. Lens subluxation following contact transscleral cyclodiode. Arch Ophthalmol (Chicago, Ill 1960). 2002;120:1393–4.

37. Shen SY, Lai JSM, Lam DSC. Necrotizing scleritis following diode laser transscleral cyclophotocoagulation. Ophthalmic Surg Lasers Imaging. 2004;35:251–3.

38. Aujla JS, Lee GA, Vincent SJ, Thomas R. Incidence of hypotony and sympathetic ophthalmia following trans-scleral cyclophotocoagulation for glaucoma and a report of risk factors. Clin Exp Ophthalmol. 2013;41:761–72.

39. Albahlal A, Al Dhibi H, Al Shahwan S, Khandekar R, Edward DP. Sympathetic ophthalmia following diode laser cyclophotocoagulation. Br J Ophthalmol. 2014;98:1101–6.

40. Kumar N, Chang A, Beaumont P. Sympathetic ophthalmia following ciliary body laser cyclophotocoagulation for rubeotic glaucoma. Clin Exp Ophthalmol. 2004;32:196–8.

41. Liao N, Li C, Jiang H, Fang A, Zhou S, Wang Q. Neovascular glaucoma: a retrospective review from a tertiary center in China. BMC Ophthalmol. 2016;16:10–5.

42. Nabili S, Kirkness CM. Trans-scleral diode laser cyclophoto-coagulation in the treatment of diabetic neovascular glaucoma. Eye. 2004;18:352–6.

43. Ness PJ, Khaimi MA, Feldman RM, Tabet R, Sarkisian SR, Skuta GL, Chuang AZ, Mankiewicz KA. Intermediate term safety and efficacy of transscleral cyclophotocoagulation after tube shunt failure. J Glaucoma. 2012;21:83–8.

44. Semchyshyn TM, Tsai JC, Joos KM. Supplemental transscleral diode laser cyclophotocoagulation after aqueous shunt placement in refractory glaucoma. Ophthalmology. 2002;109:1078–84.

45. Iliev ME, Gerber S. Long-term outcome of transscleral diode laser cyclophotocoagulation in refractory glaucoma. Br J Ophthalmol. 2007;91:1631–5.

46. Murphy CC, Burnett CAM, Spry PGD, Broadway DC, Diamond JP. A two centre study of the dose-response relation for transscleral diode laser cyclophotocoagulation in refractory glaucoma. Br J Ophthalmol. 2003;87:1252–7.

Micro-incisional Glaucoma Surgery for Neovascular Glaucoma

Jacob Kanter and Mary Qiu

1 Introduction

Reduction of intraocular pressure (IOP) is one of the core tenets of management of neovascular glaucoma (NVG), along with reducing the underlying neovascular drive. When topical and oral IOP-lowering medications prove insufficient in controlling IOP, the next step is surgical intervention. To date, surgical IOP-lowering strategies rely on either decreased aqueous production via cyclodestruction or increased aqueous outflow via *ab externo* trabeculectomy or aqueous shunt implantation. Detailed discussions on each of these surgical interventions for NVG can be found earlier in other chapters of this book.

Historically, in eyes with good ambulatory visual potential, trabeculectomy has been the IOP-lowering surgery of choice. Although it is still preferred by some, trabeculectomy has lost favor to aqueous shunts in many forms of secondary glaucomas, including NVG. Beyond the lifetime risks associated with trabeculectomy, the long-term efficacy of trabeculectomy in the setting of NVG leaves much to be desired. In a retrospective review of 101 eyes with NVG undergoing trabeculectomy, 48.3% of patients had either persistent IOP ≥ 22 mm Hg, deterioration of visual acuity (VA) to no light perception (NLP), and/or required additional glaucoma procedures at 5 years [1]. Pre- and intraoperative use of antivascular endothelial growth factor (anti-VEGF) and intraoperative use of antimetabolites such as mitomycin C have been shown to reduce complications and improve outcomes in trabeculectomy for NVG [2].

Aqueous shunts have largely become the IOP-lowering surgery of choice in NVG [3, 4]. These include the Ahmed (AGV), Baerveldt (BGI), Ahmed ClearPath, and Molteno implants. While aqueous shunts have a favorable safety profile in NVG compared to trabeculectomy, intra- or postoperative hyphema, which is more common in NVG patients, can be particularly devastating due to the potential for tube occlusion [5]. At 6–12 months, the failure rate of aqueous shunts in NVG has been reported to be approximately 25%, and at 5 years, the failure rate has been reported to be 50%, with 22% of eyes progressing to NLP [3, 4, 6].

Furthermore, it must be emphasized that IOP control is only one component of the multidisciplinary treatment goals in NVG. In some cases, early, aggressive control of the neovascular drive may obviate the need for IOP-lowering intervention [7]. Conversely, inadequate control of the neovascular drive will lead to failure of the IOP-lowering surgery via various mechanisms, e.g., recurrent neovascularization and/or

J. Kanter · M. Qiu (✉)
Department of Ophthalmology and Visual Science, University of Chicago, Chicago, IL, USA
e-mail: maryqiu@bsd.uchicago.edu

uncontrolled inflammation leading to bleb or tube failure or progressive retinal ischemia or retinal detachment leading to nonglaucomatous vision loss. For this reason, it is difficult to isolate the therapeutic effect (and thus measure a success rate) of an IOP-lowering surgery in the setting of NVG. Nonetheless, given the currently published data summarized above, there is certainly room for improvement with regard to the safety and efficacy of IOP-lowering surgery in NVG.

2   MIGS for NVG

Micro-incisional glaucoma surgeries (MIGS) have emerged as a less invasive IOP-lowering treatment option for mild-to-moderate POAG at the time of cataract surgery [8]. While some MIGS function as subconjunctival or suprachoroidal shunts, most aim to bypass, incise, or excise the trabecular meshwork (TM) via an *ab interno* approach to the iridocorneal angle. We believe that angle-based MIGS that incise/excise a large extent of the trabecular meshwork, including goniotomy and 360° *ab interno* trabeculotomy deserve consideration in NVG.

Dual-blade excisional goniotomy was first described by Seibold et al. in 2013 using the Kahook dual-blade instrument (KDB, New World Medical, Rancho Cucamonga, CA) [9]. KDB is a stainless steel blade that is used to excise a ribbon of nasal TM, extending superiorly and inferiorly for a total of 3–6 clock hours. The aqueous humor has direct access to Schlemm's canal in this area, thereby facilitating better aqueous outflow. Although it is most often used in POAG in conjunction with cataract surgery, dual-blade excisional goniotomy has been shown to be effective in angle-closure glaucoma when combined with goniosynechialysis [10]. A dual-blade excisional goniotomy can also be performed with a TrabEx (MicroSurgical Technology, Redmond, WA). Other instruments can be used to perform an *ab interno* incision of the trabecular meshwork including the SION Surgical Instrument (Sight Sciences, Menlo Park, CA), a microvitreoretinal (MVR) blade, Sinskey hook, Tanito

microhook [11], cystotome [12], or bent 30-gauge needle [13].

GATT was first described by Grover et al. in 2014 and involves creating a 360° *ab interno* trabeculotomy [14]. An initial goniotomy is made nasally, followed by the insertion of an illuminated microcatheter or suture into Schlemm's canal; the catheter is advanced for 360°, the tip is retrieved once it emerges from the other side of the initial goniotomy site, and both ends are pulled inward to perform a 360° trabeculotomy. If the nasal angle is occluded by PAS, goniosynechialysis (GSL) may be attempted to render the trabecular meshwork accessible. If PAS is present elsewhere, the catheter may lyse through them when both ends are being pulled. Although it is most widely used in open-angle glaucomas, GATT combined with goniosynechialysis (GSL) has recently been reported to be effective in chronic angle-closure glaucoma, but it was not specified whether NVG patients were excluded [15, 16]. Another device that can be used to perform a 360° *ab interno* trabeculotomy is the OMNI Surgical System (Sight Sciences, Menlo Park, CA).

Until July 2022, there had been no published reports in the English literature of any angle-based MIGS being attempted for IOP control in NVG. The reasons for this are likely due to the following.

1. The pathogenesis of NVG involves anterior advancement of a fibrovascular membrane which results in progressive synechial closure of the iridocorneal angle. To date, most KDB and GATT literature studies have been limited to open-angle glaucomas. Once the angle is synechially closed in NVG, perhaps more so than in other causes of chronic angle closure, the conventional wisdom has been that the underlying TM and Schlemm's canal is no longer salvageable, and any attempts to reopen the conventional outflow pathway in these angles would likely prove futile, especially if angle neovascularization should recur.

2. As a condition driven by neovascularization, NVG is often complicated by uncontrolled bleeding when the underlying neovascular

disease is active. Indeed, this has led to the widespread use of antivascular endothelial growth factor (anti-VEGF) and pan-retinal photocoagulation (PRP) alongside trabeculectomy and aqueous shunt implantation. Bleeding outside of the eye, as would be seen in an *ab externo* procedure, can be controlled with traditional measures such as thermocautery. But in an *ab interno* procedure, in an angle that has already been exposed to significant inflammation, uncontrolled bleeding in the immediate postoperative period could be devastating and result in surgical failure.

3. NVG is a severe condition that is notoriously difficult to control, with patients often presenting with IOPs in the 40s or higher. It may therefore seem somewhat counterintuitive or insufficient to attempt a MIGS procedure, many of which were originally conceived for mild-to-moderate glaucoma, in a circumstance that is usually far more severe.

While these are valid concerns and limitations, we propose that angle-based MIGS may have a role in surgical IOP lowering in the setting of NVG.

3   Selecting the Right Patient

There are several critical characteristics when considering angle surgery in the setting of NVG.

First, there should be some visual potential in order to consider an incisional procedure for aggressive IOP control, as opposed to a more palliative nonincisional procedure with the goal of comfort. As discussed in previous chapters of this book, accurately assessing visual potential in NVG patients can be challenging, especially in the acute setting.

Second, optimal control of the underlying neovascular drive is essential. In the case of aqueous shunt surgery, surgical outcomes are best when NVI and NVA are regressed preoperatively, which limits intraoperative and postoperative hyphema which can threaten the function of the shunt. Postoperatively, if the underlying neovascular drive is not controlled, the NVA can recur

and the angle can become synechially closed, but the IOP can remain controlled if the shunt is functioning. Compared to aqueous shunt surgery, control of the underlying neovascular drive is even more essential when attempting angle surgery for IOP control. Intraoperatively, uncontrolled bleeding will be encountered upon incising these fragile vessels if there is active NVA. Postoperatively, after angle surgery, if the underlying neovascular drive is not controlled, the NVA can recur and the angle can become synechially closed; in the absence of a functioning shunt, the IOP will become elevated again. It is of utmost importance that the patient complies with frequent follow-up visits with both the glaucoma specialist and retina specialist to monitor for IOP elevation and recurrent neovascularization, since there will be no alternate pathway for aqueous to exit the anterior chamber if NVA recurs and synechial closure occurs. Tight control of the neovascular drive will also optimally treat the underlying neovascular disease and prevent posterior segment complications such as vitreous hemorrhage and tractional retinal detachment. Indeed, even when IOP is controlled with an aqueous shunt, long-term visual outcomes in the setting of NVG are largely attributed to the underlying retinal pathology [3]. As a result, it is critical to completely suppress the underlying neovascular drive in addition to aggressively controlling the IOP.

Finally, from a technical standpoint, angle surgery is typically performed with the surgeon sitting temporally and beginning the goniotomy nasally. Therefore, for an eye with NVG to be a potential candidate for angle surgery, the nasal angle must be surgically accessible with at least part of it unobscured by peripheral anterior synechiae (PAS). The presence of synechial closure in other quadrants does not preclude the possibility of angle surgery; a GATT can physically lyse through PAS in other clock hours, as long as the catheter or suture is able to be inserted into Schlemm's canal and advanced circumferentially. If the nasal angle is already synechially closed, goniosynechialysis can be attempted to access Schlemm's canal, though this may not be physically possible in some circumstances.

Unlike PAS from primary angle closure, where goniosynechialysis with a blunt spatula can often push the iris adhesions off the trabecular meshwork, a sharper instrument may be required to incise the fibrovascular membrane covering the iris and angle structures before pushing the iris down to access Schlemm's canal. Depending on the patient's facial anatomy, it may be possible to sit superiorly or inferotemporally and begin the goniotomy inferiorly or superonasally, respectively. Of note, the angled Tanito microhook can be used to access the temporal angle with the surgeon sitting on the nasal side of the operative eye [10]. It may be prudent to consent the patient for a possible conversion to an aqueous shunt if there is extensive PAS preoperatively and the angle procedure is attempted but cannot physically be performed.

If each of these criteria is met, we believe that angle surgery may be considered an option when choosing an IOP-lowering procedure in the setting of NVG, with the goal of avoiding or at least delaying an aqueous shunt and its associated complications. Herein, we present a recently published patient case [17] from our institution to serve as an illustrative example for when angle surgery may be a viable option for IOP control in the setting of NVG and what must occur for it to be successful.

4   Patient Case

A 57-year-old African American female presented to an outside hospital with left eye ([oculus sinister], OS) pain and reduced vision. She had a past medical history of diabetes mellitus type II, as well as CRVO OS. She also had undergone cataract surgery OS 6 months previously. At the outside hospital emergency department, her IOP was reportedly elevated; IOP-lowering topical medications were administered, and she was instructed to follow up with an outpatient glaucoma specialist. Upon presentation to the glaucoma clinic, the left eye had a VA of hand motion, IOP was 45 mmHg on 0 medications, the pupil was minimally reactive with relative afferent pupillary defect by reverse, the cornea had micro-

cystic edema, the anterior chamber was deep and quiet with no hyphema, the iris had 360° of florid NVI at the pupillary margin, and a 1-piece intraocular lens implant was in the capsular bag. Gonioscopy revealed NVA and scattered focal PAS throughout approximately 75% of the angle and broad PAS in approximately 25% of the angle, but the nasal angle was open. The corneal edema precluded a clear view to the retina, but B-scan ultrasonography revealed that the retina was attached. Intravitreal bevacizumab (1.25 mg in 0.05 mL) (IVB) was promptly administered, and anterior chamber paracentesis was performed. She was started on 4 topical IOP-lowering medications OS and oral acetazolamide extended release 500 mg 3× per day. She underwent PRP OS later that week. Five weeks after the acute NVG presentation, IOP was 22 on 5 topical medications + oral acetazolamide 500 mg extended release once per day, the NVI and NVA had completely regressed, and gonioscopy revealed approximately 150°–180° of synechial closure, although the nasal trabecular meshwork was notably visible and appeared to be surgically accessible.

GATT was offered, but due to the extensive PAS, she was also consented for the possibility of converting to an aqueous shunt if the GATT could not be physically performed due to the extensive PAS. She underwent a second preoperative intravitreal bevacizumab to prevent NVA recurrence, in preparation for the upcoming GATT. Due to insurance issues, the surgery could not be performed until several weeks later, at which point it had been 8 weeks since the acute NVG presentation.

On the day of the GATT, her IOP OS was 35 mmHg on five topical medications + oral acetazolamide 500 mg extended release once per day. The stand-alone GATT procedure was performed using Healon Pro (Johnson & Johnson Vision) as the viscoelastic in the anterior chamber. At the end of the surgery, approximately 50–75% of the Healon Pro was purposely left in the anterior chamber to tamponade reflux blood from Schlemm's canal. Intravitreal triamcinolone (2 mg in 0.05 mL) was injected to reduce inflammation and prevent macular edema and PAS.

On postoperative day (POD) 1, IOP was 40 mmHg due to the Healon Pro in the anterior chamber; the paracentesis was burped and the IOP lowered to 8 mmHg. Over the subsequent 8 months, her IOP-lowering medications were able to be sequentially stopped, and she underwent 6 more intravitreal bevacizumab injections for a total of 8 injections within 9 months and 1 additional session of fill-in PRP.

By postoperative month 9, which was 11 months after the acute NVG presentation, VA OS was still stable at 20/200, IOP OS was 16 mmHg on zero IOP-lowering medications, there was no active NVI or NVA, and although there were still some areas of visible PAS on gonioscopy, more than 180° of the angle was open, and there were some areas where the back wall of Schlemm's canal was visible.

The patient then became lost to follow-up for a duration of 4 months and subsequently represented 12 months after the GATT with an IOP of 49 mmHg on 0 IOP-lowering medications, recurrent florid NVI and NVA, and a 1.5 mm layered hyphema; her angle had become 100% synechially closed. She subsequently underwent CPC followed by more serial IVBs and fill-in PRP sessions. IOP control was ultimately achieved with a Baerveldt-350 in the sulcus, 14 months after the GATT. Her final visual acuity ultimately improved to 20/150.

5 Further Considerations

Our patient achieved a physiologic IOP on 0 IOP-lowering medications 9 months after the GATT which suggests proof-of-concept that angle surgery can be a viable option for IOP control in NVG, if the underlying neovascular drive can be aggressively controlled in perpetuity. At the time of surgery, she met each of the criteria above.

First, her visual potential was deemed to be good enough that an attempt to restore physiologic IOP was warranted. Although she had NVG due to a CRVO, with prompt aggressive IOP-lowering and antineovascular therapy, her final visual acuity ended up being 20/150, which was limited by the CRVO rather than glaucomatous optic neuropathy.

Second, there was no active neovascularization at the time of GATT, having undergone two IVB injections and one session of PRP preoperatively. She was counseled extensively that she would require close follow-up in perpetuity with numerous additional serial IVBs and fill-in PRP sessions, and she appeared to be committed to adhering to the follow-up schedule.

Third, although there was scattered PAS in the majority of her angle, the nasal angle was open at presentation and remained open over the subsequent 2 months as she underwent IVB and PRP and the NVA regressed. The GATT was performed without need for goniosynechialysis and without complication. The nasal goniotomy allowed access to Schlemm's canal, the catheter was able to be advanced for 360° without obstruction, and the PAS throughout the angle was lysed when both ends of the catheter were pulled and the 360° trabeculotomy was performed. Further research is needed to quantify the success rates of angle surgery stratified by extent of PAS at the time of the acute NVG presentation and/or at the time of the angle surgery. We hypothesize that NVG eyes with a lesser extent of PAS may have a higher likelihood of achieving adequate IOP lowering with angle surgery.

Finally, this patient's relatively young age was a factor in the decision to offer an attempted GATT as a possible alternative to avoid or at least delay an aqueous shunt. Since she was only 57 years old, if her physiologic aqueous outflow pathway could be salvaged and an aqueous shunt could be deferred, this could help avoid tube-associated complications for potentially several decades. At any age, aqueous shunts have risks of hypotony-associated complications, implant-associated infections, corneal decompensation (especially if the tube is placed in the anterior chamber), and diplopia, all of which would be reduced or avoided with a successful angle surgery.

Ultimately, this patient's GATT was successful at restoring the physiologic aqueous outflow pathway and achieving IOP control for 9 months, during which time she was adherent to the close follow-up schedule including serial IVB and more fill-in PRP. Unfortunately, she was ultimately lost to follow-up for a duration of 4 months, and her neovascularization recurred, suggesting that her underlying neovascular disease was not yet quiescent. This highlights the critical importance of ongoing close follow-up, an aggressive anti-VEGF and PRP regimen, and close partnership with the retina service to ensure that the neovascular drive remains quiet in perpetuity. Although control of IOP and control of the neovascular drive are dual goals in NVG, when attempting to salvage the physiologic aqueous outflow pathway with angle surgery, the former is completely dependent on the latter.

6   Conclusion

The transient initial success of this NVG patient for 9 months after GATT demonstrates that under the right conditions, angle surgery can indeed be a viable option for IOP control in NVG. Angle surgery allows patients to maintain their physiologic aqueous outflow system and to avoid or delay an aqueous shunt and its associated complications. While further research is needed to investigate their long-term efficacy, we propose that angle surgery should be considered as a possible option for surgical IOP lowering in the setting of NVG, in carefully selected patients.

References

1. Takihara Y, Inatani M, Fukushima M, Iwao K, Iwao M, Tanihara H. Trabeculectomy with mitomycin C for neovascular glaucoma: prognostic factors for surgical failure. Am J Ophthalmol. 2009;147(5):912. https://doi.org/10.1016/J.AJO.2008.11.015.
2. Saito Y, Higashide T, Takeda H, Ohkubo S, Sugiyama K. Beneficial effects of preoperative intravitreal bevacizumab on trabeculectomy outcomes in neovascular glaucoma. Acta Ophthalmol. 2010;88(1):96–102. https://doi.org/10.1111/J.1755-3768.2009.01648.X.
3. Shalaby WS, Myers JS, Razeghinejad R, et al. Outcomes of valved and nonvalved tube shunts in neovascular glaucoma. Ophthalmol Glaucoma. 2020;4(2):182. https://doi.org/10.1016/j.ogla.2020.09.010.
4. Medert CM, Sun CQ, Vanner E, Parrish RK, Wellik SR. The influence of etiology on surgical outcomes in neovascular glaucoma. BMC Ophthalmol. 2021;21(1):440. https://doi.org/10.1186/S12886-021-02212-X.
5. Olmos LC, Lee RK. Medical and surgical treatment of neovascular glaucoma. Int Ophthalmol Clin. 2011;51(3):27–36. https://doi.org/10.1097/IIO.0B013E31821E5960.
6. Tailor R, Kinsella MT, Clarke JC. Long-term outcome of intravitreal bevacizumab followed by Ahmed valve implantation in the management of neovascular glaucoma. Semin Ophthalmol. 2018;33(5):606–12. https://doi.org/10.1080/08820538.2017.1375123.
7. Asif H, Si Z, Quan S, Amin P, Dao D, Shaw L, Skondra D, Qiu M. Neovascular glaucoma from ocular ischemic syndrome treated with serial monthly intravitreal bevacizumab and panretinal photocoagulation: a case report. Case Rep Ophthalmol Med. 2022 Jul;28(2022):4959522. https://doi.org/10.1155/2022/4959522.
8. Bar-David L, Blumenthal EZ. Evolution of glaucoma surgery in the last 25 years. Rambam Maimonides Med J. 2018;9(3):e0024. https://doi.org/10.5041/RMMJ.10345.
9. Seibold LK, Soohoo JR, Ammar DA, Kahook MY. Preclinical investigation of ab interno trabeculectomy using a novel dual-blade device. Am J Ophthalmol. 2013;155(3):524–529.e2. https://doi.org/10.1016/J.AJO.2012.09.023.
10. Dorairaj S, Tam MD. Kahook dual blade excisional goniotomy and goniosynechialysis combined with phacoemulsification for angle-closure glaucoma: 6-month results. J Glaucoma. 2019;28(7):643–6. https://doi.org/10.1097/IJG.0000000000001256.
11. Tanito M. Microhook ab interno trabeculotomy, a novel minimally invasive glaucoma surgery. Clin Ophthalmol. 2017;12:43–8. https://doi.org/10.2147/OPTH.S152406.
12. Laroche D, Okaka Y, Ng C. A novel low cost effective technique in using a 23 gauge straight cystotome to perform goniotomy: making micro-invasive glaucoma surgery (MIGS) accessible to the Africans and the diaspora. J Natl Med Assoc. 2019;111(2):193–7. https://doi.org/10.1016/J.JNMA.2018.09.006.
13. Dada T, Mahalingam K, Bhartiya S. Minimally invasive glaucoma surgery-to remove or preserve the trabecular meshwork: that is the question? J Curr Glaucoma Pract. 2021;15(2):47–51. https://doi.org/10.5005/JP-JOURNALS-10078-1299.
14. Grover DS, Godfrey DG, Smith O, Feuer WJ, Montes de Oca I, Fellman RL. Gonioscopy-assisted transluminal trabeculotomy, ab interno trabeculotomy. Ophthalmology. 2014;121(4):855–61. https://doi.org/10.1016/j.ophtha.2013.11.001.
15. Fontana L, De Maria M, Iannetta D, Moramarco A. Gonioscopy-assisted transluminal trabeculotomy for chronic angle-closure glaucoma: preliminary results. Graefes Arch Clin Exp Ophthalmol.

2022;260(2):545–51. https://doi.org/10.1007/S00417-021-05400-Z.

16. Chira-adisai T, Mori K, Kobayashi A, et al. Outcomes of combined gonioscopy-assisted transluminal trabeculotomy and goniosynechialysis in primary angle closure: a retrospective case series. Int Ophthalmol. 2021;41(4):1223–31. https://doi.org/10.1007/S10792-020-01676-Y.

17. Kanter JA, Amin P, Komati R, Mackin AG, Dao D, Shaw LT, Skondra D, Qiu M. Gonioscopy-assisted transluminal trabeculotomy in neovascular glaucoma: salvaging the conventional outflow pathway. Am J Ophthalmol Case Rep. 2022 Jul;31(28):101668. https://doi.org/10.1016/j.ajoc.2022.101668.

Advancing Care in Neovascular Glaucoma

Mary Qiu, Aakriti G. Shukla, and Catherine Q. Sun

1 Introduction

Key areas for improvement with respect to advancing care and improving outcomes in neovascular glaucoma (NVG) include the following: (1) standardizing the definition and staging of NVG, (2) detecting anterior segment neovascularization earlier, (3) increasing evidence-based research to improve outcomes, (4) determining the optimal multidisciplinary treatment approach, and (5) increasing patient adherence to treatment [1]. In this final chapter, we discuss each of these five areas and propose solutions to help address the barriers to improved outcomes.

M. Qiu (✉)
Department of Ophthalmology and Visual Science,
The University of Chicago Medicine,
Chicago, IL, USA
e-mail: maryqiu@bsd.uchicago.edu

A. G. Shukla
Bernard and Shirlee Brown Glaucoma Research
Laboratory, Department of Ophthalmology, Columbia
University Irving Medical Center,
New York, NY, USA

C. Q. Sun
Department of Ophthalmology, University of
California, San Francisco, CA, USA

Frances I. Proctor Foundation, University of
California, San Francisco, CA, USA

2 Standardizing the Definition and Staging of NVG

There is currently no consensus in the literature on how NVG is defined. We propose that standardizing the definition and staging of NVG can improve diagnosis, management, and outcomes in NVG. Potential models to mirror when developing a classification scheme for NVG include the distinction between ocular hypertension and primary open-angle glaucoma, and the classification scheme for the primary angle closure spectrum [2, 3]. The presence of optic nerve damage should be taken into account in the definition since the patient's visual potential can impact treatment decisions, but it can be difficult to assess optic nerve status during the acute presentation [4]. Consensus panels can help define and classify pre-NVG stages (anterior segment neovascularization without elevated IOP) and elucidate whether interventions should be tailored to disease stage.

3 Earlier Detection of Anterior Segment Neovascularization

The diagnosis of NVG is often delayed because patients are typically asymptomatic in the earlier stages of disease. However, the underlying disease processes that lead to NVG typically do not develop immediately. More often, NVG takes weeks to months to develop when secondary to central retinal artery occlusion or central retinal vein occlusion (CRVO), respectively, and even years in the case of proliferative diabetic retinopathy (PDR). A retrospective review reported that 25% of eyes presenting with anterior segment neovascularization without elevated IOP progressed to NVG, with the majority progressing by 6 months [5]. Therefore, there is a window of opportunity for improved outcomes if there are better systems in place to screen and identify at-risk patients and better tools for earlier diagnosis, such as identifying patients with pre-NVG.

Limited capacity and time allocation in ophthalmology clinics continue to be barriers to eye care access, potentially delaying diagnosis and treatment. In order to increase clinic efficiency, high-risk follow-up patients (many of whom have ischemic retinal disease) are often dilated by the technician before seeing the ophthalmologist if their visual acuity (VA) and IOP are within normal limits. Shortcomings of this approach include potentially missing subtle early findings of NVI postdilation and omission of gonioscopy to detect the presence of NVA and peripheral anterior synechiae (PAS) [6]. It may be unrealistic to expect comprehensive ophthalmologists and retinal specialists to examine the iris before dilation or to perform gonioscopy in all high-risk patients. Furthermore, the findings of PAS or angle closure may be challenging to detect for providers who do not frequently perform gonioscopy. As such, we need to consider alternative methods or processes that will allow earlier detection of anterior segment neovascularization without significantly increasing the burden placed on physicians and their staff.

Early detection of NVI may require the aid of diagnostic tests such as anterior segment photographs, iris or gonioscopic angiography, or noninvasive anterior segment optical coherence tomography angiography (OCTA) [7–10]. Further research is needed to elucidate the duration between subclinical presentation of anterior segment neovascularization visible on imaging and the clinical presentation of NVG. In addition, new automated parameters for iris or angle imaging need to be developed for OCTA to be feasible.

4 Additional Evidence-Based Research Needed

There are numerous areas of ongoing investigation in NVG care. These include treatment strategies for proliferative retinal pathology prior to and after the development of NVG as well as the choice of IOP-lowering procedure. While panretinal photocoagulation (PRP) and antivascular endothelial growth factor (VEGF) therapy have substantially improved outcomes in these cases, there is no standardized evidence-based approach for NVG prevention and treatment. Additionally, while the glaucoma surgical procedural landscape has expanded in the last decade, "real-world" retrospective studies remain the primary sources of data on outcomes following glaucoma surgery for NVG.

4.1 The Role of Anti-VEGF vs. PRP Before NVG Has Developed

PRP has been the mainstay treatment for ischemic retinal diseases. However, given its potential adverse effects, there has been interest in therapeutic alternatives to control the retinal ischemia driving neovascularization. Much of the work evaluating anti-VEGF agents to control ischemia has been performed in CRVO and PDR, the leading causes of NVG.

However, these studies may be underpowered to compare the incidence of anterior segment neovascularization between treatments. For example, a few RCTs have compared prompt PRP to anti-VEGF intravitreal injections for PDR and found no difference in the development of NVI or NVG [11–14]. The Diabetic Retinopathy Clinical Research Network (DRCR.net) Protocol S study reported no difference in development of NVG at 2-year (anti-VEGF 2% vs. PRP 3%) and 5-year follow-up (anti-VEGF 3% vs. PRP 4%) [11]. Another study comparing anti-VEGF (ranibizumab) with PRP to PRP alone for high-risk PDR did not report any occurrence of NVI or NVG, but "elevation in IOP" occurred in 7% of the anti-VEGF + PRP group and 9% of the PRP group at 1 year [14]. However, all of these studies were not powered to detect such a small difference (0–2%) in NVG incidence.

Since the therapeutic benefits of anti-VEGF injections are temporary and patients require frequent life-long injections, American Academy of Ophthalmology (AAO) diabetic retinopathy guidelines indicate that the decision to treat PDR with PRP versus serial anti-VEGF injections alone should be made with strong consideration of the reliability of patient follow-up and their risk for rapid progression [15]. In a real-world study using retrospective electronic health record data from a large tertiary eye hospital and private practice retina clinics, 25% of patients with PDR were lost to follow-up over 4 years [16]. The patients who did not adhere to follow-up had worse visual outcomes with anti-VEGF injections than PRP. The anti-VEGF group had higher incidence of NVI ($N = 4$, $P = 0.02$) and NVG ($N = 2$, $P = 0.15$) compared to the PRP group, in which neither NVI nor NVG occurred [17]. As such, providers are not always accurate in their assessment of follow-up reliability, and if they are wrong in their assessment, the visual consequences can be severe. Larger studies are needed to investigate NVG incidence over a longer time frame.

Similarly, updated guidelines are also needed for CRVO patients in the anti-VEGF era. The description of NVG in CRVO patients as a "90-day glaucoma" was derived from the natural history studies before anti-VEGF [18]. The current AAO Preferred Practice Pattern guidelines for retinal vein occlusion recommend PRP for individuals who develop NVI or retinal neovascularization after a CRVO [19]. This evidence is derived from the Central Vein Occlusion Study, which was conducted in patients with ischemic CRVO prior to the availability of anti-VEGF; the study determined that prophylactic PRP did not lead to a statistically significant reduction in development of NVI or NVA and "delayed but timely" PRP was effective in regressing anterior segment neovascularization [6]. The study recommended that high-risk eyes should be followed closely and prophylactic PRP should be considered in those eyes where close follow-up is not possible. However, with the change in treatment paradigm for CRVO macular edema from PRP to anti-VEGF, patients have been reported to be at highest risk for NVG development well beyond the typical 90 days and need continual monitoring after anti-VEGF discontinuation [20, 21]. An RCT compared different doses of intravitreal ranibizumab for 9 months in 20 patients with ischemic CRVO; anti-VEGF injections did not prevent the development of NVG, but delayed the onset of NVG to greater than 2 years in high-risk individuals [21]. Additional evidence is needed to determine whether or not a combination of anti-VEGF and prophylactic PRP can prevent NVG in CRVO eyes, and more work is needed to elucidate the optimal frequency and duration of follow-up to detect early signs of anterior segment neovascularization in high-risk patients who receive anti-VEGF injections.

4.2 The Role of Anti-VEGF vs. PRP After NVG Has Developed

Prior evidence demonstrates that PRP causes regression of neovascularization in patients and is associated with a higher success rate of glaucoma filtering surgeries in the setting of NVG [22, 23]. The AAO Preferred Practice Pattern guidelines for diabetic retinopathy recommend prompt PRP for high-risk PDR, which includes the presence of anterior segment neovascularization [15]. The AAO Preferred Practice Pattern guidelines for CRVO recommend PRP when NVI is present [19]. Since the FDA approval of anti-VEGF in 2004, most providers agreed that anti-VEGF is a part of the initial treatment for NVG given its rapid onset of action and that stabilized patients should receive PRP [4]. However, there is inconclusive evidence if anti-VEGF and PRP should be administered concomitantly at the onset of NVG or staged and how the timing of these treatments should occur if glaucoma surgery is needed.

The few single-center comparative studies available suggest that a combination of anti-VEGF and PRP should be given to patients with NVG [24–26]. In one study, NVG patients who received both PRP and anti-VEGF injections had fewer glaucoma surgeries than those who received anti-VEGF injections alone [24]. Another small study found regression of neovascularization at significantly higher frequency and rapidity in eyes treated with combination of anti-VEGF and PRP as compared to PRP alone [25]. This finding may be due to the rapid onset of action after anti-VEGF injections compared to PRP; as such, it has been proposed that a combination of anti-VEGF and early PRP before 4 weeks has a promising role for treating high-risk PDR without clinically significant macular edema [27]. Further multicenter prospective research is needed in this area.

4.3 The Choice of IOP-Lowering Procedure After NVG Has Developed

To date, there have been no published RCTs enrolling only NVG eyes, and data from small to medium-sized retrospective and prospective studies comparing surgical outcomes of trabeculectomy, aqueous shunts, and CPC in NVG eyes have been equivocal [28–32]. These studies define a successful surgical outcome as preservation of useful vision, adequate IOP lowering, or a combination of the two.

While there is no large RCT to serve as the basis for choosing an aqueous shunt over trabeculectomy in NVG, aqueous shunts are generally considered the treatment of choice for NVG eyes with good visual potential given the higher rates of trabeculectomy failure in the setting of anterior segment neovascularization. Valved aqueous shunts (i.e., Ahmed) are usually preferred over nonvalved aqueous shunts (i.e., Baerveldt, Molteno) given the need for immediate IOP lowering, though a recent analysis from a tertiary eye hospital of 152 NVG eyes undergoing aqueous shunts (91 Ahmed and 61 Baerveldt) reported similar failure rates at 6 months (21.6% and 25.9%, respectively) [33]. Larger, longer-term RCTs are needed to guide management.

There is no consensus among glaucoma specialists regarding the optimal IOP-lowering surgery in NVG eyes with poor visual potential, and

both aqueous shunts and CPC are commonly used [4]. CPC has traditionally been reserved for refractory glaucoma and eyes with poor visual potential due to the risk of prolonged inflammation and macular edema, so direct comparison in retrospective studies with trabeculectomy or aqueous shunts is prone to selection bias. Recent literature supports improved CPC outcomes with modified laser settings [34]. Since CPC is a fast and noninvasive procedure, further studies are needed to better characterize its utility, risk profile, and cost-effectiveness for select NVG patients.

The majority of studies pool various etiologies of NVG together, but there is evidence to suggest that the etiology of NVG may affect prognosis and outcome; for example, patients with NVG from PDR had better outcomes after incisional glaucoma surgery than patients with NVG from retinal vein occlusion [35]. Studying NVG outcomes stratified by etiology has been challenging because NVG is a relatively rare disease, so identifying a large enough cohort of patients to power studies capable of providing clinically meaningful results is a lengthy, time-intensive process. Electronic health records and larger databases or registries may be potential avenues for future research.

The currently accepted surgical strategies for IOP lowering in NVG eyes are anchored on the principle that the conventional outflow pathway has already become permanently obstructed by synechial angle closure, so the aqueous must either be shunted elsewhere (trabeculectomy of aqueous shunt) or its production must be reduced (CPC). However, in the anti-VEGF era in which intravitreal injections can be utilized to rapidly regress NVA, and with the advent of angle-based micro-incisional glaucoma surgery (MIGS) techniques in the past decade, there may be an opportunity for glaucoma specialists and retina specialists to collaborate and develop a novel NVG treatment protocol with the goal of attempting to enhance or restore aqueous outflow through the trabecular meshwork and Schlemm's canal: the physiologic conventional aqueous outflow pathway. This would challenge the widely held belief among glaucoma specialists that NVG is a contraindication to angle surgery. Further investigation into these potentially safer treatment protocols which attempt to salvage the conventional aqueous outflow pathway would have the potential to prevent or delay vision loss, or major glaucoma surgery, both of which can significantly impact vision-related quality of life.

4.4 Improving the Multidisciplinary Treatment Approach

As with any multidisciplinary condition that requires coordination of care across specialties, the management can be more challenging. To start, there is limited evidence in the literature on current real-world practice patterns for NVG in retina and glaucoma clinics. A lone 2016 survey of glaucoma and retinal specialists found that the majority of providers agreed that antivascular endothelial growth factors (VEGF) injections should be included in the initial management of NVG given its rapid onset of action and that stabilized patients should receive panretinal photocoagulation (PRP) [4]. Glaucoma specialists favored IOP-lowering surgery significantly more often than retinal specialists, though their preference for type of glaucoma procedure varied for an eye with poor vision (54% glaucoma drainage implant vs. 42% transscleral cyclophotocoagulation) [4]. There was no consensus regarding how to combine glaucoma and retinal interventions or how to manage patients after the initial acute phase.

In order to improve outcomes, we believe a paradigm shift is needed to develop a more standardized multidisciplinary treatment protocol for NVG. Central to this evolution is a commitment from the patient, the glaucoma specialist, and the retina specialist. Future domestic and international consensus panels including both retina and glaucoma specialists are needed to mitigate discrepancies in NVG management and develop care paths for more effective and efficient care delivery. Advancements in NVG treatment may also require a shift in the mindset of physicians. Glaucoma and retinal specialists may need to evaluate their current practice patterns and con-

sider adjusting their workflows. Tertiary medical centers could consider multidisciplinary visits that occur concurrently. However, discussions regarding reimbursement would need to occur to make this financially feasible for medical centers. These changes, while substantial, could potentially lead to better outcomes in this vulnerable patient population.

Evidence of this paradigm shift has been proposed in the literature. A prospective interventional case series from Peking University enrolled 51 eyes with NVG with the goal of completing PRP to preserve visual function [26]. The study aimed to establish a multidisciplinary treatment strategy for NVG where all eyes received immediate intravitreal bevacizumab upon NVG diagnosis, and if necessary, repeated anti-VEGF treatment was administered every 4 weeks until PRP could be completed; 44 eyes completed the treatment protocol. The first-line IOP-lowering surgery for eyes with uncontrolled IOP after medical management ($N = 39$ eyes) was trabeculectomy combined with cataract surgery and/or pars plana vitrectomy as needed. The second-line IOP-lowering surgery was an aqueous shunt, which was performed in seven eyes requiring additional IOP lowering after the trabeculectomy. CPC was not performed in this study. If PRP could not be completed within 4 weeks after the initial anti-VEGF injection, then anti-VEGF injections were repeated monthly until PRP could be completed. Fluorescein angiography was performed 4 weeks after PRP to determine whether supplemental PRP was needed. After the treatment protocol was completed, the IOP was ≤21 mmHg in 87% of eyes up to postoperative month 6; the IOP in the other 13% of eyes ranged from 21 to 28 mmHg. All eyes completing the treatment protocol had regression of NVI and NVA, and 93% of patients achieved stable or improved vision. The study authors emphasized that the treatment strategy for NVG must focus on the following principles: (1) lower the IOP, (2) use anti-VEGF to regress anterior segment neovascularization to optimize conditions for glaucoma surgery, and (3) perform glaucoma surgery with or without cataract surgery and vitrectomy to optimize conditions for PRP.

This study, which was performed between 2010 and 2012 (after the advent of anti-VEGF), highlights the excellent clinical outcomes that can be achieved with close collaboration between glaucoma and retinal specialists who share the patient-centric goal of preserving visual function by controlling the IOP and suppressing the underlying neovascular drive. Additional research is needed in this area in the form of randomized controlled trials in an optimal setting and pragmatic trials in a real-world setting.

5   Patient Adherence to Treatment

Engagement and education are paramount for patients with a new diagnosis of NVG. Since complex multidisciplinary care is required to adequately manage NVG, it is important that patients understand the underlying etiology of their NVG and the ophthalmic manifestations. Active patient participation is important as it is a potential indicator of patient adherence in glaucoma management [36]. Much of the research on adherence has been performed in relation to medication use. The identified barriers to medication adherence in glaucoma include cost, symptomatic side effects, poor health literacy, forgetfulness, limited trust in healthcare, busy schedules, and physical or mental limitations [37]. Furthermore, the diabetes literature reveals that patient satisfaction with physician communication, beliefs about need for medications, and level of health literacy are associated with degree of medication adherence. Factors associated with nonadherence to diabetic retinopathy screening visits include younger age, socioeconomic disparities (e.g., lower income, lower levels of education), financial burdens, less diabetes education, insulin dependence, and proxies for poor health behavior (e.g., lower adherence to other medications, smoking, hemoglobin A1c >9%) [38].

Successful mechanisms to enhance adherence and self-efficacy have focused on improving physician–patient communication [36, 39]. Studies involving video recordings of interactions between providers and patients have demon-strated that providers educate patients about glaucoma in 63% of visits; however, specific education about adherence takes place in only 18% of visits and about the purpose of medication during 17% of visits [39]. While extensive physician-led patient counseling may not be an option given time constraints in most glaucoma clinics, other providers may play a central role in offering patient education. Furthermore, cost–utility analysis of medication adherence in glaucoma using data from large clinical trials and insurance claims for adherence data found that services that improve adherence in glaucoma patients can be expanded without significant negative financial implications [40].

The participation of patient advocates and social workers has been shown to be beneficial in prior studies. A recent Cochrane review found that patient education combined with personalized one-on-one strategies had the most success in improving adherence among glaucoma patients [41]. Studies have demonstrated the need for certified patient educators in the management of glaucoma. They report a need for certified glaucoma coaches who function similarly to educators in other medical specialties and provide self-management counseling, which is reimbursable by insurance [40]. Other studies advocate involving social workers in the care of glaucoma patients specifically because of their understanding of community services and ability to counsel patients on medical and psychological needs [42]. In a 6-month intervention, a social worker intervention addressed barriers to eye care including transportation, access to low-vision resources, and patient counseling and education, and significantly decreased symptoms of depression in a population that needed follow-up eye care [42].

6   Conclusion

In conclusion, there is substantial room for future improvement in the diagnosis and management of NVG. Although great strides have been made in recent years with respect to advancements in glaucoma and retina treatment options, there have not been any standardized guidelines for NVG care. The ophthalmology community should work synergistically across specialties and with patients to surmount barriers to optimal NVG care.

References

1. Qiu M, Shukla AG, Sun CQ. Improving outcomes in neovascular glaucoma. Ophthalmol Glaucoma. 2022;5(2):125–7. https://doi.org/10.1016/J.OGLA.2021.12.001.
2. Gedde SJ, Chen PP, Muir KW, et al. Primary angle-closure disease preferred practice pattern®. Ophthalmology. 2021;128(1):P30–70. https://doi.org/10.1016/J.OPHTHA.2020.10.021.
3. Prum BE Jr, Rosenberg LF, Gedde SJ, et al. Primary open-angle glaucoma preferred practice pattern® guidelines. Ophthalmology. 2016;123:P41–P111. https://doi.org/10.1016/j.ophtha.2015.10.053.
4. Venkat AG, Singh RP, Eisengart J, Hu M, Babiuch AS. Trends in neovascular glaucoma management: practice patterns of glaucoma and retina specialists in the United States. Am J Ophthalmic Clin Trials. 2019;2:7. https://doi.org/10.25259/ajoct_11_2019.
5. Sastry A, Ryu C, Jiang X, Ameri H. Visual outcomes in eyes with neovascular glaucoma and anterior segment neovascularization without glaucoma. Am J Ophthalmol. 2021;236:1–11. https://doi.org/10.1016/J.AJO.2021.09.006.
6. A randomized clinical trial of early panretinal photocoagulation for ischemic central vein occlusion. The Central Vein Occlusion Study Group N Report. Ophthalmology. 1995;102(10):1434–44. https://doi.org/10.1016/S0161-6420(95)30848-2.
7. Li S, Wang Z, Li P, Dong Y. Application of iris fluorescein angiography combined with fundus fluorescein angiography in diabetic retinopathy with neovascular glaucoma. Zhonghua Shiyan Yanke Zazhi/Chinese J Exp Ophthalmol. 2016;34(12):1112–5. https://doi.org/10.3760/cma.j.issn.2095-0160.2016.12.013.
8. Ishibashi S, Tawara A, Sohma R, Kubota T, Toh N. Angiographic changes in iris and iridocorneal angle neovascularization after intravitreal bevacizumab injection. Arch Ophthalmol. 2010;128(12):1539–45. https://doi.org/10.1001/archophthalmol.2010.282.
9. Jia Y, Xue W, Tong X, Wang Y, Cui L, Zou H. Quantitative analysis and clinical application of iris circulation in ischemic retinal disease. BMC Ophthalmol. 2021;21(1):393. https://doi.org/10.1186/S12886-021-02165-1.
10. Roberts PK, Goldstein DA, Fawzi AA. Anterior segment optical coherence tomography angiography for identification of iris vasculature and staging of iris neovascularization: a pilot study. Curr Eye Res. 2017;42(8):1136–42. https://doi.org/10.1080/02713683.2017.1293113.
11. Gross JG, Glassman AR, Liu D, et al. Five-year outcomes of panretinal photocoagulation vs intravitreous ranibizumab for proliferative diabetic retinopathy: a randomized clinical trial. JAMA Ophthalmol. 2018;136(10):1138–48. https://doi.org/10.1001/jamaophthalmol.2018.3255.
12. Gross JG, Glassman AR, Jampol LM, et al. Panretinal photocoagulation vs intravitreous ranibizumab for proliferative diabetic retinopathy: a randomized clinical trial. JAMA. 2015;314(20):2137–46. https://doi.org/10.1001/jama.2015.15217.
13. Rani PK, Sen P, Sahoo NK, et al. Outcomes of neovascular glaucoma in eyes presenting with moderate to good visual potential. Int Ophthalmol. 2021;41(7):2359–68. https://doi.org/10.1007/s10792-021-01789-y.
14. Figueira J, Fletcher E, Massin P, et al. Ranibizumab plus panretinal photocoagulation versus panretinal photocoagulation alone for high-risk proliferative diabetic retinopathy (PROTEUS study). Ophthalmology. 2018;125(5):691–700. https://doi.org/10.1016/J.OPHTHA.2017.12.008.
15. Flaxel CJ, Adelman RA, Bailey ST, et al. Diabetic retinopathy preferred practice pattern®. Ophthalmology. 2020;127(1):P66–P145. https://doi.org/10.1016/J.OPHTHA.2019.09.025.
16. Obeid A, Gao X, Ali FS, et al. Loss to follow-up in patients with proliferative diabetic retinopathy after panretinal photocoagulation or intravitreal anti-VEGF injections. Ophthalmology. 2018;125(9):1386–92. https://doi.org/10.1016/j.ophtha.2018.02.034.
17. Obeid A, Su D, Patel SN, et al. Outcomes of eyes lost to follow-up with proliferative diabetic retinopathy that received panretinal photocoagulation versus intravitreal anti–vascular endothelial growth factor. Ophthalmology. 2019;126(3):407–13. https://doi.org/10.1016/j.ophtha.2018.07.027.
18. Hayreh SS, Rojas P, Podhajsky P, Montague P, Woolson RF. Ocular neovascularization with retinal vascular occlusion-III. Incidence of ocular neovascularization with retinal vein occlusion. Ophthalmology. 1983;90(5):488–506. https://doi.org/10.1016/S0161-6420(83)34542-5.
19. Flaxel CJ, Adelman RA, Bailey ST, et al. Retinal vein occlusions preferred practice pattern®. Ophthalmology. 2020;127(2):P288–320. https://doi.org/10.1016/J.OPHTHA.2019.09.029.
20. Rong AJ, Swaminathan SS, Vanner EA, Parrish RK. Predictors of neovascular glaucoma in central retinal vein occlusion. Am J Ophthalmol. 2019;205:201–2. https://doi.org/10.1016/j.ajo.2019.04.029.
21. Brown DM, Wykoff CC, Wong TP, Mariani AF, Croft DE, Schuetzle KL. Ranibizumab in preproliferative (ischemic) central retinal vein occlusion: the rubeosis anti-VEGF (RAVE) trial. Retina. 2014;34(9):1728–35. https://doi.org/10.1097/IAE.0000000000000191.
22. Sivak-Callcott JA, O'Day DM, Gass JDM, Tsai JC. Evidence-based recommendations for the diagnosis and treatment of neovascular glaucoma. Ophthalmology. 2001;108(10):1767–76. https://doi.org/10.1016/S0161-6420(01)00775-8.

23. Al Obeidan SA, Osman EA, Al-Amro SA, Kangave D, Abu El-Asrar AM. Full preoperative panretinal photocoagulation improves the outcome of trabeculectomy with mitomycin C for neovascular glaucoma. Eur J Ophthalmol. 2008;18(5):758–64. https://doi.org/10.1177/112067210801800516.

24. Olmos LC, Sayed MS, Moraczewski AL, et al. Long-term outcomes of neovascular glaucoma treated with and without intravitreal bevacizumab. Eye. 2016;30(3):463–72. https://doi.org/10.1038/eye.2015.259.

25. Ehlers JP, Spirn MJ, Lam A, Sivalingam A, Samuel MA, Tasman W. Combination intravitreal bevacizumab/panretinal photocoagulation versus panretinal photocoagulation alone in the treatment of neovascular glaucoma. Retina. 2008;28(5):696–702. https://doi.org/10.1097/IAE.0b013e3181679c0b.

26. Sun Y, Liang Y, Zhou P, et al. Anti-VEGF treatment is the key strategy for neovascular glaucoma management in the short term. BMC Ophthalmol. 2016;16(1):150. https://doi.org/10.1186/s12886-016-0327-9.

27. Shakarchi FI, Shakarchi AF, Al-Bayati SA. Timing of neovascular regression in eyes with high-risk proliferative diabetic retinopathy without macular edema treated initially with intravitreous bevacizumab. Clin Ophthalmol. 2018;13:27–31. https://doi.org/10.2147/OPTH.S182420.

28. Choy BNK, Lai JSM, Yeung JCC, Chan JCH. Randomized comparative trial of diode laser transscleral cyclophotocoagulation versus Ahmed glaucoma valve for neovascular glaucoma in Chinese—a pilot study. Clin Ophthalmol. 2018;12:2545–52. https://doi.org/10.2147/OPTH.S188999.

29. Shen CC, Salim S, Du H, Netland PA. Trabeculectomy versus Ahmed glaucoma valve implantation in neovascular glaucoma. Clin Ophthalmol. 2011;5(1):281–6. https://doi.org/10.2147/OPTH.S16976.

30. Liu L, Xu Y, Huang Z, Wang X. Intravitreal ranibizumab injection combined trabeculectomy versus Ahmed valve surgery in the treatment of neovascular glaucoma: assessment of efficacy and complications. BMC Ophthalmol. 2016;16(1):65. https://doi.org/10.1186/S12886-016-0248-7.

31. Sun JT, Liang HJ, An M, Wang DB. Efficacy and safety of intravitreal ranibizumab with panretinal photocoagulation followed by trabeculectomy compared with Ahmed glaucoma valve implantation in neovascular glaucoma. Int J Ophthalmol. 2017;10(3):400–5. https://doi.org/10.18240/ijo.2017.03.12.

32. El-Saied HMA, Abdelhakim MASE. Various modalities for management of secondary angle closure neovascular glaucoma in diabetic eyes: 1-year comparative study. Int Ophthalmol. 2021;41(4):1179–90. https://doi.org/10.1007/s10792-020-01673-1.

33. Shalaby WS, Myers JS, Razeghinejad R, et al. Outcomes of valved and nonvalved tube shunts in neovascular glaucoma. Ophthalmol Glaucoma. 2020;4(2):182–92. https://doi.org/10.1016/j.ogla.2020.09.010.

34. Ndulue JK, Rahmatnejad K, Sanvicente C, Wizov SS, Moster MR. Evolution of cyclophotocoagulation. J Ophthalmic Vis Res. 2018;13(1):55–61. https://doi.org/10.4103/JOVR.JOVR_190_17.

35. Mermoud A, Salmon JF, Alexander P, Straker C, Murray ADN. Motteno tube implantation for neovascular glaucoma: long-term results and factors influencing the outcome. Ophthalmology. 1993;100(6):897–902. https://doi.org/10.1016/S0161-6420(93)31557-5.

36. Sleath B, Blalock SJ, Carpenter DM, et al. Ophthalmologist-patient communication, self-efficacy, and glaucoma medication adherence. Ophthalmology. 2015;122(4):748–54. https://doi.org/10.1016/j.ophtha.2014.11.001.

37. Newman-Casey PA, Robin AL, Blachley T, et al. The most common barriers to glaucoma medication adherence: a cross-sectional survey. Ophthalmology. 2015;122(7):1308–16. https://doi.org/10.1016/J.OPHTHA.2015.03.026.

38. An JJ, Niu F, Turpcu A, Rajput Y, Cheetham TC. Adherence to the American Diabetes Association retinal screening guidelines for population with diabetes in the United States. Ophthalmic Epidemiol. 2018;25(3):257–65. https://doi.org/10.1080/09286586.2018.1424344.

39. Sleath B, Blalock SJ, Carpenter DM, et al. Provider education about glaucoma and glaucoma medications during videotaped medical visits. J Ophthalmol. 2014;2014:238939. https://doi.org/10.1155/2014/238939.

40. Newman-Casey PA, Salman M, Lee PP, Gatwood JD. Cost-utility analysis of glaucoma medication adherence. Ophthalmology. 2020;127(5):589–98. https://doi.org/10.1016/J.OPHTHA.2019.09.041.

41. Waterman H, Evans JR, Gray TA, Henson D, Harper R. Interventions for improving adherence to ocular hypotensive therapy. Cochrane Database Syst Rev. 2013;2013(4):CD006132. https://doi.org/10.1002/14651858.CD006132.PUB3.

42. Hark LA, Madhava M, Radakrishnan A, et al. Impact of a social worker in a glaucoma eye care service: a prospective study. Heal Soc Work. 2019;44(1):48–55. https://doi.org/10.1093/hsw/hly038.

Correction to: Aqueous Shunt for Neovascular Glaucoma

Wesam S. Shalaby, Dilru C. Amarasekera, and Aakriti Garg Shukla

Correction to:
Chapter 17 in: M. Qiu (ed.), *Neovascular Glaucoma*, Essentials
in Ophthalmology, https://doi.org/10.1007/978-3-031-11720-6_17

The title of Chapter 17 was printed incorrectly as "Aqueous Shunt for Neovascular Glaucoma Implant", which has been corrected as **"Aqueous Shunt for Neovascular Glaucoma"** in the Table of Contents, chapter opening page, and running heads throughout the chapter.

The updated original version of the chapter can be found at https://doi.org/10.1007/978-3-031-11720-6_17

Index

Printed in the United States
by Baker & Taylor Publisher Services